D1757300

NUTRITION AND THE CONSUMER

Issues in Nutrition and Toxicology 1

ISSUES IN NUTRITION AND TOXICOLOGY

Series Editors

Richard C. Cottrell
*Leatherhead Food Research Association,
Leatherhead, UK*

Brian A. Rolls
*AFRC Institute of Food Research,
Reading Laboratory, Shinfield, Reading, UK*

Ann F. Walker
*Department of Food Service & Technology,
University of Reading, Reading, UK*

NUTRITION AND THE CONSUMER

Issues in Nutrition and Toxicology 1

Edited by

ANN F. WALKER

Department of Food Science and Technology,
University of Reading, UK

and

BRIAN A. ROLLS

AFRC Institute of Food Research,
Reading Laboratory, Shinfield, Reading, UK

ELSEVIER APPLIED SCIENCE
LONDON and NEW YORK

ELSEVIER APPLIED SCIENCE PUBLISHERS LTD
Crown House, Linton Road, Barking, Essex IG11 8JU, England

Sole Distributor in the USA and Canada
ELSEVIER SCIENCE PUBLISHING CO., INC.
655 Avenue of the Americas, New York, NY 10010, USA

WITH 62 TABLES AND 45 ILLUSTRATIONS

© 1992 ELSEVIER APPLIED SCIENCE PUBLISHERS LTD

British Library Cataloging in Publication Data

Nutrition and the consumer. — (Issues in
nutrition and toxicology; 1)
I. Walker, Ann F.   II. Rolls, Brian A.
613.2

ISBN 1-85166-684-2

Library of Congress Cataloging-in-Publication Data

Nutrition and the consumer/edited by Ann F. Walker and Brian A. Rolls
p. cm. — (Issues in nutrition and toxicology; 1)
Includes bibliographical references and index.
ISBN 1-85166-684-2
1. Nutrition.   I. Walker, Ann (Ann F.)   II. Rolls, B. A.
III. Series.
QP141.N777   1992   91-22230
613.2 — dc20   CIP

Special regulations for readers in the USA

Phototypesetting by the Alden Multimedia, Northampton.
Printed in Great Britain by University Press Cambridge.

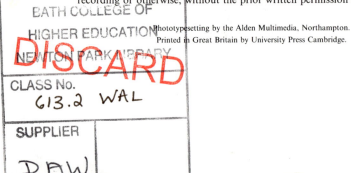

Contents

Preface

This book is the first in a series called 'Issues in Nutrition and Toxicology'. The aim of this series is to provide succinct information on important and controversial subjects in the area of nutrition, food and toxicology for a variety of interested people, including general practitioners, health professionals, technical directors, food technologists and others in the food industry, final year BSc and research students. While there are many erudite and comprehensive reviews of the scientific literature on aspects of nutrition and toxicology for specialists, often this information is not so readily available to scientific non-specialists and health specialists.

Consumer interest in nutrition has greatly increased over the last 10 years. This has been spurred on by the publication by government bodies throughout the world of dietary guidelines on eating for health. While this has concentrated the minds of many in primary health care and the food industry on the balance of the major sources of energy in the diet such as saturated fat, sugar and dietary fibre, the focus of attention has drifted away from nutrients, namely vitamins and minerals.

In the first chapter in this book a flavour of some of the controversies surrounding the setting of Recommended Daily Amounts (RDA, or Dietary Reference Values DRV, as they have come to be known recently) for nutrients is covered which should enable the reader to avoid misuse of DRVs.

Whilst various committees have deliberated on setting dietary guidelines, nutritional science has not stood still and new insights into the actions of antioxidant vitamins are emerging with the publication of data linking the prevalence of cancer and coronary heart disease to the body's status of vitamin C, A and E and β-carotene. Chapter 2 specifically deals with vitamin A and carotenoids. It is intended that other antioxidant nutrients will be covered in later volumes.

More research data on mineral nutrition are also becoming available. Chapters 3 and 4 deal with calcium and zinc nutrition, which have received particular attention more recently and Chapter 5 covers effects of mineral–

mineral interactions which may be enhanced by supplementation—a point of particular relevance for the health-conscious consumer.

The theme of the current dietary guidelines is picked up in Chapters 6 and 9 on sugar and vegetarianism respectively. Consumer concern over toxins in food also receives attention in Chapter 7 on the effects of processing fats and oils.

As one of the aims of good nutrition is health and wellbeing for all human groups, we should not forget that the best possible nutrition is also required for unfortunate people who are seriously ill or who suffer from particular dietary needs. Chapter 9 on 'Nutrition for specific disease conditions' outlines the approach illustrated with four important disease conditions, including cancer.

Finally 'Viewpoint' offers an opportunity for two scientists to discuss the debt that we owe for our knowledge of human nutrition from experiments conducted on animals. However, care must be used in the interpretation of data obtained from animal experiments, as it can never fully replace data collected in clinical trials or in the therapeutic situation.

The Editors wish to thank their respective spouses, Alan Lakin and Libby Rolls, for their support and encouragement.

A.F. Walker and B.A. Rolls

List of Contributors

A. BEAL
c/o Dr A.F. Walker, Department of Food Science and Technology, University of Reading, Whiteknights, PO Box 226, Reading RG6 2AP, UK

N. BINNS
Pfizer Limited, Ramsgate Road, Sandwich, Kent CT13 9NJ, UK

K. DEBENHAM
District Dietitian, Royal Berkshire Hospital, Reading RG1 5AN, UK

I.E. DREOSTI
CSIRO Division of Human Nutrition, Kintore Avenue, Adelaide, SA 5000, Australia

M.I. GURR
Maypole Scientific Services, Vale View Cottage, Maypole, St. Mary's, Isles of Scilly TR21 0NU, UK

T.J. HALLAS
c/o A.F. Walker, Department of Food Science and Technology, University of Reading, Whiteknights, PO Box 226, Reading RG6 2AP, UK

A.E. HARPER
Department of Nutritional Sciences, University of Wisconsin-Madison, Madison, Wisconsin 53706, USA

A.G. LOW
c/o A.F. Walker, Department of Food Science and Technology, University of Reading, Whiteknights, PO Box 226, Reading RG6 2AP, UK

B.A. ROLLS
AFRC Institute of Food Research, Shinfield, Reading RG2 9AT, UK

I.H.E. RUTISHAUSER
Department of Human Nutrition, Deakin University, Geelong, Victoria, Australia 3217

A.F. WALKER
Department of Food Science and Technology, University of Reading, Whiteknights, PO Box 226, Reading RG6 2AP, UK

G. WEBB
The Polytechnic of East London, London E15 4LZ, UK

1

Recommended Dietary Allowances of Nutrients: Basis, Policy and Politics

ALFRED E. HARPER

Department of Nutritional Sciences, University of Wisconsin-Madison, USA

BRIAN A. ROLLS

AFRC Institute of Food Research, Reading, UK

INTRODUCTION

Recommended dietary allowances (RDA) are a set of dietary standards for the planning of food supplies for population groups. They are estimates of the average daily intakes of essential nutrients that, consumed over a period, will meet the physiological needs of individuals within the specified population. They are scientifically based standards that enable qualified professionals to ensure that the diet of large groups of people is nutritionally adequate.

Recommended dietary allowances have always been controversial, increasingly so in recent years. Selection of values that ensure adequate intake and, where appropriate, adequate reserves, is a matter of scientific judgement and hence disagreement. Moreover, RDA have increasingly been used in ways for which they were not originally intended, such as formulating health and social policies, and some of these constitute a misuse.

TERMINOLOGY

The term recommended dietary allowances was coined by the Food and Nutrition Board of the US National Academy of Sciences. The corresponding term current in the UK is recommended daily amounts (which fortunately also reduces to RDA); others use recommended dietary intakes or recommended nutrient intakes. The agencies of the United Nations (FAO-WHO) use the expression safe level of intake of nutrients. These expressions are summarized in Table 1. Most countries use one or other of these terms, which all refer to recommendations for populations, and do not represent individual needs. The recommended daily allowance (USRDA, see p. 9) is, however, quite different.

HISTORICAL BACKGROUND TO RDA AND DIETARY RECOMMENDATIONS

With the exception of the British Merchant Seaman Act of 1835 (by which the provision of citrus juice to prevent scurvy was made compulsory), most early dietary recommendations, such as that of Dr Edward Smith in the UK in 1862, dealt with energy and protein (or nitrogen) intake. Their aim was to prevent starvation and its associated diseases. Smith's recommendations were based on metabolic studies, but in most cases these early proposals were based on observation rather than any scientific principle.

During the early twentieth century, more accurate estimates were made of energy and protein requirements by calorimetry and nitrogen balance studies. At the same time, the importance of the 'accessory food factors' or micronutrients, the vitamins and trace minerals, was recognized, and recommendations were aimed not simply to avoid starvation and maintain work capacity, but also to improve health.

When the Food Committee of the Royal Society reported at the end of World War I, they accepted the energy requirements of Lusk of 3000 kcal (12·6 MJ) for a 66 kg man, scaled down for women and children. These figures had been used to estimate the necessary North American food aid for war-torn Western Europe. They concluded that the diet should contain 80 g of protein a day and not less than 25% fat. For the first time the importance of 'protective' foods such as milk, fruit and vegetables was recognized, and although no quantitative figures were given, this was an important conceptual step forward. The subsequent recommendations of the British Medical Association (1933) followed the same line. The recommendations were based on energy and protein needs, again with no quantitative estimates for vitamins and minerals. Leitch (1942) has reviewed the early development of dietary recommendations in the UK; see also Harper (1985, 1990).

TABLE 1
Terminology in dietary standards

Term	User	Definition
Recommended dietary allowances (RDA)	Food and Nutrition Board, US National Academy of Sciences, 1941	Level of intake of essential nutrients to meet the known nutritional needs of practically all healthy persons
Recommended daily amounts (RDA)	Department of Health and Social Security (UK), 1979	The average amount of the nutrient that should be provided per head in a group of people if the needs of practically all members of the group are to be met
Recommended daily intakes (RDI)	Commonwealth Department of Health, Australia, 1986; also DHHS (UK) 1969–79	As above, but emphasis on intake to indicate that recommendations are for food as eaten
Recommended nutrient intakes	Department of National Health and Welfare, Canada, 1983	The level of dietary intake thought to be sufficiently high to meet the requirements of almost all individuals in a group with specified characteristics
Safe level of intake of nutrients	Agencies of the United Nations (FAO/WHO/UNU)	Amount which will meet or exceed the needs of practically all in the group specified
US Recommended daily allowances (USRDA)[a]	Food and Drug Administration, USA	Set of highest single RDA for any group for twenty nutrients

[a] Note that this is not a dietary standard; the USRDA are reference standards for nutrition information. Do not confuse this use with the use of RDA in the UK for nutrition labelling.

In the same year, however, Stiebling (1933) proposed a standard to ensure nutritional adequacy for US Department of Agriculture food programmes, and for the first time quantitative values were given for vitamins and minerals and the needs of different age groups were recognized. The League of Nations Health Organization, whose committees had examined the problem for 12 years, presented its own estimates for vitamins and minerals (League of Nations, 1937) and in 1939 the Canadian Council on Nutrition proposed intakes for different groups for energy, fat and some vitamins and minerals (Canadian Council of Nutrition, 1940). Thus, from being observation-based recommendations for alleviating starvation caused by war and economic crisis, dietary standards had become scientifically based standards for maintaining health of the population as a whole, with recognition of the special needs of children and pregnant women.

The current procedure for assessing RDA in the USA was instituted in 1940 when the National Research Council of the US Academy of Sciences set up the Committee on Food and Nutrition, later the Food and Nutrition Board (Roberts, 1944, 1958). It is the practice of the Board to put forward a tentative set of values based on current literature, seek comment from those active in the field and revise their proposals accordingly and repeat the process until reasonable agreement is achieved (Food and Nutrition Board, 1980; Harper, 1985, 1987; Truswell, 1987). This process worked successfully until 1985, when the tenth edition was rejected. This resulted in a four-year delay in publication of the tenth edition, and in two versions of the chapters on some nutrients being published. For the background to this unexpected decision, the scope of RDA must be reconsidered and, as importantly, what lies outside their scope, and this is considered later. See also the accounts by Harper (1987) and Pellett (1988) of this controversy.

Other sets of dietary standards have been proposed by various national and international bodies. The Food and Agricultural Organization of the United Nations, continuing the work of the League of Nations, have put forward recommended intakes of energy, protein and other nutrients (FAO/WHO/UNU, 1985). Some countries simply use the US or FAO values, others—including Australia, Canada (Department of National Health and Welfare, 1983), India and the UK (DHSS (UK), 1979, 1984)—compile their own. The US and UK approaches have recently been compared (Walker *et al.*, 1987). The Australian background papers are particularly full and informative (Palmer *et al.*, 1982, 1985, 1986). The UK government is currently considering the compilation of a new set of RDA (Whitehead, 1989).

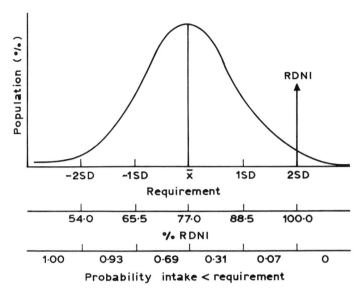

FIG. 1.   Distribution of nutrient requirements for a homogeneous population and the probability of intake being less than the requirement within given intervals below the recommended daily nutrient intake. (Reproduced, with permission, from the *Annual Review of Nutrition*, Vol. 7, © 1987 by Annual Reviews Inc.).

Truswell (1983*a*, *b*) has produced a valuable review of the dietary standards proposed by various national and international bodies. He points out that standards differ for several reasons: slightly different underlying philosophies, different definitions of physiological groups, and different criteria of adequacy—and, of course, different judgement of those on the various expert committees. In every case, however, the aim is the same: to establish a reference standard for the intakes of energy and essential nutrients to meet the needs of almost all healthy individuals or in a subset of a population.

SELECTING VALUES FOR RDA

The first step is to estimate the average requirement for a nutrient (Fig. 1). For those nutrients whose deficiency has resulted in public health problems, such as thiamin, niacin, vitamins A, C and D, iron and iodine, there is enough information from observation and experiment to make this estimation with some confidence, although more—and more accurate

—evidence is always welcome. Committees must weigh factors such as 'normal physiological function' and 'health' which are not subject to precise definition. Moreover, a mean value that, by definition, excludes 50% of the population is of little use, so the next step is to decide by how much this value should be increased to meet the needs of those with higher requirements. Increases of 50% (Stiebling, 1933), or of three times (Pett *et al.*, 1945) or twice (see Beaton, 1988) the standard deviation have been suggested; for example, the mean plus two standard deviations should meet the requirements of 97·5% of the population. Monitoring (USDA/ HHS, 1986) has suggested that this approach is satisfactory.

There is thus no absolutely correct answer: the higher the value chosen, the less the chance that an individual's needs will not be met. For obvious reasons, committees, when in doubt, tend to favour the higher of two possible values. Hence it is clear that should an individual's intake of a particular nutrient (or nutrients) fall below the RDA it does not automatically follow that his or her diet is deficient in that nutrient (although RDA is often misused in this way, and not only by non-scientists). All that can be said is that the further the intake falls below the RDA, the greater the chance that the diet is inadequate.

In setting a value for RDA, the aim is not only to prevent immediate deficiency, but to ensure that the nutrient is present in body tissues in sufficient quantity to prevent deficiency in the future, in other words to establish body reserves. This is taken into consideration in establishing the criteria for estimating the average requirement. For several nutrients the relationship between intake and body pools has been studied, but this relationship is curvilinear, and the point at which to select for an adequate body reserve is again a matter of judgement with no absolutely 'right' answer. For many nutrients the pool size has been assessed indirectly (Harper, 1978). Committees examine experimental and survey data to see whether there is any evidence that their chosen value is too low or too high. Values for some nutrients—such as vitamin A and calcium, and iron for men—have changed little over the years; for other nutrients, such as thiamin, riboflavin, protein and vitamin C, the RDA has tended to fall as more precise information becomes available and committees feel less need to incorporate an unspecified 'safety factor' to allow for possibly inaccurate data.

There are additional factors that have to be taken into account. For some nutrients there may be differences in requirement between the sexes, differences in biological availability (Beaton, 1988) of dietary sources or differences in utilization of different forms of the nutrient. If the requirements of only some of the age-sex groups have been studied, values for other groups must be estimated. The information on calcium absorption and iron utilization (for example) is extensive, whereas the availability of such nutrients as folic acid and many minerals is less exact than could be wished. Thus selection of the final values involves both knowledge and judgement, although it is an informed judgement. Despite the differences in the selection processes in different countries, the degree of agreement among different sets of RDA is encouraging.

Examples of the factors involved in reaching a final value are afforded by iron and vitamin C. Iron is the only nutrient for which the requirements of men and women exhibit differences not attributable to differences in body weight: the intakes of women of child-bearing age must take account of menstrual losses. The high RDA for iron in the USA takes account of the needs of those with very high losses, whose requirements are skewed beyond the normal distribution curve. If one were to consider that these individuals had a clinical condition requiring supplementation under medical supervision, the RDA could be much lower, and in fact in the tenth edition a move in this direction is evident. This is logical, for by definition RDA maintain health in healthy people; they are not designed to promote recovery of the sick. National committees must also take account of the bioavailability of nutrients: where most of the iron consumed is highly available (e.g. in meat) the RDA may be lower than in countries where most dietary iron comes from vegetable sources and is much less available.

In the case of ascorbic acid, a judgement must be made whether the RDA should permit a body pool of 1500 mg (close to the possible upper limit) or whether 600 mg would be acceptable. Although the former figure might be recommended for a yachtsman setting off round the world without fresh food, the latter would seem quite reasonable for someone living within reach of a supermarket.

The RDA values for calcium, iron and vitamins A and C in the USA are higher than in most other countries and probably higher than they need be (Olson & Hodges, 1987). Among the reasons are the wishes to take the safe line by assuming the lower of two possible absorptions, to ensure a more than adequate body reserve and to cater for those with unusually high requirements. Moreover, even high recommendations can be met by the US food supply without great difficulty. Committees may also be swayed by the thought that a moderate excess will do no harm in most cases but risk of a deficiency must be minimized. When the RDA are inflated by such considerations, however, the proportion of the population

estimated to have inadequate intakes will be overestimated. Although
40% of Canadians consume less than the RDA for ascorbic acid, low
serum levels are found in only 3%. A similar situation is found in the US
for iron and calcium among women (USDA/HHS, 1986).

In contrast to the RDA already discussed, the standards for energy
intake are the average requirements for that particular group. No safety
factor is considered necessary, and individuals will normally adjust their
energy intakes to take account of energy expenditure.

THE USES OF RDA

RDA have been used for many purposes other than their original intended
use as standards for planning adequate food supplies for population
groups; some are legitimate, whereas others constitute a misuse.

Nutrition information and education
If foods are grouped according to the nutrients of which they are important sources, RDA can be used to assess the numbers of servings from each
group that will meet the needs of different people (Page & Phipard, 1957).
Although the RDA reports can be used as a basis for nutrition education
(Hertzler & Anderson, 1974), they must be interpreted with care for
non-specialists.

Nutrient density
Nutrient density is the amount of a nutrient in a portion of food supplying
a standard amount of energy (e.g. 0·24 mg/100 kJ, 1 mg/100 kcal; Hansen
& Wyse, 1980; Wretlind, 1982). Then, if the RDA is expressed as the
amount needed in the total energy requirement (e.g. 25 mg/10 450 kJ,
which equals 0·24 mg/100 kJ), comparison of these two ratios gives a
useful index of the value of that food as a source of the nutrient concerned,
perhaps in comparison with another food or foods. However, this approach does assume that nutrient requirements are in proportion to
energy, which is not always true. Mineral requirements are a function of
body size and growth rate, pyridoxine requirement is a function of protein
intake, and although energy needs tend to decline with age, there is no
evidence that this is true of other essential nutrient requirements.

Nutrition labelling
The Food and Drug Administration of the USA has selected the *highest*

value for 20 nutrients from the RDA tables and called them the USRDA (in which, confusingly, D stands for daily). These are not dietary standards, they are reference standards for nutrition labelling and food fortification. These values are useful for comparing different foods, but they cannot (since only one value is used) be related to the needs for different age-sex groups.

The standard RDA are used in nutrition labelling in the UK, especially for vitamins and minerals. Their use is controlled by legislation (Food Labelling Regulations, 1984): for any claim to be made about vitamin or mineral content, the food must be capable of making an appreciable contribution to intake. Proposals being considered by the European Commission will use a similar system; however, at present member states have different RDA for some nutrients.

New, special or therapeutic foods

The RDA can appropriately be used to design products for special purposes, such as mineral and vitamin supplements or total slimming diets, to ensure that the consumer receives adequate, but not excessive, intakes. Although RDA were not intended for therapeutic diets, they can serve as a starting basis, modifications being made for the needs of the particular patient.

Evaluating nutrient intakes

Recommended daily allowances are frequently used to assess the adequacy of nutrient intakes estimated from food consumption data. Leaving aside the problems involved in obtaining accurate measurements from dietary surveys, this is not an appropriate use of RDA. If an individual should have an intake for a nutrient that falls below the RDA, neither the adequacy of that intake nor the nutritional status of that person can be assessed from RDA (see Waterlow, 1979). Nutritional status can only be assessed by clinical or biochemical measurements; whether that person has a high or low requirement for that nutrient can only be determined from metabolic studies.

It is true that statistical procedures have been proposed for estimating, from knowledge of the average requirement and intake, the probability of intake being inadequate (for reviews, see NAS, 1985; FAO/WHO/UNU, 1985; Beaton, 1986). However, these provide an estimate of risk, not an estimate of the nutritional status of individuals. At present, the proportion of people ingesting less than the RDA for a nutrient gives no information

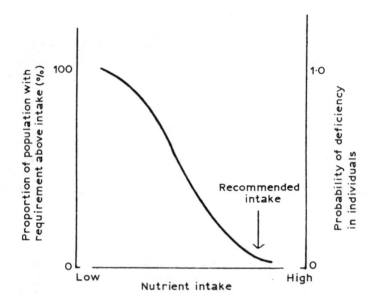

FIG. 2.   Cumulative plot of the distribution of nutrient requirements for a homogeneous population and the probability of deficiency being associated with
particular intakes. (Reproduced, with permission, from the *Annual Review of
Nutrition*, Vol. 7, © 1987 by Annual Reviews Inc.).

about the adequacy of their diet, although conclusions—generally negative—are frequently drawn in the popular media (see Fig. 2).

All that can be said—in the absence of clinical or laboratory investigation—is that if the intake is at or above the RDA then the chance of
inadequacy is remote; the further it falls below that value, the greater the
risk of deficiency. If a particular population subset—say, adolescent girls
—has a larger proportion of intakes below the recommended level, then
individuals within that group may be assessed clinically for signs of actual
harm.

For population groups the problem is even greater, since variation of
intake must be taken into account. A mean intake in excess of the RDA
may be associated with—and almost certainly will be—a part of that
group having intakes well below that mean value, for reasons that include
cultural idiosyncrasies, poverty, illness and ignorance (Harper, 1974).
These problems have led some to propose some new set of standards,
perhaps closer to the average requirement (see Truswell, (1983*a, b*) for an

account of discussions by the European Nutrition Societies), but wherever the standard is set, the only result would be to substitute a new range of probabilities. Moreover, since many are at present unclear about the correct use of RDA, further sets of standards may achieve nothing more than multiplying the opportunity for error.

DIETARY STANDARDS AND DIETARY GUIDELINES

Recommended daily allowances are often criticized because they do not serve purposes for which they were never intended. In particular, they give no guidance on the intake of fat, carbohydrate or fibre; they do not give guidance on preventing obesity and they do not deal with associations between diet and degenerative disease. The reaction seems to be to propose modification of the RDA rather than to create a new independent standard. The controversy was responsible for the delay in the publication of the tenth RDA report.

Dietary guidelines are part of general health policy: they give the public information that will enable them to select diets that are nutritious and healthy (McNutt, 1980; NACNE, 1983; DHSS (UK), 1984; Truswell, 1987; DHHS (US), 1988; NRC, 1989). In addition, reported associations between diet and degenerative diseases such as cardiovascular disease and cancer have resulted in many suggestions for diet modification. There is no conflict between dietary guidelines and RDA; indeed, they are complementary. Recommended daily allowances provide standards for population energy provision; dietary guidelines urge individuals to modify their intake to avoid obesity. Since there are no unique physiological needs for carbohydrates and the non-essential fats, RDA do not deal with their proportions in a diet; dietary guidelines do. Similarly, guidelines have recommendations about non-nutrients such as cholesterol and fibre, which by definition are given only passing attention by those compiling RDA.

There is thus little direct relationship between RDA and dietary guidelines. Populations are predictably susceptible to specific nutrient deficiencies, which can be demonstrated, and prevented by provision of the nutrient. In contrast, the associations between diet and diseases are complex and the diseases do not result predictably from a single dietary deficiency or surplus. Moreover, individuals do not have the same susceptibility to developing degenerative disease, and the chances of predicting this susceptibility are, at present, low without detailed clinical studies. To modify RDA because of uncertain associations would damage the first without advancing the cause of the second. In responding to diseases prevalent in the middle-aged male, the value of RDA for infants and pregnant women, for example, would be put into question. In addition, it should be remembered that the basis for RDA values is widely accepted, whereas dietary guidelines are based on evidence that is often still incomplete or controversial (Reiser, 1984; Ahrens, 1985; Oliver, 1986; Olson, 1986; Smith & Pinckney, 1988; Moore, 1989).

The unexpected rejection of the ninth revision of the RDA in the USA resulted from the conflict between the proposal to lower the RDA for vitamins A and C, and the proposals of a separate committee of the National Research Council that recommended increased intakes of these vitamins to help reduce cancer. This conflict, as we have seen, is more apparent than real, and based on an imperfect understanding of the purpose of RDA. If compelling evidence of prophylactic effects of certain nutrients were to be obtained, their use in amounts in excess of the RDA might be recommended as a public health measure, but this would still be inappropriate as a criterion for establishing RDA. A comparison of the USA RDA finally adopted with RDA for the UK for adults is shown in Table 2.

RDA AND DIETARY GUIDELINES: THE FUTURE

Perhaps the term 'recommended dietary allowances' leads users to believe that this is the amount that should be consumed, rather than a standard value below which the risk of inadequacy will begin to increase. If the term RDA were changed to 'safe and adequate intakes of essential nutrients' it would help stress that these are not 'desirable' or 'appropriate' intakes. It is vital that RDA continue to be as accurate as possible measures of physiological needs in the light of current knowledge, and not altered in an attempt to make them fit other, unrelated purposes. Further information about individual variation, especially about people with very high requirements, would be of great value.

Dietary guidelines have tended to focus on specific diseases, yet they are often put forward as recommendations for the general public. Perhaps because information is so incomplete, unequivocal studies are so rare and associations are often so tenuous, statements on diet–disease relationships are often characterized by emotional advocacy rather than dispassionate enquiry. If detailed background papers were prepared, as is now carried

TABLE 2
A comparison of American and British RDA for adults

	Male		Female[a]	
	USA[b] (*1990*)	*UK[c]* (*1979*)	*USA[b]* (*1990*)	*UK[d]* (*1979*)
Protein (g)	63	69	50	54
Vitamin A (μg)	1 000	750	800	750
Vitamin D (μg)	5	nr	5	nr
Vitamin E (mg)	10	nr	8	nr
Vitamin K (μg)	80	nr	65	nr
Vitamin C (mg)	60	30	60	30
Thiamin (mg)	1·5	1·1	1·1	0·9
Riboflavin (mg)	1·7	1·6	1·3	1·3
Niacin (mg)	19	18	15	15
Vitamin B_6 (mg)	2·0	nr	1·6	nr
Folate (μg)	200	nr	180	nr
Vitamin B_{12} (μg)	2·0	nr	2·0	nr
Calcium (mg)	800	500	800	500
Phosphorus (mg)	800	nr	800	nr
Magnesium (mg)	350	nr	280	nr
Iron (mg)	10	10	15	12
Zinc (mg)	15	nr	12	nr
Iodine (μg)	150	nr	150	nr
Selenium (μg)	70	nr	55	nr

[a] Non-pregnant, non-lactating.
[b] 25–50 years of age.
[c] Moderately active, aged 35–64 years.
[d] Most occupations, aged 18–54 years.
nr, no recommendation.
Compiled from DHSS (UK) (1979) and Food and Nutrition Board (1989).

out for RDA, objective information about energy sources, non-nutrients and weight control could be provided. The role of the diet could be placed in context among such other factors as lifestyle, age and sex. It may thus be possible to provide, for all age-sex groups, realistic assessments of the benefits and hazards of diet modification.

CONCLUSION

Recommended daily allowances are scientifically based standards intended for the development of certain types of food policy. Dietary guidelines are policy statements intended to maintain and improve health, and perhaps to delay the onset of disease. Both are of value only when they are kept separate and their uses and limitations are recognized. Dietary guidelines would be more soundly based if the examination of diet–disease relationships and policy recommendations were separated, as with RDA.

Note: Since this volume went to press, the new recommendations for the UK have been published.

DOH (Department of Health, UK). (1991). *Dietary Reference Values for Food Energy and Nutrients for the United Kingdom*. Report on Health and Social Subjects no. 41. London: H.M. Stationery Office.

REFERENCES

Ahrens, E.H., Jr. (1985). The diet-heart question in 1985: Has it really been settled? *Lancet* **i**, 1085–87.

Beaton, G.H. (1986). Towards harmonization of dietary, biochemical and clinical assessments; the meaning of nutritional status and requirements. *Nutrition Reviews* **44**, 349–58.

Beaton, G.H. (1988). Criteria of an adequate diet. In *Modern Nutrition in Health and Disease*, pp. 649–65 [M.E. Shils and V.R. Young, editors]. Philadelphia: Lea & Febiger.

British Medical Association (1933). Committee on nutrition. *British Medical Journal*, Suppl. 25.

Canadian Council on Nutrition (1940). The Canadian dietary standard. *National Health Reviews* **8**, 1–9.

Department of National Health and Welfare (1983). Recommended nutrient intakes for Canadians. Ottawa: Canadian Government Publishing Centre.

DHHS(US) (1988). The Surgeon General's Report on Nutrition and Health. DHHS Publication no. (PHS) 88-50210. Washington, D.C.: US Government Printing Office.

DHSS(UK) (1979). *Recommended daily amounts of food energy and nutrients for groups of people in the United Kingdom*. Report on Health and Social Subjects, no. 15. London: H.M. Stationery Office.

DHSS(UK) (1984). Committee on Medical Aspects of Food Policy (COMA). Diet and cardiovascular disease. Reports on Health and Social Subjects no. 28. London: H.M. Stationery Office.

DHSS(UK) (1985). Recommended daily amounts of food energy and nutrients for groups of people in the United Kingdom. London: H.M. Stationery Office.

FAO/WHO/UNU (1985). Energy and protein requirements. WHO Technical Report Series 724. Geneva: World Health Organization.

Food and Nutrition Board (1980). *Recommended Dietary Allowances*. 9th ed. Washington, D.C.: National Academy of Sciences.

Food and Nutrition Board (1989). *Recommended Dietary Allowances*, 10th ed. Washington, D.C.: National Academy of Sciences.

Hansen, R.G. & Wyse, B.W. (1980). Expression of nutrient allowances per 1000 kilocalories. *Journal of the American Dietetic Association* **76**, 223–7.

Harper, A.E. (1974). Recommended dietary allowances: Are they what we think they are? *Journal of the American Dietetic Association* **64**, 151–6.

Harper, A.E. (1978). Nutritional requirements and dietary allowances. *Comprehensive Therapy* **4**, 10–17.

Harper, A.E. (1985). Origin of the recommended dietary allowances—An historic overview. *American Journal of Clinical Nutrition* **41**, 140–8.

Harper, A.E. (1987). Evolution of recommended dietary allowances—New directions? *Annual Reviews of Nutrition* **7**, 509–37.

Harper, A.E. (1990). Dietary standards and dietary guidelines. In *Present Knowledge in Nutrition*, pp. 491–501 [M.L. Brown, editor]. Washington, D.C.: International Life Sciences Institute—Nutrition Foundation.

Hertzler, A.A. & Anderson, H.L. (1974). Food guides in the United States. An historical review. *Journal of the American Dietetic Association* **64**, 19–28.

League of Nations (1937). *Nutrition*. Final Report of the Mixed Committee of the League of Nations on the Relation of Nutrition to Health, Agriculture and Economic policy. Report no. A.13.II.A. Geneva: League of Nations.

Leitch, I. (1942). The evolution of dietary standards. *Nutrition Abstracts and Reviews* **11**, 509–21.

McNutt, K. (1980). Dietary advice to the public: 1957 to 1980. *Nutrition Reviews* **38**, 353–60.

Moore, T.J. (1989). *The Cholesterol Myth*. The Atlantic Monthly, September, pp. 37–70.

NACNE (National Advisory Committee on Nutrition Education) (1983). *A Discussion Paper on Proposals for Nutrition Guidelines for Health Education in Britain*. London: Health Education Council.

NAS (1985). *Nutrient Adequacy: Assessment using Food Consumption Surveys*. Washington, D.C.: National Academy Press.

NRC (1989). *Diet and Health: Implications for Reducing Chronic Disease Risk*. Washington, D.C.: National Academy Press.

Oliver, M.F. (1986). Prevention of coronary heart disease—propaganda, promises, problems, and prospects. *Circulation* **73**, 1–9.

Olson, R.E. (1986). Mass intervention vs screening and selective intervention for prevention of coronary heart disease. *Journal of the American Medical Association* **225**, 2204–7.

Olson, J.A. & Hodges, R.E. (1987). Recommended dietary intakes (RDI) of Vitamin C in humans. American Journal of Clinical Nutrition **45**, 693–703.

Page, L. & Phipard, E.F. (1957). Essentials of an adequate diet. Home Economics Research Report no. 3. Washington, D.C.: US Government Printing Office.

Palmer, N. *et al.* (1982). Recommended dietary intakes for use in Australia. *Journal of Food and Nutrition* **39**, 157–92.

Palmer, N. *et al.* (1985). Recommended dietary intakes for use in Australia. *Journal of Food and Nutrition* **41**, 109–54.

Palmer, N. *et al.* (1986). Further recommendations for dietary intakes for use in Australia. *Journal of Food and Nutrition* **42**, 47–92.

Pellett, P.L. (1988). The RDA controversy revisited. *Ecology of Food and Nutrition* **21**, 315–20.

Pett, L.B., Morrell, C.A. & Hanley, F.W. (1945). The development of dietary standards. *Canadian Journal of Public Health* **36**, 232–9.

Reiser, R. (1984). A commentary on the rationale of the diet-heart statement of the American Heart Association. *American Journal of Clinical Nutrition* **40**, 654–8.

Roberts, L.J. (1944). Scientific basis for the recommended dietary allowances. *New York State Journal of Medicine* **44**, 59–66.

Roberts, L.J. (1958). Beginnings of the recommended dietary allowances. *Journal of the American Dietetic Association* **34**, 903–8.

Smith, R.L. & Pinckney, E.R. (1988). *Diet, Blood Cholesterol and Coronary Heart Disease: A Critical Review of the Literature*. Santa Monica, CA: Vector Enterprises, Inc.

Stiebling, H.K. (1933). Food budgets for nutrition and production programs. Miscellaneous Publications no. 183. Washington, D.C.: US Department of Agriculture.

Truswell, A.S. (1983*a*). Recommended dietary intakes around the world. Part 1. *Nutrition Abstracts and Reviews* **53**, 939–1015.

Truswell, A.S. (1983*b*). Recommended dietary intakes around the world. Part 2. *Nutrition Abstracts and Reviews* **53**, 1075–1119.

Truswell, A.S. (1987). Evolution of dietary recommendations, goals and guidelines. *American Journal of Clinical Nutrition* **45**, 1060–72.

USDA/HHS (1986). *Nutrition Monitoring in the United States—A Report from the Joint Nutrition Monitoring Evaluation Committee*. DHHS Publication no. (PHS) 86-1255. Washington, D.C.: US Government Printing Office.

Walker, A.F. *et al.* (1987). RDAs—are changes necessary? *Chemistry and Industry* no. 16, August 17, 542–64.

Waterlow, J.C. (1979). Uses of recommended intakes: the purpose of dietary recommendations. *Food Policy* **4**, 107–14.

Whitehead, R.G. (1989). Recommended dietary amounts for the United Kingdom. *British Journal of Nutrition* **61**, 123–4.

Wretlind, A. (1982). Standards for nutritional adequacy of the diet: European and WHO/FAO viewpoints. *American Journal of Clinical Nutrition* **36**, 366–75.

2

Vitamin A and Carotenoids in Human Nutrition

INGRID H.E. RUTISHAUSER
Department of Human Nutrition, Deakin University, Victoria, Australia

INTRODUCTION

Vitamin A and its dietary precursors, the provitamin A carotenoids, have always played an important role in human nutrition. What has changed over the centuries is the extent of knowledge about their characteristics, sources and availability, and their biochemical and physiological functions in the human organism. In this chapter the term vitamin A is used both when referring to the vitamin in a general context and more specifically as the generic description for all β-ionone derivatives, except for provitamin A carotenoids, that exhibit the biological activity of retinol, i.e. retinol (vitamin A_1), dehydroretinol (vitamin A_2) and their respective esters, aldehydes and acids. The term provitamin A carotenoids is used when referring only to carotenoids that exhibit the biological activity of β-carotene. Provitamin A activity is found in a number of carotenoids and apo-carotenoids of which β-, α- and γ-carotene, β-cryptoxanthin and β-carotene 5, 6-epoxide are those most commonly found in food (Simpson, 1983). The term retinoids is used when referring not only to naturally occurring compounds with vitamin A activity but also to synthetic analogues of retinol with or without biological activity.

Regrettably, despite the considerable amount of knowledge now available about vitamin A and provitamin A carotenoids, the clinical manifestations of vitamin A deficiency, which are reported to be amongst the oldest recorded afflictions of mankind (Wolf, 1978; Sommer, 1982), are today still a major public health problem in many countries of the world.

For example, estimates by Sommer (1982) of the worldwide extent of deficiency severe enough to result in blindness (based on data from Bangladesh, India, Indonesia and the Philippines) suggest that every year at least 500 000 preschool children develop active xerophthalmia involving the cornea. About half of these children will become blind and an even higher proportion are likely to die. In addition, the annual prevalence of non-corneal xerophthalmia is probably of the order of 5 million cases (McLaren, 1986a).

Quite aside from the ocular manifestations of vitamin A deficiency, several recent epidemiological studies have provided evidence that vitamin A deficiency also contributes significantly to the morbidity and mortality experienced by preschool children in developing countries (Sommer, 1988). Interest in the role of vitamin A in human nutrition is, however, not confined to the problem of vitamin A deficiency. In developed nations where morbidity and mortality from degenerative diseases is high, considerable interest is focused on the possible role of vitamin A and provitamin A carotenoids in the prevention and control of cancer. From time to time concerns have also arisen in relation to the toxic effects of high doses of retinoids, both dietary and synthetic, particularly when taken during pregnancy. In order to discuss critically current views on these important aspects of the role of vitamin A in human nutrition it is necessary to look at our ability to measure the amount and availability of vitamin A and provitamin A carotenoids in the diet, to assess the validity of methods used for the assessment of vitamin A status in man and to review the basis for current recommendations for intake of vitamin A. To provide a background for current knowledge and views about vitamin A in human nutrition a brief historical review of the development of knowledge about this vitamin since the early nineteenth century is provided in Table 1.

During the nineteenth century clinical descriptions of the characteristic ocular signs of vitamin A deficiency, from night blindness to conjunctival and corneal involvement and xerophthalmia appeared in reports from Europe and Brazil and were tentatively linked with a 'faulty' diet. By the late nineteenth century the curative effects of cod liver oil for night blindness had been demonstrated and cod liver oil, meat and milk were being recommended for treatment of the corneal ulceration of keratomalacia. The twentieth century, however, proved to be the real 'age of enlightenment' with regard to knowledge about vitamin A. During the second decade of the century several investigators recognized the importance of 'accessory food factors' as a consequence of feeding 'pure' diets to animals

TABLE 1
A brief historical review of knowledge about vitamin A

1800	Dogs fed on sugar and water found to develop corneal ulcers.
1850	Clinical description of ocular signs of vitamin A deficiency from Europe, Brazil, Indonesia and Japan.
1900	Suggested link with diet and recommendations of milk, meat and cod liver oil for treatment of corneal ulceration of keratomalacia.
1910	Recognition that lipid component of foods contained substances— 'accessory food factors'—necessary for growth and eye health. Factor responsible named 'Fat-Soluble A' by McCollum in 1915, to distinguish it from 'Water-Soluble B'.
1920	Observation of morphological changes in epithelial tissues in vitamin A deficiency.
1930	Recognition of the anti-infective properties of vitamin A and of its role in reproduction in animals. Chemical characterization and isolation of β-carotene and retinol. Identification of the chromophore of visual pigment as retinene (now retinal).
1940	Synthesis of retinol and β-carotene. Experimental study of vitamin A requirements in man by Hume and Krebs.
1950	Further elucidation of the role of vitamin A in vision and of the pathology and pathophysiology of vitamin A deficiency.
1960	World wide survey of xerophthalmia by WHO. Recommendations for vitamin A intake published by FAO/WHO. Major advances in the understanding of the intermediary metabolism as well as the transport systems for vitamin A both extracellular and intracellular.
1970	Formation of the International Vitamin A Consultative Group (IVACG) and setting of recommendations for the establishment of world-wide programmes to control vitamin A deficiency. Investigation of the molecular mechanism of action of retinoids in the control of cell differentiation and proliferation. Development of new retinoids for the prevention and treatment of disease in the areas of oncology and dermatology.
1980	Epidemiological and experimental studies of the relationship between vitamin A status and the development of cancer.
1990	Prospective epidemiological studies and intervention trials of the contribution of vitamin A deficiency to the morbidity and mortality of preschool children in developing countries and of the role of vitamin A and provitamin A carotenoids in the prevention of cancer in developed countries.

and in 1915 McCollum and Davis named the active lipid soluble factor 'Fat Soluble A' to distinguish it from 'Water Soluble B'. During the 1920s vitamin A was recognized as playing an important role not only in growth and vision but also as being involved with the normal development of epithelial tissues, having anti-infective properties and necessary for reproduction in several species of animals. In the 1930s and 1940s chemical characterization, isolation and synthesis of retinol and β-carotene were achieved together with the identification of the chromophore of visual pigment as retinene. During the 1950s work was focused largely on further elucidating the role of vitamin A in vision and on detailed descriptions of the pathology and pathophysiology of vitamin A deficiency. It was, however, not until the 1960s that major advances were made in the understanding of the metabolism of vitamin A and its transport within the body both in extracellular fluids and within the cell.

In the early 1960s a world-wide survey of xerophthalmia was undertaken under the auspices of WHO which estimated that annually at least 20 000–100 000 children in the world develop compromised vision because of xerophthalmia. This led to the recognition of vitamin A deficiency as a global public health problem and eventually in 1974 to the formation of the International Vitamin A Consultative Group (IVACG) and the establishment of recommendations for a world-wide programme to control vitamin A deficiency. At about the same time considerable interest developed in the role played by retinoids in the control of cell differentiation and proliferation and in their role in the prevention and treatment of cancer and various dermatological problems. This research in turn resulted in numerous epidemiological and experimental studies of the relationship between vitamin A status and cancer and in a search for more sensitive yet practical techniques for the assessment of vitamin A status. The most recent decade has been notable principally for the effort devoted by Sommer and his colleagues to prospective epidemiological studies and intervention trials to determine the contribution of vitamin A deficiency to the morbidity and mortality of preschool children in developing countries. In developed countries similar studies have commenced in a number of countries to assess the role of vitamin A and provitamin A carotenoids in the prevention of certain types of cancer. Hopefully the coming decade will see a major impact on the control of vitamin A deficiency as a consequence of the recognition and acceptance by more governments of vitamin A supplementation as a potentially cost-effective approach both for child survival and the prevention of blindness. Similarly it is to be hoped that the intervention trials now under way of the effects of β-carotene on cancer

TABLE 2
Biological activity of vitamin A and provitamin A compounds expressed relative
to all-*trans*-retinol and β-carotene[a]

Vitamin A	Activity (%)	Provitamin A	Activity (%)
All-*trans*-retinol	100[b]	β-Carotene	100
Retinaldehyde	90	α-Carotene	50–54
13-*cis*-retinol	75	γ-Carotene	42–50
Dehydroretinol	40	β-cryptoxanthin	50–60
		α- and β-carotene	
		5,6 epoxides	21–25

[a] Compiled from Bauernfeind (1972) and Sivell *et al.* (1984).
[b] The reference standard for vitamin A activity is pure crystalline all-*trans*-retinol.

incidence will clarify whether vitamin A has an important role also in this
context or whether the active principle is some as yet unrecognized substance that occurs in foods in association with provitamin A carotenoids.

FOOD SOURCES AND BIOLOGICAL ACTIVITY

Distribution in foods
In general, preformed vitamin A is found only in animal products while
provitamin A carotenoids are found in foods of both animal and vegetable
origin. Exceptions to this general rule, however, do occur as retinal has
been isolated from the *Protista* and may, therefore, also be present in other
plant species. The carotenoids found in plants and microorganisms are the
products of biological synthesis while those found in animal products are
derived from the diet. In animal products vitamin A occurs in several
forms including the aldehyde, acid and the 3,4-dehydro form of retinol
(Vitamin A_2). Chiefly, however, vitamin A is found as retinyl esters of
longer-chain fatty acids and in particular as retinyl palmitate. The number
of naturally occurring carotenoids which have been characterized is now
close to 600 but only around 60 have provitamin A activity and of these
only five or six are commonly found in foods (Simpson, 1983). Table 2
shows the biological activity, relative to all-*trans* retinol, of the main
vitamin A and provitamin A compounds found in foods.

Biological activity
Most vitamin A activity in unfortified foods is in the form of all-*trans*
retinol esters, which have the same biological activity on a molar basis as

the free alcohol. *Cis* isomers occur to varying extents in foods. For example fish liver oils and eggs contain up to 35% and 20% respectively in this form. The most common *cis* isomer found in foods is 13-*cis* retinol which has about 75% of the activity of all-*trans* retinol. Dehydroretinol, the main form of vitamin A in the livers and flesh of some freshwater fish, has only about 40% of the activity of all-*trans* retinol. The biological activity of *β*-carotene varies with species. In humans values of 0·25 to 0·125 relative to all-*trans* retinol have been used. The most widely used value in humans, however, is 0·167. The biological activity of carotenoids other than *β*-carotene is generally taken as half that of *β*-carotene but in fact little data are available on the biological activity of these carotenoids in humans.

Stability of vitamin A compounds in foods
Both vitamin A and provitamin A carotenoids are liable to oxidation in the presence of oxygen, oxidizing agents and ultraviolet light. The rate of oxidation is accelerated by heat and the presence of trace metals. Conditions of low pH (< 4·5) and the application of heat cause some *cis–trans* isomerization but both vitamin A and provitamin A carotenoids are generally stable to cooking and processing methods in which temperatures do not exceed 100°C. The stability of vitamin A in foods under normal storage conditions is also good. Provitamin A compounds are largely stable in frozen and heat-stabilized foods but dehydrated foods must be sealed in an inert atmosphere to avoid losses. Sun drying of fruits and other foods leads to a considerable loss of vitamin A activity.

Food sources
The most concentrated sources of preformed vitamin A are liver and fish liver oils. Livers on average contain between 3 and 15 mg vitamin A/100 g while oils such as cod liver oil may contain as much as 30 mg/g oil. Significant amounts of vitamin A are also present in full cream milk and milk products, eggs, oily fish and chicken meat. Smaller amounts occur in most animal products. Table 3 gives some typical values for the retinol and *β*-carotene content of important dietary sources of vitamin A per 100 g and for overall vitamin A activity expressed as retinol equivalents per unit of energy (MJ). It is evident from this table that with the exception of fish liver oils and liver, the most concentrated sources of vitamin A activity when expressed either per 100 g of food or per MJ of energy, are the major vegetable sources such as carrots, green leafy vegetables and yellow and orange seeds, tubers and fruits. In comparison, animal products such as

TABLE 3
Foods ranked according to their vitamin A activity expressed in different ways[a]

Food	Retinol ($\mu g/100\,g$)	β-Carotene ($\mu g/100\,g$)	$RE/100\,g$[b]	RE/MJ
Fish liver oils	27 000	6 000	28 000	7 400
Beef liver	4 050	900	4 200	7 400
Carrots	—	6 000	1 000	6 000
Dark green leafy vegetables	—	3 600	600	5 100
Sweet potatoes (yellow)	—	4 200	700	1 400
Apricots	—	1 500	250	1 150
Light green leafy vegetables	—	550	92	870
Tomatoes	—	420	70	835
Mangoes	—	1 100	183	700
Eggs (hen)	200	180	230	350
Pumpkins	—	240	40	290
Butter	670	580	767	255
Milk	30	25	36	120
Maize (yellow)	—	270	45	30
Fatty fish	45	trace	45	45
Beef (mod. fat)	10	2	10	10
Lentils	—	60	10	7

[a] Compiled from Jardin et al. (1967).
[b] RE = retinol equivlent.

meats, eggs, fish, milk and butter only become important sources of vitamin A in the diet when they also contribute a significant proportion of the total dietary energy intake.

Units of vitamin A activity
It is appropriate at this stage to discuss briefly the rationale behind the units used to express the biological activity of vitamin A compounds in humans. The preferred approach is to express vitamin A activity in terms of retinol equivalents (RE), one RE being defined as equal to the vitamin A activity of 1 μg all-*trans* retinol. Table 4 illustrates the relationships between RE and the earlier system of International Units (IU) used to express vitamin A activity. For the reasons outlined above the predominant source of vitamin A activity in most diets, on a weight basis, is carotenoids. In theory one molecule of β-carotene can yield two molecules of retinal when split by intestinal β-carotene 15, 15'-dioxygenase. However, in practice it has been established from rat growth studies that 2 μg β-carotene are biologically equivalent to 1 μg retinol under conditions

TABLE 4
Units of vitamin A activity

	1 RE	1 IU[a]	1 μmol
Retinol	1 μg (3·33 IU)	0·3 μg	286 μg
Retinaldehyde	—	—	284 μg
Retinyl acetate	—	0·344 μg	328 μg
Retinoic acid	—	—	300 μg
Dehydroretinol	—	—	284 μg
β-Carotene	6 μg (10 IU)	0·6 μg	536 μg

[a] IU = International unit.

of suboptimal intake and approximately the same relationship has been observed in repletion studies in man (FAO, 1967). For example, the visual defects of vitamin A deficiency were reversed by 390 μg retinol or by 960 μg of a synthetic preparation of β-carotene, suggesting a biological efficiency ratio of about 2·5:1. In-vitro studies provide evidence for a similar efficiency of conversion as the average yield of retinol from β-carotene consumed ranges from 40 to 60%.

The IU definition of vitamin A activity is based on a 2:1 weight for weight relationship between β-carotene and retinol, one IU being defined as either 0·3 μg all-*trans* retinol or 0·6 μg all-*trans* β-carotene. This relationship between retinol and β-carotene, however, does not hold for the usual dietary sources of vitamin A and provitamin A carotenoids. Under normal conditions 70–90% of ingested retinyl esters are absorbed and there is only a slight reduction in efficiency at high doses. In contrast carotenoids are less efficiently absorbed than retinol in physiological amounts (20–50%) and at high doses the absorption is very low (< 10%). Absorption of provitamin A carotenoids in humans appears to occur by passive diffusion and varies considerably between individuals. It depends not only on normal intestinal function but also on the dose, the specific food source, the fat content of the diet and the presence of appropriate bile salts. Accurate prediction of the bioavailability of the carotenoid content of the diet is therefore difficult and it has become customary, in the absence of more specific data, to use a value of 33% for absorption of β-carotene from the diet and one half of this value for other carotenoids in the diet (FAO, 1967). Brubacher & Weiser (1985) and FAO (1988) have proposed more specific guidelines for the conversion of β-carotene to retinol in man (Table 5). For β-carotene in oily solutions Brubacher & Weiser (1985) consider a conversion factor of 1:3·33 appropriate for doses of

TABLE 5

Guidelines for the conversion of dietary β-carotene intake to retinol equivalents[a]

Intake of β-carotene (μg) per meal	Amount of β-carotene (μg) equivalent to 1 μg retinol	Conversion factor
< 1000	4	0·25
1000–4000	6	0·167
> 4000	10	0·10

[a] Source, FAO (1988).
The bioavailability of β-carotene in oil at each level of intake is up to two times higher. Conversion of β-carotene to RE is commonly done using a factor of 0·167. Because the absorption efficiency of carotenoids declines with increasing intake the factor above 4000 μg is intake-dependent.

1500–4000 μg, while with higher amounts, the factor should be decreased. For β-carotene from foods the generally accepted conversion factor of 1:6·0 is applicable to intakes of between 1000 and 4000 μg with a higher factor applicable to smaller intakes and vice versa (FAO, 1988).

Vitamin A activity expressed in RE allows for the incomplete absorption of carotenoids from foods. Thus in terms of IU, one IU of vitamin A is equated with 0·3 μg retinol and 0·6 μg β-carotene, while in terms of RE, one RE of vitamin A activity is equated with 1 μg or 3·33 IU retinol and 6 μg or 10 IU β-carotene and 12 μg of other carotenoids. The use of both IU and RE as measures of the total vitamin A activity of foods has led to considerable confusion. Firstly, the use of IU and RE essentially obscures the proportion of vitamin A activity contributed by retinol and by provitamin A carotenoids. Secondly, when expressed in terms of IU the contribution of carotenoids to total vitamin A activity appears to be greater than when expressed in terms of RE. Suppose for example that a diet provides 500 μg retinol and 1000 μg β-carotene, then in terms of IU the diet provides 3333 IU of which 50% comes from retinol and 50% comes from β-carotene. Expressed in RE, however, the diet provides 667 RE of which 75% comes from retinol and 25% from β-carotene. Given the degree of uncertainty about the availability of carotenoids from the diet, it is probably useful to identify the separate contribution of vitamin A and provitamin A carotenoids in terms of the micrograms of each in the diet.

TABLE 6

Classification of vegetables and fruits according to their pattern of provitamin A
content[a]

Group	Provitamin A Pattern	Characteristic foods
1	Mainly β-carotene	Dark green leaves, green pepper, tomato, sweet potato, snap bean musk melon, pomelo
2	Considerable amounts of α-carotene	Carrot, pumpkin
3	Carotenoids other than α- and β-carotene	Mango, pawpaw, orange, persimmon, peach, red pepper

[a] Compiled from Simpson & Tsou (1986).

A further reason for doing this is that until fairly recently the most
common method used to determine the carotenoid content of foods
measured total carotenoids rather than β-carotene specifically and consequently overestimated the vitamin A activity of some foods.

Analytical methods for carotenoids

The standard AOAC method for estimation of carotenoids involves extraction of the tissue with a suitable solvent followed by a chromatograph-
ic procedure which separates carotenoids and xanthophylls on the basis of
polarity and then quantifies the eluted carotenes by light absorption at
436 nm. The α-carotene present in the same extract co-chromatographs
with β-carotene and leads to overestimation of β-carotene if present in
significant amounts. If lycopene is also present then the extent of overestimation may be as much as tenfold. Several xanthophylls also have
provitamin A activity and these are excluded by some standard methods
if they are present as polar compounds but included if they are esterified
as in some fruits. In the newer HPLC methods individual carotenoids are
measured separately and thus it is possible to make more appropriate
calculations of the total β-carotene equivalents than before. Using HPLC
data, Simpson & Tsou (1986) have classified vegetables and fruit sources
of provitamin A activity into three categories on the basis of their carotenoid pattern (Table 6). Group 1 includes primarily green and other vegetables in which β-carotene is either the only carotene or the major carotene
present. For this group the results for β-carotene obtained by the standard

TABLE 7
Provitamin A activity (in mg β-carotene equivalent/100 g) of selected foods according to the analytical method used[a]

Method	Group 1 Spinach	Group 2 Pumpkin	Group 3 Pawpaw
AOAC	2·06	10·03	1·73
Stepwise solvent gradient elution	—	4·84	—
Saponification and solvent gradient elution	—	—	0·59
HPLC	3·32	5·09	0·52
Major carotenoids present	β-carotene	α-carotene β-carotene	β-carotene β-cryptoxanthin

[a] Compiled from Simpson & Tsou (1986).

AOAC method are similar to those obtained by HPLC. Foods in Group 2 include orange vegetables such as carrots and pumpkin, which contain considerable amounts of α-carotene or other carotenoids. The β-carotene content of these foods is overestimated by the AOAC method unless stepwise solvent gradient elution is used to separate the carotenes. Group 3 foods primarily include fruits that contain a proportion of esterified xanthophylls and require a saponification step to hydrolyse the ester linkages followed by gradient elution to separate individual compounds.

Table 7 illustrates the differences obtained using AOAC, gradient elution and HPLC methods for three individual foods representative of Groups 1, 2 and 3. For dark green leafy vegetables such as spinach the AOAC and HPLC methods give comparable results, while for pumpkin the AOAC method gives a twofold overestimation of β-carotene and for pawpaw the overestimation is even greater in the absence of a saponification step prior to elution. Earlier food composition and intake data need to be reinterpreted in the light of the different carotenoid patterns in foods and wherever possible food composition data should include not simply estimates of vitamin A equivalents but also the actual amounts of vitamin A and individual carotenoids present. In practical terms the availability of more specific data on carotenoid content will in general result in greater differences between diets 'rich' and 'poor' in vitamin A. For example, if intake values for diets of different populations in IU per head per day are recalculated based on the carotenoid patterns of the major dietary sources the effect will be relatively small for populations in whose diets animal

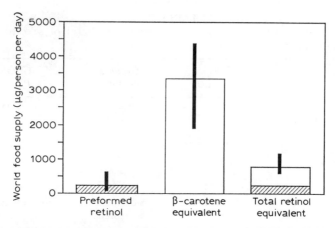

FIG. 1. Average amounts of preformed vitamin A (retinol), β-carotene equivalents and total retinol in the world food supply, expressed as μg/person per day;
▨, animal sources; □, plant sources; ■, range. (From FAO Food and Nutrition
Series no. 23: Requirements of Vitamin A, Iron, Folate and Vitamin B12 (1988);
reproduced by permission of the Food and Agriculture Organization of the United
Nations).

foods contribute a substantial proportion of the total vitamin A activity
and most marked in those populations whose diets contain significant
amounts of provitamin A activity from yellow and orange fruits, roots,
tubers and seeds.

Vitamin A availability in populations [Habitual intake]
The total amount of vitamin A available from the food supply (Fig. 1) has
been estimated as between 1000 and 1500 RE/head per day in the developed market economies of Europe, North America and Oceania and
between 500 and 1000 RE/head per day in the developing market economies of Africa, Latin America and the Near and Far East. In the developed countries 40–60% of the total vitamin A activity is estimated to
come from provitamin A carotenoids while in the majority of developing
countries over 80% comes from this source (Perisse & Polacchi, 1980). It
should be noted, however, that such estimates are very dependent on the
accuracy of the information about the most concentrated dietary sources
of vitamin A such as edible offal and red palm oil. For example, although
edible offal may contribute only 4–85 kJ (1–20 kcal)/head per day of
energy it may be the source of as much as 40% of the total available
vitamin A; and similarly palm oil may contribute only 40–170 kJ (10–

TABLE 8
Vitamin A in the food supply (RE/person per day) according to food group and source of data—Australia 1979–83

Food group	Data source			
	FAO 1984[a]	ABS 1983[b]	DCSH 1987[c]	
			Males	Females
Offal	592	421	342	932
Meat	24	24	68	44
Milk and milk products	126	243	160	129
Butter and margarine	91	279	54	44
			159	95
Vegetables	273	391	486	446
Eggs	69	85	—	—
Fish	4	5	151	131
Fruit	46	73	—	—
Cereal staples	6	1	—	—
Total	1261	1522	1420	1820
RE/MJ	99	105	129	246
Animal sources	28%	40%	51%	33%
Vegetable sources	72%	60%	49%	67%

[a] FAO, Food and Agriculture Organization of the United Nations.
[b] ABS, Apparent Food Consumption of Foodstuffs and Nutrients, Australia.
[c] DCSH, Department of Community Service and Health, Australia.

40 kcal)/head per day but may be the source of 70% of the available vitamin A. Major differences in estimates of vitamin A intake and the contribution of vegetable and animal sources also arise depending on the source of information from which they are derived. Table 8 illustrates this point with data from Australia estimated from FAO Food Balance Sheets (FAO, 1984), Apparent Food Consumption of Foodstuffs and Nutrients, Australia (Australian Bureau of Statistics, 1983) and from the National Dietary Survey of Adults, 1983 (Department of Community Services and Health, 1987). Depending on the data used estimates for the contribution of animal sources to total vitamin A intake range from 49 to 72% and are determined largely by the estimated contribution of offal which ranges from 300 to 900 RE/head per day, being three times higher in females than males.

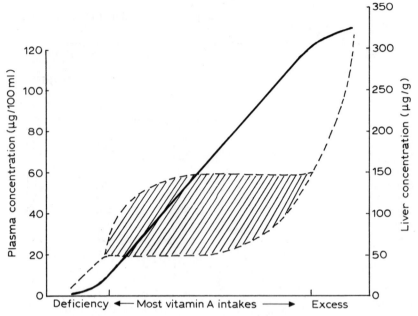

FIG. 2.   Relationship between the plasma (– – –) and liver (——) concentrations
of vitamin A at various intakes. Adapted from Rutishauser (1986).

ASSESSMENT OF VITAMIN A STATUS

Liver vitamin A
The liver is the major storage organ for vitamin A in the body and
measurement of liver vitamin A concentration provides a good measure of
vitamin A reserves. The total body reserve of vitamin A, as measured by
the total liver store, increases in an almost linear fashion with increased
dietary intake of retinol (Olson, 1984), while the relationship between liver
stores and plasma vitamin A level is more complex (Fig. 2). In well
nourished individuals the liver contains more than 90% of the total body
store of vitamin A, whereas in poorly nourished individuals the kidneys
and other tissues account for an appreciable amount of the total body
reserve (10–50%). In healthy individuals the concentration of vitamin A
in liver is very variable and median values are in the range 50–300 µg
vitamin A/g liver in well nourished populations. Total body content in a
70 kg man, with a liver vitamin A concentration of 100 µg/g and a plasma
level of 50 µg/dl, is around 200 mg with plasma and extra-hepatic vitamin

A contributing about 10% of the total. A liver retinol level of less than 20 $\mu g/g$ is associated with depleted hepatic stores and plasma vitamin A levels tend to fall; above 300 $\mu g/g$ liver plasma values tend to increase. Although a good measure of vitamin A intake and of body stores, measurement of liver vitamin A content by liver biopsy is not a practical procedure for population studies of vitamin A status.

Plasma vitamin A

Fasting plasma retinol level, although easier to measure, does not reflect liver stores of vitamin A except when these are depleted or when the liver is saturated with vitamin A as in hypervitaminosis. It is therefore not a very sensitive measure of vitamin A status within the normal range of liver vitamin A as it is homeostatically controlled (Olson, 1984). Although the plasma level of vitamin A in an individual is not a sensitive measure of vitamin A status, the distribution of plasma levels within populations can provide a useful measure of relative dietary adequacy. In apparently healthy populations consuming adequate amounts of vitamin A there is a wide range of plasma levels from 20 to 80 $\mu g/dl$ and the distribution curve is relatively normal in shape. In contrast, distribution curves for populations in which vitamin A inadequacy occurs are not always normally distributed and as the frequency of values in the lower range of the curve increases, so does the risk that this is associated with habitual 'inadequate' intakes of vitamin A (WHO, 1982). During childhood there is a positive correlation between age and serum level when diets contain adequate vitamin A and in general males have higher serum levels than females. Correct interpretation of population distribution curves for serum vitamin A thus requires a knowledge of both the age and sex distribution of the population. Serum levels of total carotenoids, in the absence of retinol levels, are not particularly useful for assessing the vitamin A status of individuals or populations because they reflect primarily the level of immediate dietary intake and because a considerable proportion of the total carotenoids may be non-vitamin A active compounds (Buzina *et al.*, 1971).

More recent data, however, suggest that in fact healthy individuals under free-living conditions maintain a characteristic carotenoid profile and that this is the result of long-term dietary patterns and is little influenced by occasional large intakes of a food high in a particular carotenoid pigment (Brown *et al.*, 1989). Thus the plasma carotenoid profile may provide a better measure of long-term carotenoid intake than previously thought but, because of the large variation in response between

Ingrid H.E. Rutishauser

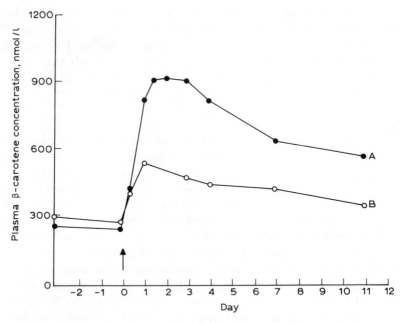

FIG. 3.   Plasma β-carotene concentration in two subjects, A and B, after ingesting 30 mg pure β-carotene at point indicated by the arrow. Adapted from Brown *et al.* (1989).

individuals to a given dose of either pure β-carotene or from a vegetable source, it is unlikely to be a good measure of the dietary intake of pro-vitamin A carotenoids (Fig. 3).

Relative dose response
This test is based on the principle that when stores of retinol are high, plasma retinol is little affected by an oral or an intravenous dose of vitamin A (Loerch *et al.*, 1979). If, however, liver stores are depleted or low the plasma retinol level following supplementation increases, reaching a peak at 5 h. During vitamin A depletion apo-RBP (retinol binding protein) accumulates in the hepatocytes, and with the oral administration of a small dose (450 μg) of vitamin A in oil the holo-RBP concentration of the plasma rapidly rises to a plateau at approximately 5 h. The percentage increase in plasma retinol values measured as the difference between plasma retinol concentrations at 0 and 5 h ($\times$ 100) divided by the value at 5 h is termed the relative dose response (RDR). Relative dose response

TABLE 9
Eye conditions classified as xerophthalmia[a]

Lesion	WHO Code	Per cent[b]
Night blindness	XN	—
Conjunctival xerosis	X1A	—
Bitot's spot	X1B	> 0·5
Corneal xerosis	X2	—
Corneal ulceration— < 1/3 cornea		
(keratomalacia)	X3A	> 0·01
Corneal ulceration— > 1/3 cornea		
(keratomalacia)	X3B	—
Corneal scar	XS	> 0·05
Xerophthalmia fundus	XF	—

[a] Taken from WHO (1982).
[b] Prevalence rates in preschool children regarded as indicative of xerophthalmia and vitamin A deficiency in a community.

values greater than 50% have been observed in vitamin A-depleted children and values above 14% in adult subjects with night blindness, which was correctable with vitamin A, or with liver vitamin A reserves of 30 μg/g or less. In contrast, subjects with liver stores above 50 μg/g had RDR values that were less than 12% (Amedee-Manesme et al., 1984). In situations where vitamin A malabsorption is likely to be a problem, such as in some forms of liver disease, administration of the vitamin A dose by intravenous injection provides an alternative means for obtaining a reliable and sensitive indicator of vitamin A status (Amadee-Manesme et al., 1987). The RDR may be inaccurate, however, in states of protein malnutrition or cirrhotic liver disease in which RBP levels may be too low to produce a response to the test dose (Russell et al., 1983).

Clinical assessment
The only clinical feature that is specifically attributable to vitamin A deficiency is xerophthalmia, the collective term used for all the eye lesions of vitamin A deficiency (Table 9). Xerophthalmia is usually indicative of advanced vitamin A depletion, so that a considerable number of biochemically deficient individuals may appear clinically normal and surveys that only examine the prevalence of eye disease will not give a true reflection of the problem of hypovitaminosis A. A history of night blindness has been found to be useful as a guide to the prevalence of vitamin A deficiency in children, especially in areas where there is a specific local name for this

symptom. Thus in Indonesia a history of night blindness, obtained by interviewing the mother, has been found to correlate well both with low plasma vitamin A values and with clinical eye signs (Sommer, 1982). Numerous other tests are available for the assessment of retinal function including dark-adaptation, rod scotometry, electroretinography, and reflective spectrophotometry. However, none of these, with the possible exception of dark-adaptation in adults, is suitable as a screening test in community surveys because of the expense of the equipment, the time taken to perform the test and the problems of compliance.

Impression cytology has been suggested as a relatively simple and also practical alternative technique for assessing the extent of physiologically significant vitamin A deficiency. The basis of the test is that vitamin A deficiency causes changes in the conjunctival epithelium characterized in part by the loss of goblet cells (Hatchell & Sommer, 1984). The test involves applying a piece of cellulose acetate filter paper to the temporal bulbar conjunctiva for 3–5 s and staining the adherent cells. Wittpenn *et al.* (1986) and Natadisastra *et al.* (1988) have used this test to differentiate between normal children and those with mild xerophthalmia. Amadee-Manesme *et al.* (1988) have shown that this test can identify individuals with physiologically significant preclinical vitamin A deficiency in children with liver disease. Gadomski *et al.* (1989) have, however, questioned the value of conjunctival impression cytology (CIC) for detecting marginal vitamin A deficiency in Guatemalan children on the basis of a low sensitivity and positive predictive value of CIC when compared with RDR ($> 20\,\mu g/dl$). The sensitivity of both the criterion measures is, however, also likely to have been limited under the conditions of this study by the high prevalence of both low RBP and plasma albumin in this population and possibly also by the administration of the oral RDR test dose together with a meal. Further field trials of standardized CIC procedures are therefore required to test the efficiency of this technique in community studies (Kjolhede *et al.*, 1989).

Dietary assessment
Assessment of dietary vitamin A intake can also be used as a crude indicator of the likelihood of vitamin A deficiency in a population, although it is clearly not a measure of vitamin A status. Table 10 shows the relationship between the different measures of assessment of vitamin A status in preschool children, the group most frequently affected by vitamin A deficiency. When vitamin A status is deficient, plasma, liver and dietary intake levels are all low, the RDR is likely to be above 50% and eye signs

TABLE 10
Indicators of vitamin A status in preschool children

Biochemical			Eye signs	Diet (RE/day)	Overall
Plasma (µg/dl)	Liver (µg/g)	RDR (%)			
< 10	< 5	> 50	Present	< 100	Poor
10–20	5–20	> 20	Present	100–300	Marginal
20–100	20–300	< 20	Absent	300–2000	Adequate
> 100	> 300	—	Absent	> 10 000	Excessive

and night blindness are present. At marginal levels eye signs and night blindness are likely to be absent but CIC is abnormal and plasma, liver and dietary intake levels are still clearly low while the RDR is greater than 20%. In contrast, adequate vitamin A status is compatible with a wide range of plasma, liver and dietary levels of vitamin A. Toxicity is encountered when plasma and liver stores are above 100 µg/dl and 300 µg/g respectively and dietary intake regularly exceeds 10 000 RE/day.

HUMAN REQUIREMENTS AND RECOMMENDED DIETARY INTAKES (RDI) FOR VITAMIN A

Past approaches
A detailed review of studies relating to vitamin A requirements in man was made some years ago by Rodriguez & Irwin (1972); however, much of the early work is difficult to interpret because of differences in the potency of vitamin A standards used and difficulties with the methods of analysis, and because studies were not carried out under carefully controlled conditions. Moreover, in the past requirements for vitamin A have often been determined on the basis of a number of different criteria. These have included:

—the amount needed to correct impaired dark adaptation;
—the amount needed to raise the concentration of plasma vitamin into the normal range and;
—the amount required to maintain a given body pool size.

The use of different criteria naturally leads to different recommended dietary intakes for vitamin A depending on the particular criterion chosen.

For example, in 1967 the Joint FAO/WHO Expert Group chose to use, as the basis for recommendations in adults, the amount of vitamin A (750 μg) needed in the Sheffield study (Hume & Krebs, 1949) to prevent any development of impaired dark adaptation and to maintain a consistent plasma vitamin A level over a period of 14–17 months. On the other hand, the Committee on Dietary Allowances of the Food and Nutrition Board of the National Research Council (Food and Nutrition Board, 1980, 1989) chose to use a level of 1000 μg based on the amount found to be required to restore plasma retinol values to 30 μg/dl in previously depleted subjects (Sauberlich *et al.*, 1974). In both the Sheffield and the American studies 400–600 μg vitamin A/day was sufficient to prevent all ocular manifestations of vitamin A deficiency but did not, in the short term (several weeks), restore blood vitamin A levels to normal after depletion.

Current principles
Because of the multiplicity of possible definitions, FAO have now adopted a 'two-tier' system of recommendations (Olson, 1988). In this system the basal dietary requirement is defined as the level that meets the following criteria:

1. Prevents the appearance of signs of vitamin A deficiency.
2. Maintains normal growth in children.
3. Cures the signs of vitamin A deficiency in depleted subjects over a specified period.

The recommended dietary intake, on the other hand, is defined as the amount that provides a specified total body reserve of the vitamin in order to minimize the effects of occasional periods of low intake, infections and other stresses. The specified level of body reserve chosen for the recommended daily intake (RDI) by FAO (1988) was a liver vitamin A concentration of 20 μg/g. At this level of liver vitamin A no clinical signs of deficiency occur, the liver is able to maintain steady state plasma vitamin A levels as determined by the relative dose response test and this level is also sufficient to protect an adult ingesting a diet free of vitamin A from a deficiency state for about 4 months as well as to meet vitamin A needs during shorter periods of stress, such as infection (Olson, 1987). This level of liver vitamin A combined with an estimate of the fractional catabolic role of vitamin A, that is the percentage of total body stores lost per day, derived from the data of Sauberlich *et al.* (1974) provides an alternative approach to estimating the vitamin A requirements of both children and adults.

TABLE 11
Calculation of the vitamin A intake required to maintain a liver vitamin A concentration of 20 μg/g in adults

---

Assumptions
1. Ratio of liver weight to body weight = 0·03 (range 0·042 in infants—0·024 in adults).
2. Ratio of total body reserve to liver vitamin A = 1·11 (assumes 90% in the liver).
3. Daily metabolic loss as a percent of body store = 0·005 (estimated from Sauberlich *et al.*, 1974.)
4. Efficiency of storage of ingested vitamin A = 0·5 (range 40–90%).
5. Estimate of individual variation in requirement = 1·4 (coefficient of variation ∼ 20%).

RDI estimate

75 kg male = 75 × 20 × 0·03 × 1·11 × 0·005 × 2 × 1·4
        = 700 μg/day.
60 kg female = 60/75 × 700
        = 560 μg/day.

Adults
Sample calculations for the vitamin A RDI for an adult male of 75 kg and an adult female of 60 kg are shown in Table 11.

The 1988 FAO approach also lends itself to the estimation of recommended dietary intakes for children and pregnant and lactating women when due allowance is made for the additional physiological needs at these times.

Pregnancy
Vitamin A is known to be required for the growth, cellular differentiation and normal development of the foetus. At term the average body weight of a newborn infant is around 3·5 kg and from the data in Table 11 it can be calculated that the total vitamin A content of the newborn is only 3·2 mg (based on a liver vitamin A concentration of 20 μg/g at birth). This compares with a maternal liver store of around 200 mg in a 60 kg woman with a liver vitamin A concentration of 100 μg/g and, therefore, constitutes only a very small proportion (less than 2%) of the maternal reserve. Moreover, since the mean retinol concentration in foetal liver appears to remain low even when the mother is given vitamin A supplements, there appears to be no advantage in recommending an increase in vitamin A intake during pregnancy in well-nourished women, particularly as vitamin A in large doses is potentially teratogenic in the early weeks of pregnancy.

From primate studies the fourth to the tenth gestational weeks are likely to be the most susceptible time for the expression of teratogenic effects of excess vitamin A intake in humans (Wallingford & Underwood, 1986) and it is, therefore, generally recommended that the intake of large doses of vitamin A should be avoided by women who might become pregnant (Underwood, 1986b). However, since there are also women in the re-productive age group who have low liver vitamin A reserves it is con-sidered advisable, at least by some authorities, to recommend an addition-al intake of 200 μg retinol daily in the last trimester of pregnancy in order to provide for the vitamin A needs of the foetus while at the same time maintaining the limited maternal vitamin A stores (Olson, 1987).

Lactation
The vitamin A content of human milk from well-nourished women ranges from 40 to 70 μg retinol/dl and the average daily output of milk between 500 and 1000 ml. On this basis, the daily additional loss of vitamin A by this route can be estimated to amount to as little as 200 μg or as much as 700 μg in lactating women but is taken to be, on average, between 400 and 450 μg daily during the first 6 months. The recommended additional intake for lactation is normally also of this order and makes no allowance for the efficiency with which ingested vitamin A is transferred to the mother's milk. However, in practical terms this is not necessary in well-nourished women in view of the size of liver vitamin A reserves. In primates, unless vitamin A intake is very high, 80–90% of the vitamin A in milk appears to be derived from the circulating retinol–RBP complex and the remaining 10–20% from lipoprotein complexes of vitamin A or its esters (Vahlquist & Nilsson, 1979). In vitamin A-depleted lactating women a large dietary supplement of vitamin A (50 000 IU) significantly increases the concentra-tion of vitamin A in the milk (Venkatchalam *et al.*, 1962). However, since relatively few studies have compared breast milk vitamin A levels with intake of retinol or retinol equivalents by lactating women there is not yet a clear picture of the relationship between intake and breast milk vitamin A level (Bates, 1983).

Infants and children
The vitamin A requirements of infants have generally been based on the assumption that during the first 2 months of life exclusive breastfeeding provides sufficient vitamin A to maintain health, permit normal growth and also allow storage of vitamin A in the liver. However, in countries where intake of vitamin A from human milk is estimated to be only

100–200 μg/day, although vitamin A deficiency and a reduced growth rate are not generally apparent in infancy there is often a high incidence of vitamin A deficiency in early childhood (Rodriguez & Irwin, 1972; Underwood, 1984) which suggests that at this level of intake liver storage of vitamin A is minimal (McLaren *et al.*, 1965). In contrast, in countries where breastfed infants receive on average, 300–450 μg vitamin A/day from human milk, vitamin A deficiency in early childhood does not occur. The vitamin A requirements of infants have therefore generally been based on the vitamin A intake of babies breastfed by well-nourished women and, in the absence of more direct evidence, the recommended intakes for children have been determined from the vitamin A intake of breastfed babies and the recommended intake for adults on the basis of body size.

Expressed per kilogram body weight per day, the average recommended intake of vitamin A in the first 6 months of life (375 μg/d) is equivalent to 75 μg/kg per day while the maintenance recommendation for adults is only 10 μg/kg per day. The requirement for growth in the first 6 months of life can therefore be estimated to be around 300 μg/day or approximately 15 μg/g of tissue gained. Applying this estimate for growth requirements throughout childhood results in the figures shown in Table 12. These are not dissimilar from the earlier FAO (1967) recommendations for vitamin A intake except for body weight-related differences between the sexes.

Elderly
Information on the vitamin A needs of older people is limited. Plasma levels in normal adults range from 30 to 90 μg/dl and do not appear to decline with age. Similarly, liver vitamin A stores of elderly people do not differ markedly from those of adults aged 40–60 years (Hoppner *et al.*, 1968). Huque (1982), in a post-mortem study, reported a definite downward trend from the fifth decade onwards, but this finding was probably influenced by the fact that subjects dying from cardiovascular disease and cancer had liver stores that were 25% lower than those of subjects dying from accidental causes and not due primarily to an age-related decrease in liver vitamin A content. Vitamin A tolerance curves in the elderly obtained with physiological doses of vitamin A show higher peak heights of retinyl esters compared with younger controls while with large doses of vitamin A no age-related differences in vitamin A tolerance were evident (Suter & Russell, 1987). Overall present evidence indicates that the elderly in North America, Europe and Australia are able to maintain body stores of vitamin A despite reported vitamin A intakes that are not infrequently lower than the RDI.

TABLE 12
Vitamin A needs during childhood calculated from estimates of maintenance and growth requirements per kg body weight

Age	Weight (kg)	Growth rate (g/day)	Vitamin A (µg/day)		
			Maintenance	Growth	Total
Children					
0– 6 months	6	20	60	315	375
7–12 months	9	15	90	225	315
1– 3 years	12	5	120	75	195
4– 7 years	17	5	170	75	245
Females					
8–11 years	30	10	300	150	450
12–15 years	48	10	480	150	630
16–18 years	57	2	570	20	590
Adult	60	—	600	—	600
Males					
8–11 years	30	10	300	150	450
12–15 years	48	15	480	225	705
16–18 years	66	10	660	150	810
Adult	75	—	750	—	750

AETIOLOGY OF VITAMIN A DEFICIENCY

Some data on the magnitude of the problem of vitamin A deficiency were provided at the beginning of this chapter. Fig. 4 shows the geographical distribution of vitamin A deficiency and xerophthalmia in the world in 1984 according to the extent to which vitamin A deficiency is considered to be a public health problem in different countries. At the present time vitamin A deficiency is encountered essentially only in developing countries, especially in Asia and in Africa. Among the most affected areas in Asia are the Indian sub-continent and South-East Asian countries. In Africa, the areas most affected are located in the Sahara region and in the eastern part of the continent, while in Latin America and the Caribbean there are pockets of xerophthalmia in Central America and in Brazil.

Aetiology
The aetiology of vitamin A deficiency is complex and although always associated with a chronically low vitamin A intake the effects of a given level of intake may be considerably modified by the physical and socio-economic environment. In general, the risk of vitamin A deficiency is

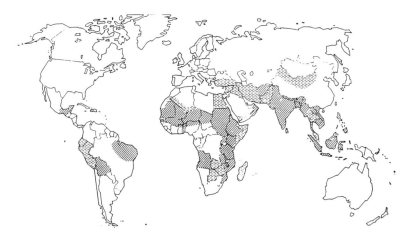

FIG. 4. World distribution of vitamin A deficiency and xerophthalmia in 1984. ▨ Vitamin A deficiency is a significant public health problem; ⊟ Vitamin A deficiency is most probably a significant public health problem; ☐ Vitamin A deficiency is not a significant public health problem. Sporadic cases may occur. (From FAO Food and Nutrition Series no. 23: Requirements of Vitamin A, Iron, Folate and Vitamin B12 (1988); reproduced by permission of the Food and Agriculture Organization of the United Nations).

greatest in countries, communities and households characterized by poverty, poor sanitation and limited access to health and social services. Within households, young children are at the greatest risk of developing xerophthalmia both because their vitamin A requirements are proportionately higher than those of older individuals and because they are much more prone to all kinds of infections.

The most dramatic impact of vitamin A deficiency is on the eye, leading in turn to night blindness, xerosis of the conjunctiva and cornea and ultimately corneal ulceration and necrosis (keratomalacia). The term xerophthalmia, which literally and opthalmologically means 'dry eye', is used in a public health context to refer to the whole range of ocular manifestations of vitamin A deficiency, which includes not only the structural changes observed in the conjunctiva, cornea and retina but also the disturbances of retinal rod and cone function attributable to vitamin A deficiency. Vitamin A deficiency, however, also affects many other physiological functions including growth, differentiation of epithelial tissues and immune responses. For example, there is now considerable evidence that morbidity and mortality due to gastrointestinal and respiratory infec-

tions is increased even in only mildly vitamin A-deficient subjects, probably as a consequence of effects on cellular differentiation and immune
function (Sommer *et al.*, 1983, 1984, 1986, 1987). Vitamin A deficiency,
like protein–energy malnutrition, with which it is not infrequently associated, haš a major impact on growth and development in early childhood
and its prevention is a matter for global concern.

Effective strategies for the prevention of vitamin A deficiency require a
clear understanding of the multiple factors that may contribute to the
vitamin A status of an individual in a given environment.

Dietary factors
Two of the most important factors affecting vitamin A status are the
adequacy of intake and the absorption of vitamin A. Given the present
day distribution of vitamin A deficiency it is not surprising, therefore, to
find a sharp distinction between the availability of both total vitamin A
and preformed vitamin A between developing and developed countries.
The latter distinction is even clearer than the former (Fig. 5). In fact, it
would appear that on a national basis the availability of vitamin A is a
good indicator not only of vitamin A status but also of income and the
stage of economic development of a country (De Maeyer, 1986).

Sources of vitamin A
Another important difference between developed and developing countries is the extent to which preformed vitamin A contributes to the total
vitamin A intake of the population. In developing countries where xerophthalmia is endemic, virtually all dietary vitamin A is derived from vegetable foods. As described earlier there is considerable variation in the
extent to which provitamin A carotenoids in foods are biologically active
and available. In contrast, preformed sources of vitamin A in the diet are
not only more completely absorbed and their absorption less influenced by
dose and other components of the diet such as fat content, but weight for
weight they also have a higher biological activity. Moreover, in general
they are also consumed on a more regular basis (e.g. milk, butter, margarine and eggs) than are the main vegetable sources of provitamin A
activity, many of which are only seasonally available (e.g. dark green leafy
vegetables and orange and yellow fruits). It is of interest in this context
that xerophthalmia rarely occurs among breastfed infants, even when
breastmilk vitamin A is low, and is seldom reported in children who
continue to be breastfed into the second year of life, presumably because

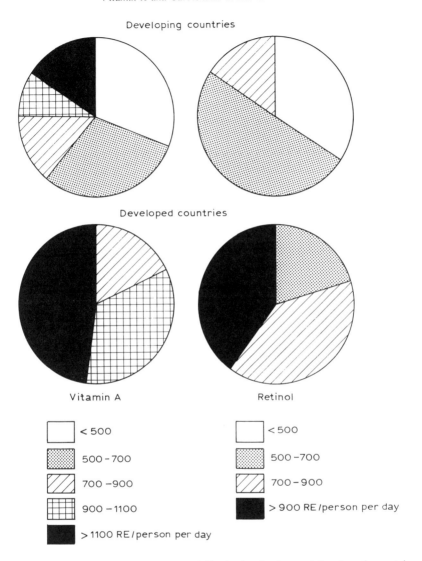

FIG. 5. Vitamin A and retinol availability in developing and developed countries in 1975. Adapted from De Maeyer (1986).

both groups receive a daily, even if small, dose of readily absorbed preformed vitamin A (Underwood, 1984).

Staple foods

When breastfeeding stops the main dietary determinant of vitamin A intake in preschool children in developing countries is often the vitamin A content of the staple food. If this contains even small amounts of vitamin A-active carotenoids, then vitamin A deficiency is less severe than when the staple food is devoid of provitamin carotenoids, as in societies eating rice, cassava and white maize. However, even if the staple food does contain small amounts of vitamin A, young children need additional sources of vitamin A in the diet to replace the small but regular intake (50–100 μg/day) previously provided by human milk. Sometimes these additional vitamin A sources, although available within a household, are not given to small children for cultural reasons.

Fat

When breastfeeding stops not only is vitamin A intake reduced but the fat intake may also drop markedly as almost 50% of the energy in human milk is derived from fat. A diet low in fat results in less efficient absorption of carotenoids while, conversely, fat given in association with foods containing carotenoids has been shown to improve their absorption and utilization (Roels *et al.* 1958; Jayarajan *et al.* 1980). It is important, therefore, not only to consider the vitamin A but also the fat content of the diet during the weaning period.

Protein

Not surprisingly, xerophthalmia is often associated with protein–energy malnutrition (PEM), although the level of association varies from country to country. In general, kwashiorkor rather than marasmus appears to be more closely associated with xerophthalmia and it is not difficult to see why this should be. In marasmus, the rate of growth is reduced and consequently also the requirement for vitamin A, which is related to growth. However, in kwashiorkor vitamin A cannot be effectively transported and utilized, even if liver stores exist, because the synthesis of transport proteins—including RBP—is impaired. Thus, keratomalacia is almost always associated with kwashiorkor rather than marasmus. Protein –energy malnutrition has also been associated with less efficient absorption of dietary vitamin A and carotenoids, but this may be as much a consequence of the low-fat diet and infections that are also associated with

PEM as of PEM *per se*. On balance, it is considered more likely that the xerophthalmia associated with mild forms of PEM is a consequence of vitamin A deficiency rather than of protein deficiency (Underwood, 1984).

Iron and zinc
Other nutrients that may influence vitamin A status are vitamin E, iron and zinc. Largely vegetable-based diets are unlikely to be limiting in vitamin E relative to their vitamin A content and therefore to interfere with vitamin A metabolism unless vitamin A is consumed in excess. Vegetable diets, however, are quite limiting in both available iron and zinc. Animal studies indicate that vitamin A is required for proper iron utilization while zinc appears to be necessary for RBP synthesis and its release from the liver. Thus anaemia can sometimes be improved by vitamin A supplementation (Mejia & Arroyave, 1982) and dark adaptation by giving zinc (Solomons & Russell, 1980).

Environmental factors
Climate, the pattern of endemic disease and cultural practices with respect to the feeding of young children are the principal environmental factors that modify susceptibility to vitamin A deficiency.

Season
Seasonal effects on the pattern of vitamin A deficiency are a consequence of both dietary and disease patterns. As indicated earlier, the most commonly available supplementary sources of vitamin A, fruits and vegetables, are often only seasonal in supply and not readily stored. For certain periods of the year, therefore, the vitamin A intake, particularly of young children, is likely to be very restricted and accompanied by an increase in the incidence of xerophthalmia. Not infrequently, however, the seasonal shortage of vitamin A sources is also accompanied by a shortage of other foods and by an increase in the incidence of PEM and diarrhoeal diseases (Blankhart, 1967; Sinha & Bang, 1973; Sommer, 1982).

Cultural practices
Vitamin A-rich foods, even when available, are frequently not given to young children and in many societies there are also food taboos, applying to women during pregnancy and lactation, which involve prohibitions on animal sources of vitamin A such as meat, eggs and milk. Since these foods tend to be minor rather than major items of the usual diet such practices, in adults, usually have no more effect than to precipitate night blindness

or conjunctival xerosis, but in children cultural practices relating to the use of dark green leafy vegetables have much more drastic consequences. Why do such apparently detrimental practices exist? Numerous reasons are given including their unpopularity with most children of this age group, the belief that they are not suitable for young children and specific cultural beliefs about the causes of other diseases such as worm infestations (Chen, 1972). Little systematic effort, however, appears to have been devoted to obtaining objective data in this area, perhaps because of the perceived problems associated with changing culturally determined food practices and the ready availability of synthetic forms of vitamin A.

Disease patterns
Diarrhoeal and other infectious diseases frequently accompany xeroph-thalmia in countries where vitamin A intakes are marginal (Oomen *et al.*, 1964). To what extent this is due to a specific depression of the immune response in vitamin A deficiency, to the co-existence of PEM or to the increased environmental opportunities for infection in such communities is not clear. Evidence on all of these aspects is often conflicting, largely because it is difficult in most studies to distinguish clearly between the effects of infections on vitamin A status, the effects of vitamin A deficiency on immune responses and the specific effects of vitamin A deficiency on the course and outcome of common childhood infections. The next section of this chapter therefore examines these different aspects of the relationship between vitamin A and infection in more detail.

VITAMIN A AND INFECTION

The non-ocular manifestations of vitamin A deficiency include reduced growth, metabolic disturbances, changes in cellular differentiation of epithelial tissues and effects on the immune system. Although clearly recognized in studies of laboratory animals, they have proved difficult to demonstrate clearly in the complex context of all the different factors that influence child health in developing cultures. Recent data, however, indicate that vitamin A deficiency does play an important role in resistance to infection and that its deficiency significantly increases a child's risk of morbidity and mortality although the specific mechanisms by which this is effected remain largely unknown. The following brief overview of current knowledge of the interactions between vitamin A and infection is based largely on a recent review of the public health aspects of this topic by West *et al.* (1989).

TABLE 13

Summary of the specific immunological effects of vitamin A deficiency and excess observed in animal and human studies[a]

Immunological function	Deficiency		Excess	
	Animal	Human	Animal	Human
Cell-mediated				
No. of lymphocytes	N/↓	—	↑	—
T- and B-cells	↓	↓	—	—
Proliferative response	↓	N	—	—
Splenic response	↓	—	↑	—
Humoral				
Primary response	↓	—	N/↑	N
Secondary response	↓	—	↑	—
Secretory IgA	—	↓	—	—
Other				
Delayed skin sensitivity	—	↓	↓	N
Monocyte	↓	—	—	—
Reticuloendothelial	—	—	N/↑	—
Complement	↑	—	↓	—
Inflammatory response	↓	—	↓	—
Host resistance	↓	↓	↑	—

[a] Adapted from Beisel *et al.* (1981).
↑, Increase; ↓, decrease; N, normal; ↑, small increase; ↓, small decrease.

Vitamin A and the immune response

Although the relationship between vitamin A deficiency and infection was first recognized more than 60 years ago it is only now that the mechanisms that underlie this association are being specifically identified. In broad terms, vitamin A appears to modify epithelial integrity and function, lymphoid tissue mass, specific immunity (both cell-mediated and humoral) and various non-specific mechanisms of host resistance (Table 13).

Epithelial integrity

Vitamin A is important in maintaining the normal development and integrity of epithelial surfaces and presumably, therefore, in the function of epithelia as a barrier to invasion by pathogens, not only in the conjunctiva and the cornea but also in the respiratory, gastrointestinal and genitourinary tracts. Experimental vitamin A deficiency leads to stratification of the cells followed by squamous metaplasia and eventual keratinization (Chytil, 1985). In the respiratory tract there is loss of mucous-secreting goblet and ciliary cells and this appears to increase susceptibility to infection by allowing micro-organisms that colonize these mucosal surfaces to invade the body. Specifically, loss of the mucociliary layer of the respiratory tract leads to impaired clearance of pathogens from the airways, to reduced secretion of mucosal antibodies such as secretory IgA and permits enhanced viral and bacterial adherence to the damaged tissue. The presence of infection in turn enhances the rate at which keratotic changes occur in vitamin A-deficient epithelia.

The gastrointestinal tract does not keratinize but impaired goblet cell differentiation and mucosal cell proliferation in the small intestine are observed early in vitamin A deficiency. These changes and others in gut-associated lymphoid tissue and local immune function all act to weaken local defences against enteric invasion. Extensive keratinization along the urinary tract and in some parts of the kidney have also been reported both in experimental vitamin A deficiency and in vitamin A-deficient children who died from infections. In vitamin A-deficient malnourished children it has been observed that the urinary tract, which is normally sterile, is subject to bacterial colonization and infection.

Lymphoid tissues
Vitamin A deficiency appears to have varying effects on lymphatic tissue mass. The thymus, which is the primary anatomic site for precursor lymphoid cell differentiation of T-lymphocytes, for example, undergoes marked atrophy in vitamin A-deficient children and animals with PEM but the effect of vitamin A deficiency alone is less clear. In animals, splenic weight also appears to be reduced while regional lymph nodes mass generally increases, apparently as a result of accumulation of cellular debris and changes in lymphocyte and macrophage activity.

Humoral immunity
Diminished antibody responses to a wide variety of antigens have been reported in vitamin A deficiency usually in the presence of normal or elevated levels of total circulating immunoglobulin levels. Work in animals suggests that vitamin A deficiency may act through a defect in antigen-specific B-cell clonal production and by impairing helper T-cell differentiation and function. Animal data on the effect of vitamin A supplementation on humoral immunity are equivocal. A recent study in children found that while antibody response to diphtheria and tetanus antigens and salivary secretory IgA were comparable between those with and without subclinical vitamin A deficiency, supplementation of the

deficient children with vitamin A enhanced antibody responses but significantly decreased salivary secretory IgA (Bhaskaram *et al.*, 1989). In the same group of children T-lymphocyte number was significantly lower in the deficient children but was restored to the same level as in the control children by vitamin A supplementation.

Cell-mediated immunity
Experimental vitamin A deficiency has been shown to impair cell-mediated immunity and this effect is most consistently observed as a depressed splenocyte blast response to T-cell mitogens such as concanavalin A, while blast transformation in the thymus does not appear to be affected in either early or late vitamin A deficiency. Region-specific variation in lymphocyte distribution may represent differences in mitogen recognition by T-cells that are mediated by vitamin A-induced changes in cell membrane glycoprotein synthesis and receptor function. The data of Bhaskaram *et al.* (1989) on the effects of subclinical vitamin A deficiency on T-lymphocyte number in children further support a specific role for vitamin A in the maintenance of normal cell-mediated immunity.

Non-specific mechanisms
Vitamin A also affects a range of non-specific mechanisms that are critical for an effective host response to infection. These include phagocytosis, peripheral blood lymphocyte trapping and localization, natural killer cell lysis, maintenance of lysozyme activity and mucosal barrier resistance to microbial penetration (Tomkins & Hussey, 1989).

Free radical scavenging
During the initial response to infection free radicals and reactive oxygen molecules are used by some types of leucocytes such as neutrophils to kill phagocytized bacteria. During this process free radicals may be overproduced and result in injury to the neutrophils as well as to neighbouring cells and tissues. β-Carotene, which has powerful free radical scavenging properties when incubated with neutrophils and bacteria, appears to protect the neutrophils from damage by their own oxidative products but does not interfere with the efficient killing of bacteria. The cells involved in the generation of specific immune responses can also be adversely affected by free radicals and oxidative products. To directly determine a carotenoid effect, separate from a provitamin A effect, on T- and B-lymphocyte functions, laboratory animals were given either β-carotene or canthaxanthin. Canthaxanthin has the same ability to quench singlet

oxygen and free radicals as β-carotene, but cannot be converted to vitamin A in mammals. Specific immune responses of laboratory animals were similarly enhanced whether they were given diets containing canthaxanthin or β-carotene (Bendich, 1989), indicating that the enhancement was due to free radical scavenging rather than to a provitamin A effect.

Effect of infections on vitamin A status

Infections adversely influence vitamin A status by interfering with vitamin A absorption and increasing vitamin A utilization and excretion in addition to their role in limiting dietary intake. Enteric infections of all kinds significantly impair the absorption of orally administered doses of vitamin A but malabsorption also occurs during systemic febrile illnesses including those of the respiratory tract. However, while infection clearly does impair vitamin A absorption, physiologically significant amounts of oral vitamin A can still be absorbed by malnourished children with diarrhoea and respiratory disease. The amount of vitamin A circulating in the blood decreases markedly during a number of severe systemic infections including pneumonia, bronchitis, septicaemia, measles and chickenpox, with the extent of the decrease closely related to the severity of the infection. These acute-phase changes, which may reflect accelerated peripheral use, depressed hepatic utilization or abnormal excretion of vitamin A, can in the longer term lead to reduced liver stores and vitamin A deficiency. Epidemiological studies from different parts of the world have frequently but not invariably reported positive associations between vitamin A deficiency and previous infections. Variations in the observed relationship between infection and vitamin A status are likely to arise not only from differences in the pattern and severity of infections and in nutritional status between populations but also from the cross-sectional nature of most studies.

Longitudinal studies, however, tend to confirm the negative effect of infections on vitamin A status. For example, in West Java the risk of developing xerophthalmia in the 3 months following an episode of diarrhoea or respiratory disease was twice that in children without these infections (Sommer et al., 1987). Similarly, an outbreak of chicken pox in Brazilian children was found to be associated with accelerated depletion of hepatic vitamin A reserves as demonstrated by the RDR test (Campos et al., 1987). Measles has a particularly severe effect on vitamin A status and remains a life-threatening disease for children in many developing countries. Typically between 25 and 75% of children presenting to hospitals with corneal xerophthalmia report having had measles during the previous 3 months, while in one study measles raised the risk of developing corneal xerophthalmia more than ten times (Sommer, 1982).

Effect of vitamin A on infection
In animals raised in a conventional environment infection is often an early complication of vitamin A deficiency and may lead to substantial mortality prior to the development of xerophthalmia. On the other hand, vitamin A-deficient animals raised under germ-free conditions continue to survive despite developing the classic lesions of vitamin A deficiency. These findings suggest that since vitamin A plays a crucial role in maintaining resistance to infection in animals, a similar situation is likely to exist in human populations. Data from two large longitudinal studies in Asia provide some insight into this relationship in children. In Indonesia children with mild xerophthalmia at any two consecutive three-monthly examinations were 1·78 and 2·7 times more likely to develop respiratory and diarrhoeal infections respectively during the interval than were children with clinically normal eyes (Sommer *et al.*, 1984). In addition, an Indian study found that children with mild xerophthalmia at the outset of a six month interval were twice as likely to develop a respiratory infection as were non-xerophthalmic children, although there was no relationship with diarrhoea (Milton *et al.*, 1987).

These studies suggest that pre-existing vitamin A deficiency may increase a child's risk of developing respiratory infection and under some circumstances possibly also diarrhoeal disease. If this is the case then supplementation of children at risk of vitamin A deficiency should reduce not only the incidence of xerophthalmia in the population but also the incidence of respiratory infections and diarrhoea. At the present time no such information is available from any large scale trial in a developing country, but two randomized double-blind clinical trials carried out in Australia and the USA provide some evidence for the role of physiological doses of vitamin A in reducing morbidity from respiratory conditions in selected groups of susceptible individuals (Pinnock *et al.*, 1986; Shenai *et al.*, 1987). Rather more information is available on the effect of vitamin A deficiency and vitamin A supplementation on mortality in preschool children.

Vitamin A and early childhood mortality
The high mortality associated with severe xerophthalmia cannot be separated from the effects of co-existing PEM, which independently reduces resistance to infection. There is now, however, also evidence that

milder forms of xerophthalmia are similarly associated with an increased risk of death from the two main causes of early childhood mortality in developing countries, respiratory infections and diarrhoeal diseases. For example, in the longitudinal study of Indonesian preschool children already referred to (Sommer *et al.*, 1983), children with mild xerophthalmia (night blindess and/or Bitot's spots) had on average a mortality rate that was four times the rate of children without xerophthalmia. Mortality rose with the severity of xerophthalmia and the effect was consistent when stratified on the basis of weight for age as a measure of concurrent PEM.

Two large field trials, both in Indonesia, have assessed the effect of vitamin A supplementation on mortality at the community level. In the first, a randomized controlled trial in 450 villages in northern Sumatra, semiannual distribution of a 60 000 RE capsule of vitamin A reduced preschool child mortality by 34% over the course of a year (Sommer *et al.*, 1986). In the second, vitamin A-fortified monosodium glutamate, distributed through normal market channels, was tested for its effectiveness in improving child health in more than 11 000 children in 10 communities (Muhilal *et al.*, 1988). Over a one-year period the vitamin A status in the recipient population improved, haemoglobin levels and growth rates increased and overall mortality decreased by 31% relative to that in control villages. The fact that neither of these field trials met the strict methodological criteria for a randomized double-blind controlled intervention trial, in which treatment allocation is randomized and treatment is masked, has led to some criticism of the interpretation of the findings as solely due to the effects of vitamin A supplementation. It would be quite inappropriate, however, to allow methodological criticisms to overshadow the impact these trials have had, not simply on health and morbidity in Indonesia but also in highlighting the need for, and importance of, well-conducted trials of intervention strategies for the prevention of vitamin A deficiency worldwide.

STRATEGIES FOR THE PREVENTION OF VITAMIN A DEFICIENCY

Historically, the disappearance of vitamin A deficiency has occurred in conjunction with economic development, increasing affluence and a consequent improvement in the overall quality of the diet and an increased intake of vitamin A. Clearly this is the desirable long-term solution to the problem of vitamin A deficiency but not one that can be quickly or easily achieved in those countries in which vitamin A deficiency is currently a major public health problem. There is therefore a need for short- and medium-term strategies that can be successfully implemented even in countries with depressed economies and primitive marketing, distribution and communication infrastructures.

Such strategies have included programmes to provide the most vulnerable segments of the population with massive periodic doses of vitamin A, to fortify food products accessible to the whole population with vitamin A, to increase the availability and use of inexpensive sources of vitamin A and to introduce public health measures to reduce morbidity.

Periodic massive dosing
The administration to vulnerable groups of single, large doses of vitamin A on a periodic basis can be initiated relatively quickly and with a minimum of additional infrastructure.

The dosing of children with large amounts of vitamin A (usually 60 000 RE as retinyl palmitate or retinyl acetate in oil with 40 mg vitamin E) as a prophylactic measure every 4–6 months was first tried on a pilot scale in Jordan and introduced in India in the early 1970s. Several other countries including Bangladesh and Indonesia now have vitamin A deficiency prevention programmes that employ this strategy and currently over 100 million oral doses of vitamin A are distributed annually. In Lombok in Indonesia an evaluation of periodic massive dosing during the period 1977–82 found a dramatic reduction in the prevalence of xerophthalmia (De Maeyer, 1986). More recently, reports of improved growth (West *et al.*, 1988) and reduced mortality have also appeared (Sommer *et al.*, 1986) from a large community trial designed to assess the impact of vitamin A supplementation on childhood xerophthalmia, mortality and growth in the northern Sumatran province of Aceh.

Although this programme clearly had a significant impact on xerophthalmia, growth and mortality, the authors suggest that the impact may have been even greater if programme coverage had been more complete. Factors related to the receipt of vitamin A were therefore investigated in order to increase the effectiveness and efficiency of the program (Tarwotjo *et al.*, 1989). Coverage was found to be better in rural villages and the best performance was achieved by village distributors who were representative of the majority of the local population (farmers or others with minimum education) rather than more upwardly mobile, more highly educated residents. Information such as this is clearly important for the planning of future community-based programmes, in Indonesia and elsewhere (Darnton-Hill *et al.*, 1988).

Fortification

Fortification of inexpensive, commonly used foods with vitamin A has been in use for over 50 years in the Western world for milk products and margarine. This approach is not as easy to initiate as periodic massive dosing and is only feasible given an inexpensive, commonly used, centrally processed and distributed food that can conveniently be fortified with vitamin A. In Central America fortification of sugar at the national level effectively improved vitamin A status in a number of countries (De Maeyer, 1986) but this approach is not practical in South and East Asia where small scale local processing units limit the feasibility of controlled fortification. In these areas alternative food vehicles for vitamin A fortification that have been considered or tried include bread, salt, tea, fish sauces and monosodium glutamate. Of these, fortification of monosodium glutamate appears to be the most promising (Muhilal *et al.*, 1988).

Although, in theory, food fortification appears to provide a relatively simple and low-cost solution to the problem of vitamin A deficiency, in practice there are often social, political and economic constraints that make this solution impractical at a national level.

Other measures

Increased production and consumption

Increasing the production and consumption of inexpensive vitamin A- and β-carotene-containing foods involves the collaborative efforts of agriculture, education and health workers with communities and families in a number of different ways.

For example, assistance with the development of 'backyard gardens' planted with appropriate fruits and vegetables can increase the availability of vitamin A-rich foods in some areas. In others, where utilization rather than availability is the main constraint on vitamin A consumption, educational programmes to overcome traditional beliefs that operate against giving vitamin A-rich foods to children (Chen, 1972) or that provide information or equipment for preparing and/or processing suitable foods in appropriate ways for young children may be more relevant.

The effectiveness of programmes of this type is not well documented mainly because they are usually relatively small in population terms as well as being community-specific and therefore not amenable to evaluation in the short term in the same way as national and regional programmes of prophylactic dosing or food fortification. Programmes aimed at increasing vitamin A consumption are, nevertheless, an important component of the long-term process of reducing vitamin A deficiency.

Public health measures
The introduction of measures directed towards the prevention and spread of, in particular, gastrointestinal and respiratory infections, constitute another longer-term strategy that can usefully be combined with community programmes aimed at increasing vitamin A intake in order to improve vitamin A status in young children. Appropriate measures include the introduction of hygiene practices designed to ensure a microbiologically safer food and water supply, proper waste disposal and immunization.

Socioeconomic measures
Although overall improved socioeconomic development is the long-term solution to the problem of vitamin A deficiency, Underwood (1984) has pointed out that raising the social and economic status of women is particularly important in alleviating the problems of malnutrition in young children. If poor women have access to additional money, they, more than men, tend to use it for improving the diet of their children. In addition to an improved diet, added income is usually also associated with an improvement in environmental conditions and in turn with less morbidity. However, when mothers remain illiterate this sequence does not necessarily follow and highlights the need for a high priority to be given to the education of women in the overall context of socioeconomic development strategies.

VITAMIN A AND CANCER

Treatment of this topic is confined in this chapter to the role of natural vitamin A compounds in the development of human cancer. A better understanding of the role that vitamin A compounds play in the prevention of cancer is potentially of major significance both in developed and developing countries of the world. At the present time, although there is a significant body of evidence that suggests that cancer induction may be inversely related to vitamin A status (Peto *et al.*, 1981), it is not clear whether an increased consumption of vitamin A within the physiological range will decrease cancer incidence either in those individuals whose

vitamin A status is marginal or in those whose vitamin A status is currently regarded as adequate. Nor is it clear which, if any, dietary vitamin A
compounds are most effective, or if indeed vitamin A activity is an essential feature of the effective compounds.

The relationship between vitamin A deficiency and metaplastic changes
in the epithelia of the respiratory, gastrointestinal and genitourinary tracts
was first reported in animals in the 1920s. Since metaplasias are considered
to be the first step in the transformation process from normal to neoplastic
tissue and there are many similarities between the histological features of
epithelial tissues in vitamin A-deficient animals and those seen in some
precancerous lesions of skin and mucous membranes, it is not unreason-
able to postulate a role for vitamin A in cancer prevention (Sporn &
Roberts, 1983). Indeed, in-vivo animal studies have demonstrated a
prophylactic effect of vitamin A on the induction of precancerous conditions such as benign epithelial tumours and metaplasias, as well as of
some carcinomas (Bollag, 1983). A relationship between vitamin A status
as measured by plasma vitamin A level and human gastrointestinal cancer
was reported in 1941 (Abels *et al.*, 1941), and since that time an extensive
literature has accumulated about the role of vitamin A in human cancer.

Clinical use of vitamin A for cancer prevention and therapy has mainly
been limited by the fact that therapeutically active doses are frequently
accompanied by the undesirable side-effects of vitamin A toxicity. As a
consequence, considerable effort has been devoted to the development and
synthesis of retinoids that are therapeutically effective but non-toxic when
given in therapeutic doses (Sporn, 1977). At first sight, the need for
therapeutic doses that are clearly above the physiological level of vitamin
A intake would seem to make it unlikely that there is a role for dietary
levels of preformed vitamin A in cancer prevention, at least in adequately
vitamin A nourished individuals. However, this has not deterred investigators from examining the relationships between vitamin A intake and/
or vitamin A status and the incidence of various cancers in human populations. Because of the methodological problems inherent in what are essentially observational rather than experimental studies, it is not possible
from such studies to do more than identify possible risk or protective
factors for cancer. Demonstration of a definite cause–effect relationship
requires large controlled clinical trials and although a number of these are
now in progress the results are not yet available. Observational studies
among varied populations have not provided consistent evidence for an
inverse association between vitamin A status and the prevalence of cancer
(Table 14). In most of these studies either serum levels of retinol and/or

TABLE 14
Summary of evidence for links between vitamin A and cancer

Animals—experimental evidence		
Vitamin A deficiency	⟶	Squamous metaplasia Keratinization Papillomas Frank carcinomas
Large doses of retinoids and carotenoids	⟶	Prevention and regression of chemically induced tumours
Man—epidemiological evidence		
↓ Blood retinol	⟶	? Association with cancer
↓ Blood beta-carotene ↓ Intake of preformed	⟶	↑ Incidence of some cancers
vitamin A	⟶	? Association with cancer
↓ Intake of total vitamin A ↓ Intake of fruits and	⟶	Weak association with cancer
vegetables	⟶	↑ Incidence of some cancers
Man—clinical evidence		
Large doses of retinoids (etretinate and isotretinoin)	⟶	↑ Regression, remission and recurrence of some malignant conditions

β-carotene or dietary questionnaires have been used as the measure of vitamin A status.

Serum vitamin A studies

The majority of these studies have been retrospective and have compared the serum level of retinol and/or β-carotene in a group of recently diagnosed cancer cases with those in a matched group of controls. A number of such studies from different parts of the world have reported significantly lower serum vitamin A levels in cases than controls (Peto *et al.*, 1981; Palgi, 1984). However, these findings need to be interpreted with caution since in these studies blood samples were taken from people with cancer whose appetites and dietary patterns may have altered or in whom the tumour itself may have lowered retinol or β-carotene levels. Because of these potential problems the results of retrospective studies are difficult to interpret and prospective studies of serum vitamin A levels are more likely to provide useful information about the role of vitamin A status in the development of cancer. Only a small number of such studies have been reported to date and in most of these, the number of cases and controls are likely to have been too small to provide reproducible trends.

A combined analysis of the results from three large prospective studies provides no evidence for a relationship between serum retinol level and the risk of cancer at all sites combined or of the lung. The combined data does, however, suggest a possible relationship between serum retinol level and the risk of gastrointestinal cancer (Seigel, 1984). In contrast, prospective studies of serum or plasma β-carotene and cancer have consistently found a significant negative association between lung cancer and β-carotene level, although not for cancer at other sites (Ziegler, 1988). One prospective study that measured total serum carotenoids found no association with incidence of either all cancer or cancer of the lung alone (Willett *et al.*, 1984). The overall findings of the serum studies do not yet provide a clear picture of the influence of blood retinol and/or carotenoid levels on the subsequent risk of neoplasia. Future prospective serum studies need to consider a larger number of cancer cases and also to control adequately for other factors that may influence blood vitamin A levels, such as smoking.

Dietary vitamin A studies
Studies relating vitamin A intake and cancer have assessed intake in a variety of ways and thus do not make it easy to compare data from different studies directly. Some studies, for example, have assessed the total dietary intake of vitamin A as retinol equivalents while others have evaluated dietary preformed and precursor vitamin A separately. Still others have created a vitamin A index or vegetable index based on food groups. In general, dietary intake studies have not found a consistent association between cancer and preformed vitamin A intake and only a weak negative relationship with total vitamin A intake. The most consistent relationship has been with indices of green and/or yellow fruit and/or vegetable intake (Underwood, 1986). More recently, cancer epidemiologists have begun to treat β-carotene and preformed vitamin A as distinct dietary exposures that should be evaluated separately. This approach is likely to help in clarifying the protective role of retinol, if any, as distinct from that of carotenoids, some of which do not have vitamin A activity.

A recent review of nine retrospective studies of diet and cancer of the lung found that all nine studies observed a significantly decreased risk of lung cancer with increased intake of carotenoid or green or yellow–orange vegetables (Ziegler, 1988). In seven of these studies the effect of retinol intake was evaluated separately but was not found to be related to lung cancer risk. Other dietary factors concentrated in vegetables and fruits were only rarely investigated. Inverse associations with risk of lung cancer were noted for vitamin C in two studies and for dietary fibre in one study but the associations were weaker than with carotenoids. Non-nutrient constituents of vegetables and fruits, such as indoles and phenols, were not evaluated.

Retrospective dietary studies, like retrospective serum studies, need to be viewed with caution. Recall bias due to selective memory in either cases or controls may be a significant source of error, and the changes in taste and appetite produced by cancer may alter an individual's perception of his or her usual diet prior to the onset of disease (Palgi, 1984). Despite these caveats, prospective studies of diet and cancer have provided essentially similar findings to those of the retrospective studies for cancer at all sites and for lung cancer. Of six prospective studies reviewed by Palgi (1984) and Ziegler (1988), four out of five studies that examined lung cancer risk and three out of four studies that examined the risk for all cancers combined found a significant decrease in risk with increased intake of fruit and vegetables or carotenoids. Unfortunately, only one study systematically investigated the relationship of intake of all major nutrients to cancer risk (Shekelle *et al.*, 1981). This study found that carotenoid intake alone was significantly associated with risk of lung cancer. The only other study that used a qualitative measure of carotenoid intake rather than an index based on fruit and vegetable intake, however, found no association with lung cancer and only a non-significant inverse association with all cancer. No increase in risk of lung cancer with low retinol intake was found in two studies while a third study did suggest such a relationship.

The finding of a lower cancer risk with increased consumption of fruit and vegetables, but not necessarily with retinol or a qualitative index of provitamin A carotenoid intake, strongly suggests that the active carotenoids do not first have to be metabolized to vitamin A to be protective and also the possibility that the effect observed could be due to a non-carotenoid constituent of fruit and vegetables such as fibre, vitamin C, indoles or phenols. It should be recognized, however, that the different dietary indices used to measure vitamin A and carotenoid intake make it difficult to compare the results of these studies (Palgi, 1984). Other limitations of existing prospective dietary studies include small numbers of cases and potential confounding of the results by cancer inhibitors other than vitamin A or carotenoids in the foods studied. Since intake of vegetables and fruits is decreased in smokers and smokers also have lowered blood levels of carotenoids, uncontrolled confounding by smoking could also generate an apparent protective effect for diet in studies of lung and other smoking-related cancers.

Summary of epidemiological findings
Low intake of fruit and vegetables and carotenoids is consistently associated with an increased risk of lung cancer in both prospective and retrospective studies. In addition, low levels of serum or plasma β-carotene are consistently associated with a subsequent increased risk of developing lung cancer. The simplest explanation for these findings is that β-carotene is protective. Since retinol does not seem to be related to cancer risk in the same way, it is possible that β-carotene plays a role that does not require its conversion into vitamin A. The importance of other carotenoids, and other nutrient and non-nutrient constituents of vegetables and fruit has not yet been widely explored. Epidemiological studies also suggest that carotenoids may be associated with a reduced risk of some cancers other than lung cancer, but at present there are too few studies with adequate data to evaluate the consistency of this effect.

Experimental studies of carotenoids
Since β-carotene is essentially non-toxic in humans the potential utility of carotenoids for the prevention of cancer in human populations is considerable. Animal studies of carotenoids as chemopreventive agents are relatively few in number since rodents, which are commonly used as experimental models for cancer studies, only absorb dietary β-carotene poorly and therefore require large amounts of carotenoids in the diet to obtain significant blood and tissue levels. Despite this problem a number of animal studies have indicated that dietary carotenoid supplements, both with (β-carotene) and without vitamin A activity (canthaxanthin) can inhibit the process of cancer induction (McCormick & Moon, 1986). The doses of carotenoids required for chemoprevention in rodents are much higher than those required for retinoids, but this may be a function of poor absorption rather than a lower anticarcinogenic activity.

A number of intervention trials of β-carotene and other carotenoids are also under way in humans. For example, a large co-operative study is currently evaluating the potential of β-carotene in lowering cancer incidence in 20 000 male physicians over the age of 40 years. Other smaller intervention studies focused on specific high risk groups for certain cancers such as UV-induced skin cancers, lung cancer and colorectal cancer are also in progress.

VITAMIN A TOXICITY

In the overall context of the role of vitamin A in human nutrition, toxicity is a very minor problem as compared with vitamin A deficiency. For example, the worldwide incidence of hypervitaminosis A is estimated to be less than 200 cases annually compared with estimates in excess of a million cases of vitamin A deficiency (Bauernfeind, 1980; McLaren, 1986). In general, vitamin A toxicity can therefore be regarded as a potential but unlikely problem except in unusual circumstances. The potential for vitamin A toxicity exists because excess amounts of the vitamin are stored rather than excreted. Under most circumstances this is an advantage rather than a disadvantage since it protects individuals against the effects of seasonal and even longer shortages of vitamin A intake. In a few special situations, however, it can lead to toxicity. In particular, there has been concern in recent years that the ready availability of vitamin A in large doses and the increased use of vitamin supplements by populations in Western countries might lead to an increased incidence of vitamin A toxicity. However, despite the significant growth in production and use of vitamin A supplements over the last 50 years, the number of reported cases of hypervitaminosis A has remained relatively constant (Bendich & Langseth, 1989).

Hypervitaminosis A can be divided into acute toxicity, which results from ingestion of a very high dose over a short period of time, and chronic toxicity, which results from continued ingestion of high amounts over a period of months or years. Ingestion of carotenoids as opposed to preformed vitamin A does not lead to toxicity, both because the absorption of carotenoids decreases as intake increases and because the conversion of carotenoids to vitamin A is regulated in a way that prevents the absorption of excess vitamin A from carotenoids.

Acute toxicity
Acute hypervitaminosis A may occur after a short period of ingestion of 100 000 μg or more vitamin A daily, or between 100 and 200 times the recommended daily allowance (RDA) for adults and children respectively. Symptoms of toxicity occur when the amount of vitamin A ingested exceeds the capacity of the liver to produce RBP to bind it. The most common symptoms include nausea and vomiting, fatigue, headaches, bulging fontanelle (in infants), elevated serum vitamin A level and anorexia. All these symptoms disappear when vitamin A intake returns to a normal level. Acute vitamin A toxicity occurs only rarely as a consequence

of the consumption of natural foods. When it does, it is almost exclusively attributable to the consumption of the livers of carnivorous animals or large fish, which may contain up to 10 000 μg vitamin A/g liver. More frequently, however, acute toxicity occurs as a result of the overuse of vitamin A supplements either because of misuse by the consumer or from over-prescription by a physician. Reasons for overuse by the public include the belief that if a little is good more must be better, a lack of appreciation of the high potency of vitamin A preparations and self-medication. Prescription-related overuse has also occurred when the dangers of high doses have not been adequately explained or when patients have continued to take high doses for longer than the prescribed period.

Chronic toxicity
Chronic hypervitaminosis A is more common than acute hypervitaminosis A and occurs when relatively large amounts of vitamin A are consumed over a long period of time. Its symptoms are highly varied and it may go unrecognized unless a careful history is taken or the serum vitamin A level determined (Bendich & Langseth, 1989). In both children and adults chronic vitamin A toxicity is uncommon unless the daily dose exceeds 20 times the RDA for at least several months. The appearance of chronic hypervitaminosis is dependent on a number of factors apart from the dose. These include the physical form in which the vitamin is taken, the general health status of the individual and interactions with other dietary components including protein, vitamins C, D, E and K, and alcohol. In most cases when excess vitamin A intake is discontinued virtually all of the symptoms of chronic hypervitaminosis A are relieved within a week. Longer-term or irreversible effects of chronic toxicity include some bone changes and possibly cirrhosis of the liver (Bendich & Langseth, 1989).

Teratogenic effects
In animals both vitamin A deficiency and very high doses of vitamin A during pregnancy result in birth defects in the offspring. A small number of cases of birth defects have also been reported in the infants of women exposed to high intakes of vitamin A during early pregnancy (10 times the RDA). The defects resembled those observed in animal studies and those that have occurred in the foetuses of women ingesting therapeutic doses of 13-*cis*-retinoic acid (isotretinoin) during the first trimester of pregnancy (Costas *et al.*, 1987; Miller *et al.*, 1987). In consequence of these findings the FAO/WHO Joint Expert Consultation on vitamin A requirements (FAO, 1988) recommends that women who are or who might become

pregnant should limit their total daily vitamin A intake to a maximum of 3000 RE (retinol equivalent) to minimize the risk of foetal malformations, and a number of national committees no longer recommend an additional allowance for vitamin A during pregnancy.

REFERENCES

Abels, J.C., Gerham, A.T., Pack, G.T. & Rhoads, C.P. (1941). Metabolic studies in patients with cancer of the gastrointestinal tract 1. Plasma vitamin A levels in patients with malignant neoplastic disease particularly of the gastrointestinal tract. *Journal of Clinical Investigation* **24**, 749–64.

Amadee-Manesme, O., Anderson, D. & Olson, J.A. (1984). Relation of the relative dose response to liver concentrations of vitamin A in generally well-nourished surgical patients. *American Journal of Clinical Nutrition* **39**, 898–902.

Amadee-Manesme, O., Mourey, M.S., Hanck, A. & Therasse, J. (1987). Vitamin A relative dose response test: validation by intravenous injection in children with liver disease. *American Journal of Clinical Nutrition* **46**, 286–9.

Amadee-Manesme, O., Luzeau, R., Wittpenn, J.R., Hanck, A. & Sommer, A. (1988). Impression cytology detects subclinical vitamin A deficiency. *American Journal of Clinical Nutrition* **47**, 875–8.

Australian Bureau of Statistics (1983). *Apparent consumption of Foodstuffs and Nutrients, Australia, 1982–83*. Canberra: AGPS.

Bates, C.J. (1983). Vitamin A in pregnancy and lactation. *Proceedings of the Nutrition Society* **42**, 65–79.

Bauernfeind, J.C. (1972). Carotenoid vitamin A precursors and analogs in foods and feeds. *Journal of Agricultural and Food Chemistry* **20**, 456–73.

Bauernfeind, J.C. (1980). *The safe use of vitamin A: a report of the International Vitamin A Consultative Group*. Washington, D.C.: The Nutrition Foundation.

Beisel, W.R., Edelman, R., Nauss, K. & Suskind, R.M. (1981). Single-nutrient effects on Immunologic Functions (Report of a Workshop sponsored by the Department of Food and Nutrition and its nutrition advisory group of the AMA). *Journal of the American Medical Association* **245**, 53–8.

Bendich, A. (1989). Carotenoids and the immune response. *Journal of Nutrition* **119**, 112–5.

Bendich, A. & Langseth, L. (1989). Safety of vitamin A. *American Journal Clinical Nutrition* **49**, 358–71.

Bhaskaram, P., Jyothi, S.A., Rao, K.V. & Rao, B.S.N. (1989). Effects of subclinical vitamin A deficiency and administration of vitamin A as a single large dose on immune function in children. *Nutrition Research* **9**, 1017–25.

Blankhart, D.M. (1967). Individual intake of food in young children in relation to malnutrition and night blindness. *Tropical and Geographical Medicine* **19**, 144–53.

Bollag, W. (1983). Vitamin A and retinoids: from nutrition to pharmacotherapy in dermatology and oncology. *Lancet* **i**, 860–3.

Brown, E.D., Micozzi, M.S., Craft, N.E., Bieri, J.G., Beecher, G., Edwards, B.K., Rose, A., Taylor, P.R. & Smith, C. (1989). Plasma carotenoids in normal men after a single ingestion of vegetables or purified beta-carotene. *American Journal of Clinical Nutrition* **49**, 1258–65.

Brubacher, G.B. & Weiser, H. (1985). The vitamin A activity of beta-carotene. *International Journal of Vitaminology and Nutrition Research* **55**, 5–15.

Buzina, R., Jusic, M., Brodarec, A., Milanovic, N., Brubacher, G., Vuilleumier, J.P., Wiss, O. & Christeller, S. (1971). The assessment of dietary vitamin intake of 24 Istrian farmers: II Comparison between the dietary intake and biochemical status of ascorbic acid, vitamin A, thiamine, riboflavin and niacin. *International Journal of Vitaminology and Nutrition Research* **41**, 289–300.

Campos, F.A.C.S., Flores, H. & Underwood, B.A. (1987). Effect of an infection on vitamin A status of children as measured by the relative dose response (RDR). *American Journal of Clinical Nutrition* **46**, 91–4.

Chen, P.C.Y. (1972). Sociocultural influences on vitamin A deficiency in a rural Malay community. *Journal of Tropical Medicine and Hygiene* **75**, 231–6.

Chytil, F. (1985). Function of Vitamin A in the respiratory tract. *Acta Vitaminologica et Enzymologica* **7** (Supplement), 27–31.

Costas, K., Davis, R., Kim, N., Stark, A.S., Thompson, S., Vallet, H.L. & Morse, D.L. (1987). Use of supplements containing high dose vitamin A—New York State, 1983–1984. *Journal of the American Medical Association* **257** 1292–7.

Darnton-Hill, I., Sibanda, F., Mitra, M., Ali, M., Drexler, A.E., Rahman, H. & Samad Khan, M.A. (1988). Distribution of vitamin A capsules for the prevention and control of vitamin A deficiency in Bangladesh. *Food and Nutrition Bulletin* **10**, 60–70.

De Maeyer, E.M. (1986). The WHO programme of prevention and control of vitamin A deficiency, xerophthalmia and nutritional blindness. *Nutrition and Health* **4**, 105–12.

Department of Community Services and Health (1987). *National Dietary Survey of Adults: 1983. no. 2 Nutrient Intakes*. Canberra: AGPS.

FAO (1967). Requirements of vitamin A, thiamine, riboflavine and niacin. Report of a Joint FAO/WHO Expert Group. *FAO Nutrition Meetings Report Series*. no. 41. Rome: FAO.

FAO (1984). *Food Balance Sheets. 1979–1981 Average*. Rome: FAO.

FAO (1988). Requirements of vitamin A, iron, folate, and vitamin B12. Report of a Joint FAO/WHO Expert Consultation. *FAO Food and Nutrition Series* no. 23. Rome: FAO.

Food and Nutrition Board (1980). *Recommended Dietary Allowances*, 9th ed. Washington, D.C.: NAS/NRC.

Food and Nutrition Board (1989). *Recommended Daily Allowances*, 10th ed. Washington, D.C.: NAS/NRC.

Gadomski, A.M., Kjolhede, C.L., Wittpenn, J., Bulux, J., Rosas, A.R. & Forman, M.R. (1989). Conjunctival impression cytology (CIC) to detect subclinical vitamin A deficiency: comparison of CIC with biochemical assessments. *American Journal of Clinical Nutrition* **49**, 495–500.

Hatchell, D. & Sommer, A. (1984). Detection of ocular abnormalities in experimental vitamin A deficiency. *Archives of Opthalmology* **102**, 1389–93.

Hoppner, L., Phillips, W.E.J., Murray, T.K. & Campbell, J.S. (1968). Survey of liver vitamin A stores of Canadians. *Canadian Medical Association Journal* **99**, 983–6.

Hume, E.M. & Krebs, H.A. (1949). Vitamin A requirements of human adults. An experimental study of vitamin A deprivation in man. *MRC Special Report Series* no. 254 London: H.M. Stationery Office.

Huque, T. (1982). A survey of human liver reserves of retinol in London. *British Journal of Nutrition* 47, 165–72.

Jardin, C., Adrian, J. & Perisse, J. (1967). Hierarchy in the nutritive value of foods calculated on an isocaloric basis. *Tropical Medicine* 27, 27–42.

Jayarajan, P., Reddy, V. & Mohanram, M., (1980). Effect of dietary fat on absorption of β-carotene from green leafy vegetables in children. *Indian Journal of Medical Research* 71, 53–6.

Kjolhede, C.L., Gadomski, A.M., Wittpenn, J., Bulux, K.H. & Forman, M.R. (1989). Conjunctival impression cytology: feasibility of a field trial to detect subclinical vitamin A deficiency. *American Journal of Clinical Nutrition* 49, 490–4.

Loerch, J.D., Underwood, B.A. & Lewis, K.C. (1979). Response of plasma levels of vitamin A to a dose of vitamin A as an indicator of hepatic vitamin A reserve in rats. *Journal of Nutrition* 109, 778–86.

McCormick, D.L. & Moon, R.C. (1986). Vitamin A status and cancer induction. In *Vitamin A Deficiency and its Control*, pp. 245–84 [J.C. Bauernfeind, editor]. New York: Academic Press.

McLaren, D.S., Shirajian, E., Tchalian, M. & Khoury, G. (1965). Xerophthalmia in Jordan. *American Journal of Clinical Nutrition* 17, 117–30.

McLaren, D.S. (1986a). Global occurence of vitamin A deficiency. In *Vitamin A Deficiency and Its Control*, pp. 1–18 [J.C. Bauernfeind, editor]. New York: Academic Press.

McLaren, D.S. (1986b). Pathogenesis of vitamin A deficiency. In *Vitamin A Deficiency and Its Control*, pp. 153–76 [J.C. Bauernfeind, editor]. New York: Academic Press.

Mejia, L.A. & Arroyave, G. (1982). The effect of vitamin A fortification of sugar on iron metabolism in preschool children in Guatemala. *American Journal of Clinical Nutrition* 36, 87–93.

Miller, R.K., Brown, K., Cordero, D., Dayton, D., Hardin, B., Greene, M., Grabowsk, C., Hendrick, A., Hook, E. & Jensh, R. (1987). Position paper by the Teratology Society: vitamin A during pregnancy. *Teratology* 35, 267–75.

Milton, R.C., Reddy, V. & Naidu, A.N. (1987). Mild vitamin A deficiency and childhood morbidity—an Indian experience. *American Journal of Clinical Nutrition* 46, 827–9.

Muhilal, Permeisih, D., Idjradinata, Y.R., Muherdiyantini-Ngsih, Karyadi, D. (1988). Vitamin A-fortified monosodium glutamate and health, growth, and survival of children: a controlled field trial. *American Journal of Clinical Nutrition* 48, 1271–6.

Natadisastra, G., Wittpenn, J.R., Muhilal, West, K.P., Mele, L. & Sommer, A. (1988). Impression cytology: a practical index of vitamin A status. *American Journal of Clinical Nutrition* 48, 695–701.

Olson, J.A. (1984). Serum levels of vitamin A and carotenoids as reflectors of nutritional status. *Journal of the National Cancer Institute* 73, 1439–44.

Olson, J.A. (1987). Recommended dietary intakes (RDI) of vitamin A in humans. *American Journal of Clinical Nutrition* 45, 704–16.

Olson, J.A. (1988). Vitamin A, Retinoids and Carotenoids. In _Modern Nutrition in Health and Disease_ 7th ed, pp. 292–312 [M.E. Shils and V.R. Young, editors]. Philadelphia: Lea & Febiger.

Oomen, H.A.C., McLaren, D.S. & Escapini, H. (1964). Epidemiology and public health aspects of hypovitaminosis A. A general survey on xerophthalmia. _Tropical and Geographical Medicine_ 16, 271–315.

Palgi, A. (1984). Vitamin A and lung cancer: a perspective. _Nutrition and Cancer_ 6, 105–20.

Perisse, J. & Polacchi, W. (1980). Geographical distribution and recent changes in world supply of vitamin A. _Food and Nutrition_ 6, 27–7.

Peto, R., Doll, R., Buckley, J.D. & Sporn, M.B. (1951). Can dietary beta-carotene materially reduce human cancer rates? _Nature_ 290, 201–8.

Pinnock, C.B., Douglas, R.M. & Badcock, W.R. (1986). Vitamin A status in children who are prone to respiratory tract infection. _Australian Paediatrics Journal_ 22, 95–9.

Rodriguez, M.S. & Irwin, M. (1972). A conspectus of research on vitamin A requirements of man. _Journal of Nutrition_ 102, 909–68.

Roels, O.A., Trout, M. & Dujacquier, R. (1958). Carotene balances on boys in Ruanda where vitamin A deficiency is prevalent. _Journal of Nutrition_ 65, 115–27.

Russell, R.M., Iber, F.L., Krasinski, S.D. & Miller, P. (1983). Protein–energy malnutrition and liver dysfunction limit the usefulness of the relative dose response (RDR) test for predicting vitamin A deficiency. _Human Nutrition: Clinical Nutrition_ 37C, 361–71.

Rutishauser, I.H.E. (1986). Vitamin A. _Journal of Food and Nutrition_ 42, 48–59.

Sauberlich, H.E., Hodges, R.E., Wallace, D.L., Kolder, H., Canham, J.E., Hood, J., Raica, N. & Lowry, L.K. (1974). Vitamin A metabolism and requirements in the human studied with the use of labelled retinol. _Vitamins and Hormones_ 32, 251–75.

Seigel, D. (1984). Discussion of case-control studies of Peleg, Stahelin and Willett. _Journal of the National Cancer Institute_ 73, 1469–70.

Shekelle, R.B., Liu, S., Raynor, W.J., Lepper, M., Maliza, C., Rossof, A.H., Oglesby, P., Shryrock, A. & Stamler, J. (1981). Dietary vitamin A and risk of cancer in the Western Electric Study. _Lancet_ ii, 1185–90.

Shenai, J.P., Kennedy, K.A., Chytil, F. & Stahlman, M.T. (1987). Clinical trial of vitamin A supplementation in infants susceptible to bronchopulmonary dysplasia. _Journal of Pediatrics_ 111, 269–77.

Simpson, K.L. (1983). Relative value of carotenoids as precursors of vitamin A. _Proceedings of the Nutrition Society_ 42, 7–17.

Simpson, K.L. & Tsou, S.C.S. (1986). Vitamin A and provitamin A composition of foods. In _Vitamin A Deficiency and Its Control_, pp. 461–78 [J.C. Bauernfield, editor] New York: Academic Press.

Sinha, D.P. & Bang, F.B. (1973). Seasonal variation in signs of vitamin A deficiency in rural West Bengal children. _Lancet_ ii, 228–30.

Sivell, L.M., Bull, W.L., Buss, D.H., Wiggins, R.A., Scuffam, D. & Jackson, P.A. (1984). Vitamin A activity in foods of animal origin. _Journal of the Science of Food and Agriculture_ 35, 931–9.

Solomons, N.W. & Russell, R.M. (1980). The interaction of vitamin A and zinc:

implications for human nutrition. *American Journal of Clinical Nutrition* **33**, 2031–40.

Sommer, A. (1982). *Nutritional blindness, Xerophthalmia and Keratomalacia.* Oxford: Oxford University Press.

Sommer, A. (1988). New imperatives for an old vitamin. *Journal of Nutrition* **119**, 96–100.

Sommer, A., Tarwotjo, I., Hussaini, G. & Susanto, D. (1983). Increased mortality in children with mild vitamin A deficiency. *Lancet* **ii**, 585–8.

Sommer, A., Katz, J. & Tarwotjo, I. (1984). Increased risk of respiratory disease and diarrhoea in children with pre-existing mild vitamin A deficiency. *American Journal of Clinical Nutrition* **40**, 1090–5.

Sommer, A., Tartwotjo, I., Djunaedi, E., West, K.P., Loeden, A.A., Tilden, R., Mele, L. & the ACEH Study Group (1986). Impact of vitamin A supplementation on childhood mortality. *Lancet* **i**, 1169–73.

Sommer, A., Tarwotjo, I. & Katz, J. (1987). Increased risk of xerophthalmia following diarrhoea and respiratory disease. *American Journal of Clinical Nutrition* **45**, 997–1080.

Sporn, M.B. (1977). Retinoids and carcinogenesis. *Nutrition Reviews* **35**, 65–9.

Sporn, M.B. & Roberts, A.B. (1983). Role of retinoids in differentiation and carcinogenesis. *Cancer Research* **43**, 3034–9.

Suter, P.M. & Russell, R.M. (1987). Vitamin requirements of the elderly. *American Journal of Clinical Nutrition* **45**, 501–12.

Tarwotjo, I., West, K.P., Mele, L., Nur, S., Nendrawati, H., Kraushaar, D., Tilden, R. & the ACEH Study Group (1989). Determinants of community-based coverage: periodic vitamin A supplementation. *American Journal of Public Health* **79**, 847–9.

Tomkins, A. & Hussey, G. (1989). Vitamin A, immunity and infection. *Nutrition Research Reviews* **2**, 17–28.

Underwood, B.A. (1984). Vitamin A in animal and human nutrition. In *The Retinoids*, Vol. 1, pp. 282–392 [M.B. Sporn, A.B. Roberts and D.S. Goodman, editors]. New York: Academic Press.

Underwood, B.A. (1986*a*). Vitamin A status, carotene and cancer prevention. In *Proceedings of the XIIIth International Congress of Nutrition*, pp. 474–7 [T.G. Taylor and W.K. Jenkins, editors]. London: John Libbey.

Underwood, B.A. (1986*b*) *Recommendations for safely improving the vitamin A status of pregnant and lactating women and the nursing infant.* International Vitamin A Consultative Group, Washington, D.C.: The Nutrition Foundation.

Vahlquist, A. & Nilsson, S. (1979). Mechanisms for vitamin A transfer from blood to milk in rhesus monkeys. *Journal of Nutrition* **109**, 1456–63.

Venkatchalam, P.S., Belavady, B. & Gopalan, C. (1962). Studies on vitamin A nutritional status of mothers and infants in poor communities in India. *Journal of Pediatrics* **612**, 262–8.

Wallingford, J.C. & Underwood, B.A. (1986). Vitamin A deficiency in pregnancy, lactation and the nursing child. In *Vitamin A Deficiency and its Control*, pp. 101–52 [J.C. Bauernfeind, editor]. New York: Academic Press.

West, K.P., Djunaedi, E., Pandji, A., Kusdiono, Tarwotjo, I., Sommer, A. and the ACEH Study Group (1988). Vitamin A supplementation and growth: A randomized community trial. *American Journal of Clinical Nutrition* **48**, 1257–64.

West, K.P., Howard, G.R. & Sommer, A. (1989). Vitamin A and infection: Public Health Implications. *Annual Reviews of Nutrition* **9**, 63–86.

WHO (1982) *Control of Vitamin A Deficiency and Xerophthalmia.* Geneva: WHO.

Willett, W.C., Polk, B.F., Underwood, B.A. & Hames, C.G. (1984). Hypertension detection and follow-up program study of serum retinol, retinol binding protein, total carotenoids and cancer risk. A summary. *Journal of the National Cancer Institute* **73**, 1459–62.

Wittpenn, J., Tseng, S. & Sommer, A. (1986). Detection of early xerophthalmia by impression cytology. *Archives of Ophthalmology* **104**, 237–9.

Wolf, G. (1978). A historical note on the mode of administration of vitamin A for the cure of night blindness. *American Journal of Clinical Nutrition* **31**, 290–2.

Ziegler, R.G. (1988). A review of epidemiological evidence that carotenoids reduce the risk of cancer. *Journal of Nutrition* **119**, 116–22.

3

Calcium Nutrition

Brian A. Rolls

AFRC Institute of Food Research, Reading UK

INTRODUCTION

Calcium is an essential dietary nutrient, quantitatively the most prevalent mineral, and the standard 70 kg man will contain about 1·2 kg calcium, the overwhelming majority of which is in the bones and teeth. It is tempting to think of these as inert structures, but bone is a metabolically active tissue undergoing continual renewal under hormonal control to permit growth, repair and response to activity. The rate of renewal slows with age, but even in an adult replacement will be complete over about 10 years.

In contrast, the metabolic calcium in soft tissues and body fluids is only about 6–10 g, yet it is a vital intracellular messenger, essential for a range of regulatory functions, controlling hormone secretion and nerve and muscle function (Table 1). Calcium also acts as a cofactor in several enzyme systems and is involved in blood clotting. For a review of the two major roles of calcium, see Nordin (1988).

Blood calcium is controlled by powerful homeostatic mechanisms: if the concentration should fall, calcium is mobilized from bone, absorption from the intestine is increased and urinary calcium is reduced (Fig. 1). Bone acts as a reserve, absorbing or releasing calcium to ensure that these vital functions remain undisturbed. Control of this process is largely under the control of parathyroid hormone (PTH, from the parathyroid glands), calcitonin (CT, from the thyroid gland) and calcitriol (see Fig. 2). Blood calcium occurs in three forms, ionic, protein-bound and complexed; it is the ionic form that is so closely controlled.

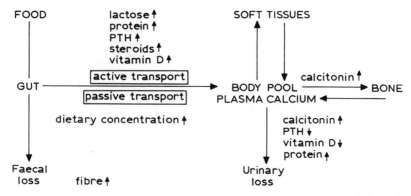

FIG. 1.   Influences on calcium balance. This diagram shows some of the influences on calcium excretion and balance, and demonstrates how, whatever the balance, the calcitropic hormones (parathyroid hormone (PTH), calcitonin and calcitriol (the active form of vitamin D)) act to keep the concentration of calcium in the plasma within narrow limits (2·2–2·7 mm).

There has been a revival of interest in calcium in recent years, and several useful reviews have been produced, aimed at the professional (NDC, 1984; BNF, 1989), communicators (NDC, 1985) and the lay person (NDC, 1985; NOS, 1989a).

This chapter will consider first the requirements for and the sources of calcium, the mechanisms of absorption and regulation and finally the roles of calcium in osteoporosis and—more controversially—such conditions as hypertension and colon cancer. There are questions that remain to be answered in all aspects of calcium metabolism.

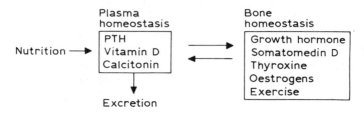

FIG. 2.   Some factors effecting calcium homeostasis in plasma and bone.

TABLE 1
Functions of calcium

Hard tissues: bones and teeth ~1·2 kg	Soft tissues and body fluids ~7 g
Formation of bones and teeth Repair and replacement	Nerve function Muscle function Enzyme activation Blood clotting

REQUIREMENT FOR CALCIUM

Recommended dietary allowances (recommended daily amounts, RDAs) are discussed in detail in another chapter, but briefly the RDA for calcium is that intake that would meet the nutritional needs of almost every healthy person. As such, the actual intake recommended can change in either direction as knowledge is refined or new aspects are considered.

To assess the requirement, that is, the amount of calcium that will satisfy all the body's needs and allow for the inevitable losses, is particularly difficult. The calcium stores in the skeleton are so large that any deficiency is hard to demonstrate. The normal balance method is unreliable because people adapt to changes in intake at different rates and over a long time-scale, and the calcium requirement is usually assessed as the sum of requirements in the body, to cover excretory losses and any output (for instance, as milk), taking into account that only part of the calcium eaten is actually absorbed (Fig. 3, Table 2).

Even assuming complete information, it would not be possible to give a single RDA for calcium, for the body's requirements vary with age, pregnancy and lactation, smoking, obesity, activity and current calcium

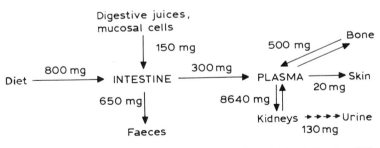

FIG. 3. Calcium balance of a (non-pregnant, non-lactating) adult eating 800 mg calcium/day.

TABLE 2
Calcium needs of a lactating woman

	Calcium needs (mg/day)
Calcium in milk	280
Urine loss	100
Skin loss	20
Total	400
Assuming absorption of 40–50%, intake = 800–1000	
RDA (intake + 2 SD) ~ 1200	

and vitamin D status. The reasons for some of these differences are clear: the need for calcium will obviously be greater in infants and children (rapid growth and bone mineralization), in adolescents (growth spurts followed by increasing bone density) and in pregnancy and lactation (building the skeleton of the growing baby).

The foetus lays down half its calcium in the last 8 weeks before birth, and the lactating mother, in producing milk of 330 mg calcium/kg, may have to provide 150–200 mg/day, either from her diet or her own body. The newborn baby contains about 25 g calcium, at six months this has trebled. If this output is not replaced by the diet, peak bone mineralization —which is achieved during the reproductive years—may be adversely affected, with possibly impaired subsequent bone health. For this reason, lactating teenagers are at particular risk.

The recommended daily calcium intake for an adult varies widely in different countries, being 500 mg in the UK, 800 mg in the US and many EC states and lower in developing countries (Table 3). These recommended values are increased slightly for infants and children and markedly during pregnancy and lactation; some countries suggest higher intakes for postmenopausal women and the elderly, others do not.

Many—and especially those concerned with osteoporosis—are convinced that the RDA is inadequate even in Western countries, and have urged that the RDA should be increased (National Institute of Health, 1984; Spencer et al., 1984; NOS, 1989b). Typical suggested daily intakes are a minimum of 800 mg for adults with higher intakes for adolescents (1100 mg), lactating women (1200 mg) and postmenopausal women (1500 mg). Others can see no valid scientific reason for increasing the current values, since there are no indications (such as deficiencies) that they are inadequate (Anon, 1987; Kanis & Passmore, 1989). Bearing in

TABLE 3
Recommended daily amounts/recommended dietary allowances for calcium in different countries

RDA (mg/day for an adult)			
450	*500*	*600*	*800*
Greece	Columbia	Denmark	Australia
India	Indonesia	Italy	France
Malaysia	Mexico	Japan	West Germany
Thailand	Philippines	New Zealand	Netherlands
Venuzuela	UK	Spain	Poland
			USA
			USSR

These recommended values vary more widely than do the figures for most nutrients. This variation reflects the problems associated with assessing calcium requirements, and the greater or lesser willingness of national committees to give weight to the possible beneficial effects of intakes in excess of the physiological requirements. Some also take account of the possibility of achieving the intake.

mind that diet is only one factor in the development of osteoporosis (see below) and that RDAs are intended as population requirements for *healthy* groups (see Chapter 1), the balance seems in favour of leaving the RDA for calcium at its present value in the absence of conclusive evidence that it is too low.

As mentioned before, the RDAs in many developing countries are much lower than the 'Western' figures, and there are indications that even these lower recommended group intakes are often not achieved. Nonetheless, signs of overt calcium deficiency are rare, and this presents an interesting challenge to present views on calcium nutrition. Indeed, some argue that these observations show that the current RDAs in developed countries are not only adequate but an overestimate. However, it should be remembered that there are large differences in total diet and lifestyle involved.

CALCIUM SOURCES

Although calcium is present in a range of foods (Table 4), the relatively high intakes in Western countries depend heavily on dairy produce, which supplies 50–75% in a highly available form. The calcium content of milk is high, and it is retained in semi-skimmed and skimmed milk. Calcium concentration in cheese is particularly high. (See Paul & Southgate, 1978).

Brian A. Rolls

TABLE 4
Calcium contents of food

Food	Calcium content (mg/100 g)
Cheese	400–1200
Cottage cheese	73
Whole milk	115
Semi-skimmed milk	120
Skimmed milk	120
Yoghurt	150
Apples, potatoes	4–10
Oranges	41
Water	up to 16
White bread	110
Wholemeal bread	54
Eggs	50–60
Poultry	7–10
Meat	6–18
Cabbage	38
Watercress	220

(Values from Paul & Southgate, 1978)

Although the intakes of calcium in the Western world vary among countries, the proportion coming from dairy foods is similar (Fig. 4). Smaller amounts come from cereal foods, fish and hard water. Some cereal foods may be calcium-enriched, such as fortified white bread (UK) and calcium-enriched breakfast cereals (US). An unknown number of people consume supplements, particularly in the US (Kolata, 1986).

Since more than a third of this intake comes from a single source—milk —calcium intake in western countries is vulnerable to the negative image that dairy foods have acquired in recent years. Indeed, daily calcium intake has fallen (e.g. from 1010 mg in 1975 to 890 mg in 1985 in the UK) largely because less milk is drunk. This trend is greater among younger (under 35) women and especially in teenage girls, who according to one viewpoint are the very group who should be encouraging peak bone mineralization. Moreover, although the mean calcium intake in developed countries is still above the RDA, the range is considerable, and substantial numbers are failing to meet this target.

It is at least arguable that those who reduce their intake of dairy foods because of concern about saturated fat intake may be exposing themselves

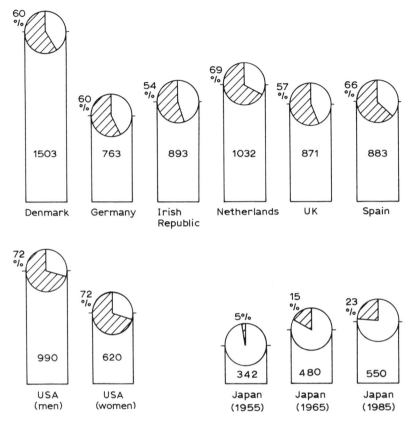

FIG. 4. Calcium intake in industralized countries (intake in milligrams and pro-portion of this coming from milk products). In most 'Western' nations, dairy produce accounts for about $\frac{2}{3}$ of the calcium intake, even though the absolute amount varies. In most Third World nations, where dairying is not traditional, the intake is much lower (≈ 150–$400\,mg/day$) and milk products account for ≈ 5–10%. Japan is a particularly interesting case: industrialized but culturally a mixture of Western and non-Western traditions.

to other risks. Assuming at least some basis for the current RDA values, it would be more difficult to achieve the intakes consistent with good health if dairy foods were eliminated altogether, although some in-dividuals certainly manage it.

It would not be reasonable to extend this argument to state that dairy foods are essential for an adequate calcium intake, since many who do not eat them remain perfectly healthy. It is more convincing to propose that milk products contribute to sound general nutrition, which is as important to, say, bone health as calcium intake alone (e.g. Schaafsma, 1983). For this reason, although calcium salts given as supplements are quite adequately absorbed (Recker *et al.*, 1988), they do not contribute to the general nutrition of the consumer in other ways and are less desirable than obtaining calcium (or other nutrients) from a sound diet (see Kolata, 1986).

Calcium intakes in many parts of the world, particularly in developing countries where dairying is not traditional and may not be practical, are often about half those in Western countries. Despite this, disorders associated with calcium metabolism are no more, and often less, prevalent. It is difficult to put forward an entirely convincing reason why this should be so, and this problem will be considered later.

CALCIUM ABSORPTION AND BIOAVAILABILITY

Calcium is absorbed from the gut by two separate mechanisms, one of which is passive and depends only on concentration differences (see Fig. 1). In the other, calcitriol is involved. The inactive vitamin D_3 (cholecalciferol), which is derived either from the diet or manufactured from cholesterol in the liver and then the skin under ultraviolet light, is converted into its active form, calcitriol (1,25-dihyroxycholecalciferol). Calcitriol controls the manufacture of intestinal calcium-binding protein which promotes the absorption of calcium even against a concentration gradient. As vitamin D acts at a particular target organ (or group of cells), it is perhaps better described as a hormone rather than a vitamin.

Active transport predominates at low calcium intakes, the less efficient passive absorption at high intakes. Hence, as intake rises, the proportion absorbed falls, although of course the total amount absorbed also rises. For useful reviews, see Allen (1982) and Nordin (1988). In addition, people adapt to low calcium intakes (Malm, 1958), although some do so more readily than others.

Since ultraviolet light is involved, calcium deficiency is often associated with lack of sunlight (Loomis, 1967). People of African or Asian origin living in northern Europe, whose dark skins (and perhaps cultural habits) reduce such benefits as may be derived from the feeble northern sun, are at particular risk from rickets and osteomalacia (its adult equivalent). This involves the accumulation of inadequately mineralized bone due to vitamin D deficiency. The active component of calcium absorption is known to become less efficient with age, so another group at risk is the elderly, especially if they are housebound and unable to benefit from the effects of sunlight on the skin. Such people may benefit from calcium and vitamin D supplements, although as with all fat-soluble vitamins these must be given with caution, since an excess of vitamin D is harmful.

Not all the calcium eaten is available to the body for structural or metabolic purposes. Some is lost in the urine or faeces, or through the skin (Fig. 1). The intake corrected for faecal loss gives the proportion that enters the body: this is the concept of bioavailability. Generally, about 25–30% of the calcium intake is available to the body (Allen, 1982), although this figure must not be applied universally. Absorption is higher in infancy (50–70%) and pregnancy ($\sim$ 40%, see below) and there is considerable variation. Moreover, calcium absorption changes from day to day (Heaney *et al.*, 1988*a*), can adapt to high or low calcium intakes, status or requirements, and can be affected considerably by other nutrients and even non-dietary factors such as exercise and stress. Thus, it is not possible to derive a single bioavailability value (see Allen, 1982). Many measurements have been made in the rat, which handles some minerals differently from man. However, recent estimates in human subjects using double-tracer stable isotopes or neutron activation are probably more reliable.

Many interactions between calcium and other nutrients have been recorded. The metabolism of phosphorus and calcium is intimately connected and has received considerable attention. In general, phosphorus stimulates calcium retention in man and the calcium: phosphorus ratio does not seem to matter provided that phosphorus intake is adequate. High dietary phosphate may decrease calcium absorption at high calcium intakes (> 2000 mg/day) but may actually enhance absorption at low intakes (< 500 mg/day). On the other hand, high-phosphate diets reduce calcium absorption in rats and dogs are very sensitive to the calcium: phosphorus ratio. This is a reminder of the necessity of applying results obtained from animal models to the human condition with caution.

The consumption of high-protein diets reduces the absorption of minerals in general, including calcium, largely by increasing urinary loss (Linkswiler *et al.*, 1981; Yuen *et al.*, 1984). Since a similar effect is seen in short-term starvation, it has been suggested that this is due to enhanced renal acid secretion (and a consequent need of more calcium salts for buffering). Meat consumption, which promotes a more acid urine, results in greater calcium loss than eating soya protein. It has been reported that bone losses in vegetarians tend to be less than in omnivores. This may not be the whole story, and it is possible that insulin, stimulated by protein consumption, directly affects renal absorption. Postmenopausal women are affected more than men.

It is conceivable that at least part of the ability of those in the Third World to cope with lower calcium intakes may be connected with the generally lower protein intakes, much of which will be vegetable in origin.

The proteins in milk have a less negative effect on absorption, and some may even enhance availability (Lee *et al.*, 1983), although the high protein content of dairy foods may partly reduce this effect (Recker & Heaney, 1985). In addition, it is known that lactose enhances calcium absorption and this contributes to the high availability of the calcium from dairy products, as does the vitamin D (where present). The beneficial effect of these milk constituents do not seem to be affected by processing (Porter, 1980; Smith *et al.*, 1985).

Dietary fibre, phytate (*myo*-inositol hexaphosphoric acid; present in cereals, legumes and oilseeds, including wheat and soya) and oxalic acid (present in green vegetables such as spinach) have long been known to affect mineral availability by increasing faecal loss. These effects are probably secondary to changes in bile acid and salt secretion and resorption. The 'soluble' fibre found in fruit and other sources has less effect. The effects of fibre may be less harmful than was originally supposed, and may be confined to conditions in which the fibre : calcium ratio is high (> 0·2?) and calcium and vitamin D status is poor. Nonetheless, recent studies have found markedly lower calcium bioavailability from plant foods (Heaney *et al.*, 1988; Fairweather-Tait *et al.*, 1989). This is not, of course, to deny the beneficial effects of an adequate fibre intake in protecting against a range of disorders, including diverticular disease and colon cancer. The effects of fibre vary with dietary concentration, physicochemical properties and the response of the individual. For example, metal-fibre complexes may be more or less resistant to digestion and the human gut may adapt to a high fibre intake.

Calcium loss is known to occur in steatorrhoea (a fatty diarrhoea typical of severe malabsorption), but it is also possible that calcium bioavailability is decreased by high-fat diets, although the results are not clear-cut. The effect seems to increase with concentration, chain length and degree of saturation; indeed, medium-chain and polyunsaturated fats may enhance absorption (Tantibhedhyangkul & Hashim, 1978).

Many interactions have been recorded between calcium absorption and metabolism and that of other minerals, in many cases because they share absorption sites or mechanisms or body storage compartments (see also Chapter 5). High dietary zinc causes, at least in rats, a decrease in bone calcium, probably by shifting phosphorus excretion from the urine to the faeces and increasing faecal calcium loss. Fluoride probably improves calcium retention by promoting bone formation, although the results are vary. Excess phosphate interferes with calcium absorption in infants (Barltrop *et al.*, 1977) although this seems less important in adults. Some medical conditions, including stress, reduce calcium retention or increase losses.

In many of the above instances, calcium status can be protected or restored by giving calcium supplements with or without vitamin D.

OSTEOPOROSIS

During childhood and the early adult years the body will—assuming sound diet and lifestyle—achieve positive net calcium balance and the skeleton will grow, thicken and reach peak mineralization and bone density during the thirties. Each part of the skeleton consists of two types of bone, compact and trabecular. As already mentioned, bone is not inert, it is a living tissue consisting of a protein similar to collagen set in a mineral similar to hydroxyapatite (calcium phosphate, $Ca_{10}(PO_4)_6(OH)_2$) but with

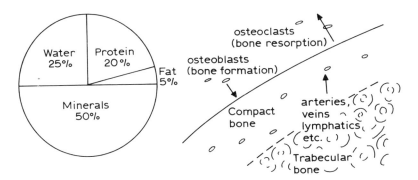

FIG. 5(a). Bone.
Protein: similar to collagen
Mineral: crystals similar to hydroxyapatite, $3Ca_3(PO_4)_2 \cdot Ca(OH)_2$.

FIG. 5(b). Bone consists of mineral crystals surrounding long, collagen-like fibres. The ratio of compact to trabecular bone is 4:1, but this varies in different bones.

inclusions of other minerals. It is undergoing continuous turnover, with specialized cells building up (osteoblasts) or removing (osteoclasts) bone, a process known as remodelling (Fig. 5). Bone grows on the outside, but is lost inside, producing a cavity. It has been claimed that a high calcium intake can increase peak bone mass or ameliorate osteoporosis (Nordin, 1961; Matkovic et al., 1979; Heaney et al., 1982; Kanders et al., 1984; Sandler et al., 1989), but accurate assessment of diet—particularly in retrospect—is difficult and others have found no effect (Garn et al., 1969; Hegsted, 1967; Garn, 1970; Nilas et al., 1984).

In early life, growth induces an accumulation of calcium: a positive calcium balance. Eventually, however, the body will in later life move into negative calcium balance: parathyroid hormone concentrations will rise, resorption will occur and the bones will suffer a net mineral loss. The process is inevitable and a natural part of ageing: although measures can be taken to slow it, it will take place, regardless of diet, activity, lifestyle, sex or race. Calcium in the teeth is relatively inaccessible, even under conditions of negative calcium balance, and the old wives' tale of losing a tooth for each child seems to be just that. To damage the teeth, a poor diet at the formative stage is probably necessary.

At the age of 50, men will be losing about 10 mg calcium a day and women about twice this; however, when the latter reach the menopause the loss can accelerate to 40–100 mg/day, apparently as a result of the withdrawal of the protective action of oestrogen. This rate does eventually fall, presumably as the body adjusts to the loss of the hormone. Both smoking (Jick et al., 1977) and alcoholism (Saville, 1965) exacerbate the loss by inducing early menopause, although smoking has a similar effect on men (Seeman et al., 1983).

If the calcium loss upon ageing is severe, the bones eventually thin and lose structural strength, a condition known as osteoporosis; sufferers are likely to experience backache, compression fractures of the vertebrae (especially in the dorsal and lumbar regions) and acute fractures, typically at the femoral neck, hip and wrist. The condition is widespread: probably 25% of women experience it to some degree in Western countries, and it has been claimed that up to 20 000 deaths a year in the UK result from the consequences of the fractures or subsequent surgery. Such fractures are slow to heal, for the bones are in a state of calcium loss and accretion is slow.

Whether osteoporosis develops depends on many influences, such as genetic background, overall nutrition, calcium malabsorption, vitamin D deficiency, renal malfunction, immobility, endocrine factors and possible

TABLE 5
Factors affecting bone loss

Increase	Reduce
Smoking	Moderate exercise
Leanness	Hormone replacement
Lack of exercise	Diuretics
Excessive exercise	Being male
Diet (?)	Obesity

side-effects of medication. Larger people lose bone more slowly, in fact the rate of loss is inversely related to body mass index (weight/height^2), the influence being greater on cortical than trabecular bone. This may be because of increased exercise demands or a greater oestrogen production (fat women have later menopauses). An interesting example is that of black South African women, who are usually very active and often overweight. Despite extended breastfeeding and calcium intakes of only 150–200 mg/day, they rarely suffer from osteoporosis. For reviews of the risk factors for osteoporosis (Table 5), see Heaney (1984), Aloia *et al.*, (1985) and Anon. (1985).

Investigation of osteoporosis is difficult. Radiographic appearance is not a good indicator of bone density (bone loss can reach 40% before it becomes obvious on X-rays), although recently introduced procedures, single and dual photon absorptiometry give estimates of bone density within 1–4% (Krølner & Pors Nielsen, 1980; Al Azzawi *et al.*, 1987). Fasting hydroxyproline excretion gives a measure of current (although not past) calcium loss.

Can anything be done to avoid or delay osteoporosis? First, it must be repeated that some loss is inevitable. Blacks have a higher bone mass than whites, but both lose calcium; athletes lose bone as do the sedentary, although more slowly. It is arguable that bone health is affected by heredity (Lutz, 1986), environment, lifestyle and nutrition (some would suggest that heredity is the only factor) and achieving a high peak bone mass is a sound investment for old age. It is widely accepted (although not always on sound grounds, see above) that bone density is sensitive to calcium availability—assuming adequate intake of other nutrients—and a high intake of calcium as part of a good general nutrition in early life, together with an active lifestyle, avoiding smoking and drinking only in moderation are advisable. Good nutrition during pregnancy and lactation is especially important because of the large calcium output to the foetus and the milk.

It has to be admitted, however, that much of the basis for this view of the importance of diet is by inference, since few longitudinal studies have been carried out and retrospective studies of osteoporotic patients may not give an accurate impression of their diet when their bone was being deposited.

Moreover, osteoporosis is very much a disease of advanced societies. Rural Bantu women have a tenth of the incidence of hip fracture despite a calcium intake half that of Western women (200–400 mg/day) and greater demands for childbearing and lactation. (It is true that more frequent pregnancies can confer extra oestrogen protection.) Any coherent theory of the relationship between bone health and calcium intake must account for such anomalies.

Age-related and postmenopausal bone loss cannot be prevented by a high-calcium diet alone (see Kolata, 1986), although it is possible that it may be slowed by a suitable lifestyle, including a sound diet. The role of calcium supplements and high-calcium diets is controversial, and any who conduct studies in this field must expect their methodology to be given considerable critical attention.

Oestrogen therapy (hormone replacement therapy, HRT) reduces bone resorption, arrests postmenopausal bone loss and reduces fracture sites (Horsman *et al.*, 1977; Lindsay *et al.*, 1980; Riggs *et al.*, 1982; Ettinger *et al.*, 1985; Civitelli *et al.*, 1988; Horowitz *et al.*, 1988), but does carry a slightly increased risk of endometrial cancer. Some investigators have found no benefit from calcium supplements alone; some claim a reduction in bone resorption only when phosphorus is given with calcium; others have found advantages only with high intakes (1400–2000 mg/day). There does seem to be agreement, from studies of calcium balance and the healing of microfissures in bone surfaces, that calcium intakes of about 1000 mg/day (giving total intakes of about 1800–2000 mg/day) with oestrogen at 0·3 mg/day can replace oestrogen alone at 0·6 mg/day, thus reducing the risk of endometrial stimulation. Responses to treatment can differ for different bone sites, perhaps reflecting their content of compact or trabecular bone.

Exercise is generally beneficial to bone health. This may be a piezo-electric effect: muscle tension produces a minute electrical current that promotes the deposition of bone. Thus, an active lifestyle both increases peak bone density in youth (Nilsson & Westlin, 1971) and slows bone loss in later years (Krølner *et al.*, 1983). Those in sedentary occupations—astronauts are an extreme example—suffer greater bone loss than do active people. Mineral loss is consequent to bone loss, which also occurs in unexercised muscles. Postmenopausal bone loss cannot be prevented by exercise alone, but it is a useful adjunct to oestrogen therapy and calcium supplementation.

It is clear that elderly housebound people suffer several disadvantages. Appetite may be poor and calcium intake may decline (Krehl, 1974) with total food intake, for less energy is required, and the adaptability of the gut to reduced intake also falls with age (Ireland & Fordtran, 1973). The active component of calcium absorption becomes less effective with age (Aviolo *et al.*, 1965; Bullamore *et al.*, 1970), perhaps due to impaired hydroxylation of vitamin D_3 (Slovik *et al.*, 1981), and the beneficial effects of exercise and sunlight are reduced. This results in poor calcium and calcitriol status, negative calcium balance, a rise in parathyroid hormone, bone resorption and accelerated weakening of bone.

An exception to the general rule about exercise is afforded by amenorrhoeic women athletes, who can have reduced spinal mineral density and may develop back trouble. The explanation may lie in the relationship between bone density and body fat, since the final activation of oestrogen takes place in fat, and suggests that oestrogens have a greater influence than exercise. In this, as in other aspects of lifestyle, moderation is the prudent option.

HYPERTENSION

Hypertension, that is, chronically raised blood pressure, carries increased risks of stroke, congestive heart disease, myocardial infarction, renal and retinal damage and enlargement of the heart. In pregnancy, hypertension increases risks for both mother and infant (Lindheimer & Katz, 1985).

Hypertension is difficult to define, since blood pressure is a continuous variable, but in recent years the pressure at which the benefits of treatment (less possible side-effects) are considered to outweigh the risks of inaction have tended to move to lower values. Two figures are quoted: the systolic or maximum pressure, reached when the heart contracts, and the diastolic pressure when the heart relaxes. Treatment now aims to keep pressures (in mm Hg) below 140/90 for those below 65 (BMJ, 1981).

Some forms of hypertension are consequent upon known disease ('secondary' hypertension) but most ('essential' hypertension) is of unknown aetiology. Although the dangers of very high blood pressures

TABLE 6
Possible risk factors for hypertension

Non-dietary	Dietary
Smoking	High sodium
Alcoholism	Low potassium
Being male	High saturated fat
Being black	Low magnesium
Lack of exercise	Low fibre
Stress (?)	High protein
Obesity	Low calcium
Drugs	Low essential fatty acid

('malignant' hypertension) are so unequivocal that immediate treatment is essential, problems arise with marginal hypertension (diastolic pressures of 90–100 mm Hg). Even the mild first-line drugs have side effects some of which actually tend to increase the risk of cardiovascular disease (Flamenbaum, 1983; Schiff & Schollmeyer, 1985) and their use does not necessarily lead to a reduction in mortality (MRFIT, 1982).

The developed world, and particularly countries such as Finland and the UK, have unenviable positions in the tables of premature deaths from heart disease, although figures in the US have recently begun to fall. The factors of diet and lifestyle associated with hypertension and heart disease (Table 6) have received considerable attention (for reviews, see Bulpitt, 1985; Huttunen et al., 1985; Elliot et al., 1987). They interact, so the diagnosed hypertensive is wise not to be an obese, unfit smoker. When diet and cardiovascular disease are discussed, it is well to remember that dietary factors are only part of the story (e.g. Anon., 1983).

Over recent years, many claims have been made that the consumption of an excess (or a deficiency) of this or that nutrient results in the development or the exacerbation of hypertension (e.g. Klatsky et al., 1977; Puska et al., 1983; Anon., 1984; Harlan et al., 1984; Khaw & Barrett-Connor, 1984; Saudie et al., 1984; Hodges & Rebello, 1985; Malhotra et al., 1985; Melby et al., 1985; Pacy & Dodson, 1985; Verlangieri et al., 1985; Weinsier & Norris, 1985; Berry, 1986; Norris et al., 1986; Krotkiewski, 1987; Webster & Dyckner, 1987; Wright et al., 1979; and the reviews of Bulpitt, 1985; Elliot et al., 1987 and Huttunen et al., 1985 cited previously). The evidence for this comes from three sources: epidemiology, animals models and direct intervention studies; all these have their deficiencies. For every nutrient possibly implicated in hypertension there are studies that support the possibility and others that fail to demonstrate any effect. The problem is not in amassing evidence, but in judging how valid and relevant the studies may have been. Measurement of nutrient intake is notoriously difficult (Marr, 1965, 1971), animal studies have to be interpreted with caution and it is difficult to make changes in the consumption of the nutrient under investigation without affecting others. It is not even known whether the alleged ill-effects of excess of a particular nutrient are direct or the result of increased demand for other nutrients.

Primitive peoples with low salt intake are admirably free from cardiovascular disease, nor do their blood pressures rise with age. But before we conclude that a high salt diet 'causes' hypertension we should reflect that such people are likely to be small, active, lean and eating a completely different diet, high in vegetable foods and low in protein and fat. Studies of sodium within, rather than between, countries have been rather disappointing, and measurements of sodium intake without stringent precautions are unreliable.

Yet even studies that fail to show any link between salt and hypertension are not conclusive. Hypertension is almost certainly multifactorial and heterogeneous, and individuals differ in their sensitivities. The results from a section of the population sensitive to sodium may be masked by those from unresponsive subjects. Moreover, equivocal trials in which salt intake has been reduced to no effect do not remove the possibility that a lifetime of high intake is a factor. (For some idea of the controversy generated, see Altschul *et al.*, 1981; Various, 1984; MacGregor, 1985; Swales, 1988.)

The earliest evidence that calcium intake may be a factor in heart disease came from studies that indicated a lower incidence of cardiovascular disease in hard-water areas (for review, see Kesteloot, 1985). Interest in calcium has been revived by the work of McCarron and his colleagues, who used the HANES 1 survey to show that hypertensives had lower intakes of calcium and also of potassium, vitamin A and vitamin C (McCarron *et al.*, 1984; McCarron, 1985). The study has been criticized, particularly with regard to its statistics and nutrient assessment (Feinleib *et al.*, 1984; MacGregor, 1985); see also McCarron & Morris (1987).

Subsequent studies have provided some support for these claims. High blood pressure has been shown to be inversely related to the consumption of dairy products (Ackley *et al.*, 1983; Garcia-Palmiera *et al.*, 1984; Sowers *et al.*, 1985) and freedom from hypertension of pregnancy is associated with a higher calcium intake (Belizan & Villar, 1980). There is a higher incidence of hypertension among osteoporosis sufferers, who are thought to have (or to have had) an inadequate intake or excessive losses of calcium. As a group, hypertensives excrete more calcium in their urine. Diets high in protein and sodium, which promote calcium loss, can be associated with higher blood pressure. Blacks have a higher incidence of hypertension and also of lactase deficiency, which would make them avoid milk products (for reviews, see Bulpitt, 1985; McCarron, 1985). It is sometimes difficult to judge whether calcium or an associated nutrient is involved (e.g. Reed et al., 1985). Studies of the relationship between hypertension and blood ionized calcium concentrations have, however, been contradictory (e.g. Ackley et al., 1983; Hunt et al., 1984; Richards et al., 1984; Hvarfner et al., 1987; Kesteloot, 1987).

The most convincing evidence comes from intervention studies in which calcium supplements (1000–2000 mg/day) were given to groups of hypertensives and normotensive controls. Various trials have shown reduced blood pressure in: hypertensives but not normotensives, more in hypertensives than normotensives, or only in certain groups of hypertensives. Other trials have shown no effect. (See Belizan et al., 1983a, b; Resnick & Laragh, 1983; Johnson et al., 1985; McCarron & Morris, 1985; Grobbee & Hofman, 1986; Lyle et al., 1987; Vinson et al., 1987.) The situation is not unlike that with low-sodium diets (cf. Resnick, 1987), and reinforces the concept of hypertension as a heterogeneous disorder.

The spontaneously hypertensive rats (in fact, there are several strains of hypertensive rat) provides a useful model for human hypertension (Ganten, 1987). With these animals, a low-calcium diet exacerbates hypertension, whereas a high-calcium diet (even one that is also high-sodium) attenuates the rise in blood pressure. This rat has been shown to share many biochemical and physiological abnormalities with human hypertensives, many of which involve defects in calcium absorption, transport and control (McCarron et al., 1981). Calcium is intimately involved with muscle function, and various mechanisms have been proposed for the way smooth muscle cell function may be affected by defects in calcium metabolism, although at present these remain speculative (for reviews, see Haddy, 1983; Swales, 1983; Wasserman & Fullmer, 1983; Robinson, 1984).

There is evidence that at least some cases of hypertension may be associated with low calcium intake, and for most people a moderate increase in dietary calcium would do no harm. (In some medical conditions it would be dangerous.) More clinical studies are necessary before calcium supplements can be recommended unreservedly to the general public (Zawanda & Brautbar, 1985; Anon, 1986, 1987).

TABLE 7
Factors affecting colon cancer

Increase risk	Decrease risk
Fat	Vitamin A
Protein	Vitamin C
Cholesterol	Fibre
Alcohol	Calcium (?)

The attractions of the calcium hypothesis, as with any concerned with diet and/or lifestyle, are that drugs may be discontinued or reduced (e.g. Stamler *et al.*, 1987) and that even a small reduction in blood pressure in the population would substantially reduce hypertension and heart disease, especially among those with mild or marginal hypertension.

COLON CANCER

In most Western countries, around 12% of cancer deaths are due to colorectal cancer. The incidence of colon cancer is positively correlated with intakes of fat, protein, cholesterol and alcohol, but negatively associated with fibre and vitamins A and C (Table 7). It has recently been suggested (Newmark *et al.*, 1984; Garland *et al.*, 1985; Slattery *et al.*, 1988) that calcium may also act protectively.

As with the possible link between calcium intake and hypertension, there are studies that support and contradict this theory. Within the US, regions and social groups consuming more calcium or more milk products tend to have a lower incidence of colon cancer. This is also true for some comparisons between countries, but Japan has a low calcium intake and little colon cancer while Australia has both high calcium intakes and high colon cancer rates. Clinical studies are similarly equivocal; again, susceptibility to a disease will depend on other nutrients, sex, heredity and lifestyle. Exposure to sunlight is corrrelated with vitamin D status (Garland & Garland, 1980), so the calcium effect may be mediated through the vitamin (see also Pence & Baddengh, 1988). It is also possible that a nutrient in milk other than calcium is responsible for any effect.

A confounding factor in these studies is that fat intake is known to be correlated with colonic cancer and, at least in Western countries, most of the calcium consumed comes from dairy produce, which is often a source of saturated fat. It has been proposed that a high-fat diet increases the concentrations of free fatty acids and bile acids in the colon, which in turn increases epithelial cell turnover, increasing susceptibility to carcinogens. Calcium, it is argued, inhibits these toxic effects by rendering these irritating agents insoluble (Newmark et al., 1984) and reduces cell proliferation (Wargovich et al., 1983; Lipkin & Newmark, 1985).

An elegant series of in-vitro and in-vivo experiments (van der Meer, R., pers. comm.) has cast some light on possible mechanisms for the beneficial effect of calcium. Both fatty acids and deoxycholates are cytotoxic (in the case of deoxycholates, there appears to be a threshold concentration), the more so when they are present together. For fatty acids alone, both soluble calcium and insoluble calcium phosphate decrease cytotoxicity. For deoxycholate, however, only insoluble calcium phosphate is effective. This suggests that insoluble calcium salts in particular act by binding bile salts and decreasing soluble (but not total) bile acids in the lower gut.

Unfortunately, fibre is also negatively correlated with colon cancer, and fibre reduces calcium absorption (see above) and if anything increases free fatty acids in the lower gut. Moreover, there are suggestions that the protective effect of calcium against bowel tumours operates in low-fat but not high-fat diets (Bull et al., 1987).

Although there is some interesting evidence to suggest that a high calcium intake may reduce the risk of colonic cancer, it is by no means conclusive at present.

CONCLUSIONS

Many aspects of calcium nutrition remain uncertain or controversial, although it does seem that a high calcium intake may have a place in the treatment of osteoporosis and perhaps hypertension. Most probably this will be as an adjunct to other treatment, perhaps enabling lower drug dosages to be used. Even minor improvements along these lines would reduce suffering and be of economic benefit.

Perhaps the greatest challenge to the conventional view of calcium metabolism is to explain why less developed countries, with much lower calcium intakes, have so much less hypertension, cardiovascular disease and osteoporosis. The body can certainly adapt to lower intakes, and the gut can become more efficient at calcium absorption (in pregnancy and lactation, for instance), but in that case why do Western osteoporosis sufferers not adapt? Is it simply that they live longer, and have time to show evidence of degenerative diseases? Is it a question of lifestyle, exercise, heredity or the whole dietary context? No explanation seems entirely satisfactory.

REFERENCES

Ackley, S., Barrett-Connor, E. & Suarez, L. (1983). Dairy products, calcium, and blood pressure. *American Journal of Clinical Nutrition* **38**, 457–61.

Al Azzawi, F., Hart, D.M. & Lindsay, R. (1987). Long-term effect of oestrogen replacement therapy on bone mass as measured by dual photon absorptiometry. *British Medical Journal* **294**, 1261–2.

Allen, L.H. (1982). Calcium absorption and bioavailability: a review. *American Journal of Clinical Nutrition* **35**, 783–808.

Aloia, J.F., Cohn, S.H., Vaswani, A., Yeh, J.K. & Ellis, K. (1985). Risk factors for postmenopausal osteoporosis. *American Journal of Medicine* **78**, 95–100.

Altschul, A.M., Grommet, J.K., Slotkoff, L. & Ayers, W.R. (1981). Sodium sensitivity. In *Nutritional Factors: Modulating Effects on Metabolic Processes*, pp. 45–62 [R.F. Beers, Jr and E.G. Bassett, editors]. New York: Raven Press.

Anon. (1983). Genetics, environment and hypertension. *Lancet* **i**, 681–2.

Anon. (1984). Diet and hypertension. *Lancet* **ii**, 671–3.

Anon. (1985). Risk factors in postmenopausal osteoporosis. *Lancet* **i**, 1370–2.

Anon. (1986). Hypertension: is there a place for calcium? *Lancet* **i**, 359–61.

Anon. (1987). Calcium supplements: does the milkman know best? *Lancet* **i**, 370–1.

Avioli, L.V. McDonald, J.E. & Lee, S.W. (1965). The influence of age on the intestinal absorption of ^{47}Ca in women and its relation to ^{47}Ca absorption in post-menopausal osteoporosis. *Journal of Clinical Investigation* **44**, 1960–7.

Barltrop, D., Mole, R.H. & Sutton, A. (1977). Absorption and endogenous faecal excretion of calcium by low birthweight infants on feeds with varying contents of calcium and phosphates. *Archives of Diseases in Childhood* **52**, 41–9.

Belizan, J.M. & Villar, J. (1980). The relationship between calcium intake and edema-, proteinuria- and hypertension-gestosis: an hypothesis. *American Journal of Clinical Nutrition* **33**, 2202–10.

Belizan, J.M., Villar, J., Zalazar, A., Rojas, L., Chan, D. & Bryce, G.F. (1983*a*). Preliminary evidence of the effect of calcium supplementation on blood pressure in pregnant women. *American Journal of Obstetrics and Gynecology* **146**, 175–80.

Belizan, J.M., Villar, J., Pineda, O., Gonzalez, A.E., Sainz, E., Garrera, G. & Sibrian, R. (1983*b*). Reduction of blood pressure with calcium supplementation in young adults. *Journal of the American Medical Association* **249**, 1161–5.

Berry, E.M. (1986). Does dietary linolenic acid influence blood pressure? *American Journal of Clinical Nutrition* **44**, 336–40.

BMJ (1981). *ABC of Hypertension*. London: British Medical Association.

BNF (1989). *Calcium. The Report of the British Nutrition Foundation's Task Force*. London: British Nutrition Foundation.

Bull, A., Bird, R.P., Bruce, W.R., Nigro, N. & Medline, A. (1987). Effect of calcium on ozoxymenthane induced intestinal tumors in rats. *Gastroenterology* **92**, 1332.

Bullamore, J.R., Gallagher, J.C., Wilkinson, R., Nordin, B.E.C. & Marshall, D.H. (1970). Effect of age on calcium absorption. *Lancet* **ii**, 535–7.

Bulpitt, C.J. (Editor) (1985). *Handbook of Hypertension, Vol. 6: Epidemiology of Hypertension*. Amsterdam: Elsevier.

Civitelli, R., Agnusdei, D., Nardi, P., Zacchei, F., Avioli, L.V. & Gennari, C. (1988). Effects of one year treatment with estrogens on bone mass, intestinal calcium absorption and 25-hydroxyvitamin D_1 hydroxylase reserve in postmenopausal osteoporosis. *Calcified Tissue International* **42**, 77–86.

Elliott, P., Fehily, A.M., Sweetnam, P.M. & Yarnell, J.W.G. (1987). Diet, alcohol, body mass, and social factors in relation to blood pressure: the Caerphilly Heart Study. *Journal of Epidemiology and Community Health*. **41**, 37–43.

Ettinger, B., Genant, H.K. & Cann, C.E. (1985). Long-term oestrogen replacement therapy prevents bone loss and fractures. *Annals of Internal Medicine* **102**, 319–24.

Fairweather-Tait, S.J., Johnson, A., Eagles, J., Ganatra, S., Kennedy, H. & Gurr, M.I. (1989). Studies on calcium absorption from milk using a double label stable isotope method. *British Journal of Nutrition* **62**, 379–88.

Feinleib, M., Lenfant, C. & Miller, S.A. (1984). Hypertension and calcium. *Science* **226**, 384; 386–8.

Flamenbaum, W. (1983). Metabolic consequences of antihypertensive theory. *Annals of Internal Medicine* **98**, 875–80.

Ganten, D. (1987). Role of animal models in hypertension research. *Hypertension* **9**, 2–4.

Garcia-Palmieri, M.R., Costas, R., Cruz-Vidal, M., Sorlie, P.D., Tillotson, J. & Havlik, R.J. (1984). Milk consumption, calcium intake, and decreased hypertension in Puerto Rico. *Hypertension* **6**, 322–8.

Garland, C.F. & Garland F.C. (1980). Do sunlight and vitamin D reduce the likelihood of colon cancer? *International Journal of Epidemiology* **9**, 227–31.

Garland, C., Shekelle, R.B., Barrett-Connor, E., Criqui, M.H., Rossof, A.H. & Paul, O. (1985). Dietary vitamin D and calcium and risk of colorectal cancer: A 19-year prospective study in men. *Lancet* **i**, 307–9.

Garn, S.M. (1970). *The Earlier Gain and Later Loss of Cortical Bone in Nutritional Perspective*. Springfield: C.C. Thomas.

Garn, S.M., Rohmann, C.G., Wagner, B., Davila, G.H. & Ascoli, W. (1969). *Clinical Orthopaedics* **65**, 51–60.

Grobbee, D.E. & Hofman, A. (1986). Effect of calcium supplementation on diastolic blood pressure in young people with mild hypertension. *Lancet* **ii**, 703–7.

Haddy, F.J. (1983). Abnormalities of membrane transport in hypertension. *Hypertension* **5** (Suppl. V), 66–72.

Harlan, W.R., Hull, A.L., Schmouder, R.L., Landis, J.R., Larkin, F.A. & Thompson, F.E. (1984). High blood pressure in older Americans. *Hypertension* **6**, 802–9.

Heaney, R.P. (1984). Risk factors in age-related bone loss and osteoporotic fracture. In *Osteoporosis. Proceedings of the Copenhagen International Symposium on Osteoporosis*, pp. 245–53 [C. Christiansen, C.D. Arnaud, B.E.C. Nordin, A.M. Parfitt, W.A. Peck and R.L. Riggs, editors]. Copenhagen: Aalbord Stistsbogtrykkeri.

Heaney, R.P., Gallagher, J.C., Johnston, C.C., Neer, R., Parfitt, A.M. & Whedon, G.D. (1982). Calcium nutrition and bone health in the elderly. *American Journal of Clinical Nutrition* **36**, 986–1013.

Heaney, R.P., Recker, R.R. & Hinders, S.M. (1988*a*). Variability of calcium absorption. *American Journal of Clinical Nutrition* **47**, 262–4.

Heaney, R.P., Weaver, C.M. & Recker, R.R. (1988*b*). Calcium absorbability from spinach. *American Journal of Clinical Nutrition* **47**, 707–9.

Hegsted, D.M. (1967). Mineral intake and bone loss. *Federation Proceedings* **26**, 1747–54.

Hodges, R.E. & Rebello, T. (1985). Dietary changes and their possible effect on blood pressure. *American Journal of Clinical Nutrition* **41**, 1155–62.

Horowitz, M., Need, A.G., Morris, H.A., Wishart, J. & Nordin, B.E.C. (1988). Biochemical effects of calcium supplementation in post menopausal osteoporosis. *European Journal of Clinical Nutrition* **42**, 775–8.

Horsman, A., Gallagher, J.C., Simpson, N. & Nordin, B.E.C. (1977). Prospective trial of oestrogen and calcium in postmenopausal women. *British Medical Journal* ii, 789–92.

Hunt, S.C., McCarron, D.A., Smith, B.J., Ask, K.D., Bristow, M.R. & Williams, R.R. (1984). The relationship of plasma ionized calcium to cardiovascular disease end point and family history of hypertension. *Clinical and Experimental Hypertension* **6**, 1397–414.

Huttunen, J.K., Pietinen, P., Nissinen, A. & Puska, P. (1985). Dietary factors and hypertension. *Acta Medica Scandinavica (Suppl.)* **701**, 72–82.

Hvarfner, A., Bergström, R., Mörlin, C., Wide, L. & Ljunghall, S. (1987). Relationships between calcium metabolic indices and blood pressure in patients with essential hypertension as compared with a healthy population. *Journal of Hypertension* **5**, 451–6.

Ireland, P. & Fordtran, J.S. (1973). Effect of dietary calcium and age on jejunal calcium absorption in humans studied by intestinal perfusion. *Journal of Clinical Investigation* **52**, 2672–81.

Jick, H., Porter, J. & Morrison, A.S. (1977). Relation between smoking and age of natural menopause. *Lancet* i, 1354–5.

Johnson, N.E., Smith, E.L. & Freudenheim, J.L. (1985). Effects on blood pressure of calcium supplementation of women. *American Journal of Clinical Nutrition* **42**, 12–17.

Kanders, B., Lindsay, R., Dempster, D., Markhard, L. & Valiquette, G. (1984). Determinants of bone mass in young healthy women. In *Osteoporosis. Proceedings of the Copenhagen International Symposium on Osteoporosis*, pp. 337–9 [C. Christiansen, C.D. Arnaud,, B.E.C. Nordin, A.M. Parfitt, W.A. Peck and R.L. Riggs, editors]. Copenhagen:Aalborg Stistsbogtrykkeri.

Kanis, J.A. & Passmore, R. (1989). Calcium supplementation of the diet—I. Not justified by present evidence. *British Medical Journal* **298**, 137–40.

Kesteloot, H. (1985). Blood pressure, calcium and water hardness. In *Handbook of Hypertension, Vol. 6: Epidemiology of Hypertension*, pp. 216–29 [C.J. Bulpitt, editor]. Amsterdam: Elsevier.

Kesteloot, H.E.C. (1987). Dietary calcium and blood pressure. *ISI Atlas of Science: Pharmacology* **1**, 295–8.

92   *Brian A. Rolls*

Khaw, K.-T. & Barrett-Connor, E. (1984). Dietary potassium and blood pressure in a population. *American Journal of Clinical Nutrition* **39**, 963–68.

Klatsky, A.L., Friedman, G.D., Siegelaub, A.B. & Gerard, M.J. (1977). Alcohol consumption and blood pressure. *New England Journal of Medicine* **296**, 1194–200.

Kolata, G. (1986). How important is calcium in preventing osteoporosis? *Science* **233**, 519–20.

Krehl, W.A. (1974). The influence of nutritional environment on aging. *Geriatrics* **29**, 65–76.

Krølner, B. & Pors Nielsen, S. (1980). Measurement of bone mineral content (BMC) of the lumbar spine. 1. Theory and application of a new two-dimensional dual-photon attenuation method. *Scandinavian Journal of Clinical and Laboratory Investigation* **40**, 653–63.

Krølner, B., Toft, B., Pors Nielsen, S. & Tøndevold, E., (1983). Physical exercise as prophylaxis against involutional vertebral bone loss: a controlled trial. *Clinical Science* **64**, 541–6.

Krotkiewski, M. (1987). Effect of guar gum on the arterial blood pressure. *Acta Medica Scandinavica* **222**, 43–9.

Lee, Y.S., Noguchi, T. & Naito, H. (1983). Intestinal absorption of calcium in rats given diets containing casein or amino acid mixture: the role of casein phosphopeptides. *British Journal of Nutrition* **49**, 67–76.

Lindheimer, M.D. & Katz, A.I. (1985). Current concepts in hypertension and pregnancy. *New England Journal of Medicine* **313**, 675–80.

Lindsay, R., Hart, D.M., Forrest, C. & Baird, C. (1980). Prevention of spinal osteoporosis in oophorectomised women. *Lancet* **ii**, 1151–4.

Linkswiler, H.M., Zemel, M.B., Hegsted, M. & Shuette, S. (1981). Protein-induced hypercaliuria, *Federation Proceedings* **40**, 2429–33.

Lipkin, M. & Newmark, H. (1985). Effect of added dietary calcium on colonic epithelial-cell behavior of subjects at high risk for familial colonic cancer. *New England Journal of Medicine* **313**, 1381–4.

Loomis, A.B. (1967). Skin pigment regulation of Vitamin D: biosynthesis in man. *Science* **157**, 501–6.

Lutz, J. (1986). Bone mineral serum calcium and dietary intakes of mother/daughter pairs. *American Journal of Clinical Nutrition* **44**, 99–106.

Lyle, R.M., Melby, C.L., Hyner, G.C., Edmondson, J.W., Miller, J.Z. & Weinberger, M.H. (1987). Blood pressure and metabolic effects of calcium supplementation in normotensive white and black men. *Journal of the American Medical Association* **257**, 1772–6.

MacGregor, G.A. (1985). Sodium is more important than calcium in essential hypertension. *Hypertension* **7**, 628–37.

Malhotra, H., Mathur, D., Mehta, S.R. & Khandelwal, P.D. (1985). Pressor effects of alcohol in normotensive and hypertensive subjects. *Lancet* **ii**, 584–86.

Malm, O.J. (1958). Calcium requirements and adaptations in adult men. *Scandinavian Journal of Clinical and Laboratory Investigation, Suppl. 36* **10**, 1–289.

Marr, J.W. (1965). Individual weighed dietary surveys. *Nutrition* **19**, 18–24.

Marr, J.W. (1971). Individual dietary surveys: purposes and methods. In *World Review of Nutrition and Dietetics, Vol. 13*, pp. 105–64. Basel: Karger.

Matkovic, V., Kostial, K., Simonovic, I., Buzina, R., Broarec, A. & Nordin, B.E.C. (1979). Bone status and fracture rates in two regions of Yugoslavia. *American Journal of Clinical Nutrition* **32**, 540–9.

McCarron, D.A. (1985). Is calcium more important than sodium in the pathogenesis of essential hypertension? *Hypertension* **7**, 607–27.

McCarron, D.A. & Morris, C.D. (1985). Blood pressure response to oral calcium in persons with mild to moderate hypertension. *Annals of Internal Medicine* **103**, 825–31.

McCarron, D.A. & Morris, C.D. (1987). The calcium deficiency theory of hypertension. *Annals of Internal Medicine* **107**, 919–22.

McCarron, D.A., Yung, N.N., Ugoretz, B.A. & Krutzik, S. (1981). Disturbances of calcium metabolism in the spontaneously hypertensive rat. *Hypertension* **3**, 162–7.

McCarron, D.A., Morris, C.D., Henry, H.J., & Stanton, J.L. (1984). Blood pressure and nutrient intake in the United States. *Science* **224**, 1392–8.

Melby, C.L., Hyner, G.C. & Zoog, B. (1985). Blood pressure in vegetarians and non-vegetarians: a cross-sectional analysis. *Nutrition Research* **5**, 1077–82.

MRFIT (1982). Multiple risk factor intervention trial research group: multiple risk factor intervention trial. Risk factor changes and mortality results. *Journal of the American Medical Association* **248**, 1465–77.

National Institutes of Health. (1984). Osteoporosis: consensus conference. *Journal of the American Medical Association* **252**, 799–802.

NDC (1984). *Calcium. A Summary of Current Research for the Health Professional.* Rosemont, IL: National Dairy Council.

NDC (1985). *Diet and Health. The Fresh Approach.* London: National Dairy Council.

Newmark, H.L., Wargovich, M.J. & Bruce, W.R. (1984). Colon cancer and dietary fat, phosphate and calcium: A hypothesis. *Journal of the National Cancer Institute* **72**, 1323–5.

Nilas, L., Christiansen, C. & Rodbro, P. (1984). Calcium supplementation and postmenopausal bone loss. *British Medical Journal* **289**, 1103–6.

Nilsson, B.E. & Westlin, N.E. (1971). Bone density in athletes. *Clinical Orthopaedics and Related Research* **77**, 179–82.

Nordin, B.E.C. (1961). The pathogenesis of osteoporosis. *Lancet* **i**, 1011–14.

Nordin, B.E.C. (1988). *Calcium in Human Biology.* London: Springer Verlag.

Norris, P.G., Jones, C.J.H. & Weston, M.J. (1986). Effect of dietary supplementation with fish oil on systolic blood pressure in mild essential hypertension. *British Medical Journal* **293**, 104–5.

NOS (1989*a*). *Calcium Guide.* London: National Osteoporosis Society.

NOS (1989*b*). *Calcium: Recommended Daily Allowances.* [Submission by the National Osteoporosis Society to the Minerals Working group of the Committee on the Medical Aspects of Food Policy (COMA)] London: National Osteoporosis Society.

Pacy, P.J. & Dodson, P.M. (1985). Nutrition and hypertension. *Annals of Nutrition and Metabolism* **29**, 129–37.

Paul, A.A. & Southgate, D.A.T. (1978). *McCance and Widdowson's The Composition of Foods, 4th edn.* London: H.M. Stationery Office.

Pence, B.C. & Baddengh, F. (1988). Inhibition of dietary fat-promoted colon carcinogenesis in rats by supplemental calcium or vitamin D_3. *Carcinogenesis* **9**, 187–90.

Porter, J.W.G. (1980). The role of milk and milk constituents in the human diet. *International Dairy Federation Bulletin* Document No. 125. Brussels: FIL/IDF.

Puska, P., Iacono, J.M., Nissinen, A., Korhonen, H.J., Vartiainen, E., Pietinen, P., Dougherty, R., Leino, U., Mutanen, M., Moisio, S. & Huttunen, J. (1983). Controlled, randomised trial of the effect of dietary fat on blood pressure. *Lancet* **i**, 1–10.

Recker, R.R. & Heaney, R.P. (1985). The effect of milk supplements on calcium metabolism, bone metabolism and calcium balance. *American Journal of Clinical Nutrition* **41**, 254–63.

Recker, R.R., Bammi, A., Barger-Lux, J. & Heaney, R.P. (1988). Calcium bioavailability from milk products, an imitation milk and calcium carbonate. *American Journal of Clinical Nutrition* **47**, 93–5.

Reed, D., McGee, D., Yano, K. & Hankin, J. (1985). Diet, blood pressure and multicollinearity. *Hypertension* **7**, 405–10.

Resnick, L.M. (1987). Dietary calcium and hypertension. *Journal of Nutrition* **117**, 1806–8.

Resnick, L.M. & Laragh, J.H. (1983). The hypotensive effect of short-term oral calcium loading in essential hypertension. *Clinical Research* **31**, 334A (abstract).

Richard, S.R., Nelson, D.M. & Zuspan, F.P. (1984). Calcium levels in normal and hypertensive pregnant patients. *American Journal of Obstetrics and Gynecology* **149**, 168–71.

Riggs, B.L., Seeman, E., Hohgson, S.F., Taves, D.R. & O'Fallon, W.M. (1982). Effect of the fluoride/calcium regime on vertebral fracture occurrence in postmenopausal osteoporosis. *New England Journal of Medicine* **306**, 446–50.

Robinson, B.F. (1984). Altered calcium handling as a cause of primary hypertension. *Journal of Hypertension* **2**, 453–60.

Sandler, R.B., Slemenda, C.W., La Porte, R.E., Cawley, J.A., Schramm, M.M. & Barresi Kriska, A.M. (1989). Post-menopausal bone density and milk consumption in childhood and adolescence. *American Journal of Clinical Nutrition* **42**, 270–4.

Saudie, E., Grosslight, G.M. & Adena, M.A. (1984). Relation of alcohol and cigarette consumption to blood pressure and serum creatinine levels. *Journal of Chronic Diseases* **37**, 617–23.

Saville, P.D. (1965). Changes in bone mass with age and alcoholism. *Journal of Bone and Joint Surgery* **47A**, 492–9.

Schaafsma, G. (1983). The significance of milk as a source of dietary calcium. *International Dairy Federation Bulletin* Document No. 166. Brussels: FIL/IDF.

Schiff, H. & Schollmeyer, P. (1985). Metabolic consequences of long-term thiazide-based antihypertensive treatment of renal hypertension. *Cardiology* **72** (Suppl.), 54–6.

Seeman, E., Melton, L.J., O'Fallon, W.M. & Riggs, B.L. (1983). Risk factors for spinal osteoporosis in men. *American Journal of Medicine* **75**, 977–83.

Slattery, M.L., Sorenson, A.W. & Ford, M.H. (1988). Dietary calcium intake as a mitigating factor in colon cancer. *American Journal of Epidemiology* **128**, 504–14.

Slovik, D.M., Adams, J.S., Neer, R.M., Holick, M.F. & Potts, J.T. (1981).

Deficient production of 1,25-dihydroxyvitamin D in elderly osteoporotic patients. *New England Journal of Medicine* **305**, 372–4.

Smith, T.M., Kolars, J.C. & Savaiano, D.A. (1985). Absorption of calcium from milk and yoghurt. *American Journal of Clinical Nutrition* **42**, 1197–200.

Sowers, M.R., Wallace, R.B. & Lemke, J.H. (1985). The association of intakes of vitamin D and calcium with blood pressure among women. *American Journal of Clinical Nutrition* **42**, 135–42.

Spencer, H., Kramer, L., Lesniak, M., De Bartolo, M., Norris, C. & Osis, D. (1984). Calcium requirements in humans. *Clinical Orthopaedics* **184**, 270–9.

Stamler, R., Stamler, J., Grimm, R., Gosch, F.C., Elmer, P., Dyer, A., Berman, R., Fishman, J., Van Heel, N., Civinelli, J. & McDonald, A. (1987). Nutritional therapy for high blood pressure. *Journal of the American Medical Association* **257**, 1484–91.

Swales, J.D. (1983). Abnormal ion transport by cell membranes in hypertension. In *Handbook of Hypertension*, Vol. 1, pp. 239–66 [J.I.S. Robertson, editor]. Amsterdam: Elsevier.

Swales, J.D. (1988). Salt saga continued. Salt has only small importance in hypertension. *British Medical Journal* **297**, 307–8.

Tantibhedhyangkul, P. & Hashim, S.A. (1978). Medium-chain triglyceride feeding in premature infants: effects on calcium and magnesium absorption: *Pediatrics* **61**, 537–45.

Various authors (1984). Correspondence. *Lancet* **ii**, 456, 634, 1333–4.

Verlangieri, A.J., Kapeghian, J.C., el-Dean, S. & Bush M. (1985). Fruit and vegetable consumption and cardiovascular mortality. *Medical Hypotheses* **16**, 7–15.

Vinson, J.A., Mazur, T. & Bose, P. (1987). Comparison of different forms of calcium on blood pressure of normotensive young males. *Nutrition Reports International* **36**, 497–505.

Wargovich, M.J., Eng, V.W.S., Newmark, H.L. & Bruce, W.R. (1983). Calcium ameliorates the toxic effect of deoxycholic acid on colonic epithelium. *Carcinogenesis* **4**, 1205–7.

Wasserman, R.H. & Fullmer, C.S. (1983). Calcium transport proteins, calcium absorption and vitamin D. *Annual Reviews of Physiology* **45**, 375–90.

Webster, P.-O. & Dyckner, T. (1987). Magnesium and hypertension. *Journal of the American College of Nutrition* **6**, 321–8.

Weinsier, R.L. & Norris, D. (1985). Recent developments in the etiology and treatment of hypertension: dietary calcium, fat and magnesium. *American Journal of Clinical Nutrition* **42**, 1331–8.

Wright, A., Burstyn, P.G. & Gibney, M.J. (1979). Dietary fibre and blood pressure. *British Medical Journal* **2**, 1541–3.

Yuen, D.E., Draper, H.H. & Trilok, G. (1984). Effect of dietary protein on calcium metabolism in man. *Nutrition Abstracts and Reviews* **54**, 447–59.

Zawanda, E.T. & Brautbar, N. (1985). Calcium therapy of hypertension—has the time come? *Nephron* **41**, 129–31.

4

Zinc Nutrition

Ivor E. Dreosti
Division of Human Nutrition CSIRO, Adelaide, South Australia

INTRODUCTION

Zinc (atomic No. 30, atomic weight 65·38) occurs widely in nature and is found to some extent in most foodstuffs. The human body contains between 1 and 2 g of zinc, which is distributed throughout the tissues and is especially concentrated in the prostate gland and eye membranes, where it occurs at levels around 200 μg/g (Underwood, 1977). Although less concentrated in muscle (30 μg/g) and bone (100 μg/g), the greater mass of these tissues results in most zinc in the body being located in the musculo-skeletal system. However, unlike most other micronutrients, body zinc deposits, including those in the liver (30–70 μg/g) are generally not mobilized to any significant extent during times of nutritional inadequacy, with the result that labile zinc stores are limited and optimal zinc nutriture requires a regular dietary intake of the element (Dreosti, 1982*a*).

Zinc is associated with more than 100 metalloenzymes of widely differing function, in which it is generally found located at the active catalytic site of the molecule (Vallee & Galdes, 1984). Many deficiency symptoms of zinc impoverishment can be related directly to its role in cellular biochemistry, which would include the importance of zinc in the synthesis of the nucleic acids and proteins, the metabolism of carbohydrates and fats, the stabilization of cell membranes and its emerging involvement in immunocompetence and neurophysiology.

The present chapter will review zinc nutrition in general, but will focus particularly on dietary aspects of zinc nutriture and on the detrimental effects zinc impoverishment may have on human health and well-being.

UNITS AND MEASUREMENT OF ZINC

The concentration of zinc in biological tissue is variously expressed as mg/g, ppm or mmol. Factors for their interconversion are given below:

1 mmol = 65·38 mg
1 mg = 0·0153 mmol
1 ppm = 1 mg/kg
1 ppm = 0·0153 mM

In the past, zinc was routinely assayed colorimetrically, following reaction with dithiozone. Nowadays, it is most commonly measured using atomic absorption spectroscopy (AAS), either in the flame mode or with a carbon furnace attachment, which provides a greater level of sensitivity. Recently, use of a high resolution polychromator and wavelength modulation of a continuum light source has led to the development of simultaneous multi-element atomic absorption spectroscopy (SIMAAC). Also, but less widely used are the techniques of inductively coupled plasma optical emission spectrometry (ICP-OE), and inductively coupled plasma mass spectrometry (ICP-MS). Both employ an argon plasma flame to generate ions which are then determined using either optical emission or mass spectrometry (Fell & Lyon 1988; Janghorbani *et al.*, 1988). An alternative technique, thermal ionization mass spectrometry (TIMS) is less widely used as also is X-ray fluorescence spectrometry, although recent modifications involving more powerful synchrotron X-ray sources and scanning at the edge of absorption spectra (XANES) have greatly improved sensitivity (Gordon, 1987). Neutron activation analysis (NAA) and more recently particle-induced X-ray emission (PIXIE) provide useful nuclear analytical techniques, but are limited in their applicability due to the need for a source of a neutron or proton beam (Jones & Pounds, 1987; Janghorbani *et al.*, 1988).

ZINC IN FOODS

Although zinc is widespread in nature, the level at which it occurs and its availability from the diet are variable. Seafood, especially shell-fish, and

TABLE 1

Zinc content of several common natural and processed human foods (Sandstead, 1973; Mertz, 1974; Paul & Southgate, 1978).

Foodstuff	Zinc content (μg/g fresh wt)
Oysters, shell fish	100–1000
Meat (lean)	20–50
Cheese (cheddar-type)	40
Whole-grains, legumes, nuts	10–30
Fish, poultry	10–20
Maize, rice (unpolished)	10–25
Eggs	12
Vegetables, potatoes	2–20
Cows milk	2
Fruits	< 1

meat generally contain in excess of 20 μg zinc/g food (fresh wt) and the zinc from these sources is readily available. With the exception of nuts and legumes, vegetable foods are commonly low in zinc, and the bioavailability of the metal may be reduced due to the presence of substances which bind to zinc and reduce its absorption from the intestine. More will be said about factors which affect zinc bioavailability in the next section. Listed in Table 1 are several of the more common human foodstuffs which have been arranged in decreasing order of their zinc content. Highly relevant to this table is the observation by Mertz (1980) that calculations based on a mean dietary energy density of 2 kcals (8·4 kJ)/g (wet wt) reveal that the average zinc concentration of the constituent foods would have to be about 15 μg/g in order to meet the American Recommended Dietary Intake (RDA) of 15 mg/day (Food and Nutrition Board, 1980). However, only meats, seafoods and certain selected whole grains, nuts and legumes are able to do this (Casey & Hambidge, 1980), while the bulk of food sources, especially the staple foodstuffs, provide an average rather less than 5 μg zinc/g. Not surprisingly, these observations, together with evidence of low zinc intakes from dietary surveys and some clinical evidence of suboptimal zinc status in humans has led to speculation that marginal zinc deficiencies in the human population may be more widespread than is generally recognized. These issues will be discussed in greater detail later in this paper.

As with most micronutrients, food processing can have a significant effect on the final zinc content of the prepared food. In particular, since most of the zinc in grains and cereals is found in the outer layers of the seed, refinement of the flour to low extraction rates results in large losses (75%) of zinc (Schroeder, 1967). Cooking foods in water rich in zinc from galvanized plumbing may increase the zinc content of foods, but on the other hand, considerable amounts of zinc can be lost into cooking water when it is discarded (Mertz, 1974).

BIOAVAILABILITY OF ZINC

A variety of factors in the diet seem able to alter the efficacy of absorption of zinc from the intestine. Most commonly, metal chelating ligands in the gut lumen tend to decrease absorption, but some act oppositely. Competition by other minerals for carriers or uptake sites may sometimes occur and would depress bioavailability. The subject has been widely studied, but the actual relevance of the interactions to human nutrition remains uncertain. Most studies on animals models have involved concentrations of these factors in the food at levels highly unlikely to occur naturally in the human diet, and in many cases factors are added to the diet as purified chemicals, and not in the form in which they occur naturally in foodstuffs.

Nevertheless, several compounds seem at least potentially capable of promoting or depressing zinc absorption in humans and need to be considered. Foremost as a promoter must be the actual zinc intake in the diet, as the capacity for intestinal uptake to improve significantly when zinc intakes are low is now well established in man (King, 1986; King & Turnlund, 1989). Several low-molecular-mass ligands; notably citrate and picolinate have been proposed but not satisfactorily demonstrated to enhance zinc bioavailability (Sandström & Lönnerdal, 1989).

Antagonists of zinc absorption occur rather more widely in food, and include the controversial iron/zinc interaction, metal binding by insoluble protein, and interference by phytate and insoluble non-starch polysaccharides. With respect to iron, several workers have reported that absorption of zinc from the intestine is reduced by the presence of high intakes of iron (Aggett et al., 1983; Solomons, 1988), and the suggestion has been made that when more than 25 mg of total ions are involved and the molar ratio of iron:zinc exceeds 2:1, zinc absorption may be reduced (Solomons, 1986). Not surprisingly, since iron supplementation occurs routinely during pregnancy and in infant formula, considerable attention has recently been focused in this area. However, the precise extent of the problem in humans has not been established, and several workers are of the opinion that while the effect may be real with respect to a single oral dose of the metals unaccompanied by food, moderate iron supplementation is unlikely to depress zinc availability when taken at mealtimes (Flanagan & Valberg, 1988).

Dietary protein has attracted attention because of the high affinity zinc displays to bind to undigested protein and to become largely insoluble at the physiological pH of the small intestine (Sandström & Lönnerdal, 1989). Thus it has been speculated that zinc may be less available to infants from cows milk than from breast milk because of the high levels of zinc bound to casein (Lönnerdal *et al.*, 1980), and that lower absorption of the metal from soybean-based foods may arise from a lower intestinal digestion of soy-protein than meat protein (Sandström & Lönnerdal, 1989). Total protein intake also seems to play a role with diets providing more than 100 g of protein/day, apparently enhancing intestinal uptake of zinc (Greger & Snedeker, 1980).

Probably of most practical dietary significance is the effect of plant fibre and other associated cell wall constituents (e.g. phytate) on mineral bioavailability. Despite the many positive benefits associated with an increased intake of dietary fibre, concern exists that the practice may lead to reduced bioavailability of some essential minerals, especially if high fibre levels occur in diets providing only marginal intakes of the elements concerned. This concern may be especially relevant to the developing countries where diets tend to include higher levels of plant fibre, and calcareous supplements, which aggravate phytate-mineral binding, are often made during cooking (Mills, 1989). Several studies, both *in vivo* and *in vitro* have pointed to reduced bioavailability of zinc (Sandström & Lönnerdal, 1989) due primarily to binding with the various constituents of dietary fibre, although entrapment of zinc ions within the fibre matrix, together with decreased transit time through the gut may also contribute to reduced absorption. Most investigations on animals and humans indicate significantly depressed bioavailability of zinc by increased intakes of bran, cellulose, hemicellulose and phytate (inositol hexaphosphate). Binding of zinc to phytate is much stronger than to cellulose and the effect of bran is much reduced if phytate levels are reduced by prior acid washing or by the action of phytase enzymes during leavening. Particularly high levels of phytate are found in seeds where it serves as a phosphate reserve for the seedling, which accounts for the special emphasis on cereals in many bioavailability studies. Based on animals studies, a molar ratio of phytate: zinc in the diet greater than 12–15:1 has been proposed to adversely affect zinc availability, although recent findings with humans do not support this view at normal dietary zinc intakes (Smith *et al.*, 1983). The phytate/zinc interaction is greatly enhanced by elevated intakes of calcium, although calcium on its own has no effect on zinc uptake (Dawson-Hughes *et al.*, 1986).

In summary, the absorption of zinc from the small intestine can be influenced by dietary factors to rise as high as 60% or to fall to less than 10%. From the average diet, bioavailability is around 25–30%. Many of the dietary constituents reported to affect the efficiency of absorption appear to be of more theoretical than practical significance and are of limited concern in actual human nutrition. Nevertheless, the extent to which plant fibre and phytate interfere with zinc absorption remains unresolved, and signals caution when diets very high in natural fibre or supplemented with processed fibre are consumed.

ZINC REQUIREMENTS AND THE RECOMMENDED DIETARY ALLOWANCE

The dietary requirement for zinc in humans has been estimated from balance studies and from investigations with stable and radioactive isotopes. Most balance studies have indicated that a dietary intake of 6–12 mg of zinc/day will maintain zinc equilibrium in healthy adults (Halsted *et al.*, 1974), although very recent data obtained with young men fed on a low zinc intake for several weeks (King & Turnlund, 1989) suggests that it may be possible for human adults to adapt to be in zinc equilibrium on zinc intakes as low as 5·5 mg/day. In the past, radioisotope data have suggested a body zinc turnover rate of about 6 mg/day (Halsted *et al.*, 1974), while factorial estimates of the zinc requirement, which represent the sum of obligatory losses on an essentially zinc-free diet, have also been of this order, and have set the requirement at around 6 mg/day (WHO, 1973). These latter estimates are supported by data from balance studies with patients on total parenteral nutrition (TPN) which estimate the daily infusion rate required for an adult at about 2 mg zinc/day (Phillips, 1982), and from zinc turnover rates of 2·7 mg/day (King & Turnlund, 1989) which, assuming about 30% availability of zinc from food, provides a similar estimate of the dietary zinc requirement as the other methods.

Of the 42 countries and organizations with Recommended Dietary Allowances (RDAs) only 10 have included recommendations for zinc with a mean adult value of 13·2 mg/day (Table 2).

TABLE 2
Recommended dietary allowance for zinc (mg/day) from several countries

Group	Australia[a]	Canada[b]	USA[b]	USSR[b]	WHO[b]
		Country			
Children	4·5–12	5–12	10–15	—	5–9
Women	12	10	15	—	7
Men	12	10	15	10–15	7
Pregnancy	+4	+3	+5	—	+3
Lactation	+6	+7	+10	—	+11

[a] Dreosti (1982[b]).
[b] Truswell & Chambers (1983).

Most recommendations have been based on an estimated zinc requirement of around 10 mg/day together with allowances to cover differences in bioavailability of zinc from various foods, and to accommodate the variance in zinc metabolism and utilization of most individuals within the community. Additional intakes are recommended to cover the demands of growth, pregnancy and lactation, which generally reflect the amount of zinc present in the new tissue, together with consideration of bioavailability and individual variation. It is of particular interest that the Australian advisory group on RDAs has recently recommended that they reduce their adult RDA from 12–16 mg of zinc/day to 12 mg/day, on account of the accumulating evidence of improved absorptive efficiency of zinc and reduced endogenous excretion at lower dietary intakes (King & Turnland, 1989), and since many communities within Australia and elsewhere in the world consume diets providing less zinc than many current RDAs with no apparent biochemical or clinical signs of zinc deficiency.

ZINC INTAKES AROUND THE WORLD

Daily intakes of zinc from diets around the world tend to be remarkably similar, ranging between about 5 and 20 mg/day with a mean consumption of the order of 10–12 mg/day. The main difference in intake lies in the high proportion of zinc obtained from animal protein sources, approximately 70% in industrialized countries from which about 30% could be expected to be absorbed, to the predominantly vegetable-based diets in many Third World countries, from which probably only about 10–20% of zinc is

TABLE 3
Dietary zinc intakes for adults from countries around the world

Country	Zinc intake (mg/day)	Reference
Australia	Women 10·9	
	Men 12·3	Baghurst et al. (1987)
Belgium	15·0	Buchet et al. (1983)
Brazil	7·3	Shrimpton (1984)
China (Linxian)	12·0	Thurnham et al. (1985)
Egypt	20·0	FAO (1984)
Finland	16·0	Varo & Kovistoinen (1980)
Holland	14·0	Van Dokkum et al. (1989)
India	16·1	Soman et al. (1969)
Sweden	9·0	Slorach et al. (1983)
Tokelau Islands	4·5	McKenzie et al. (1978)
UK	9·0	Hazell (1985)
UK	9·0	Lewis & Buss (1988)
USA	8.5–13.0	Sandstead (1973)
USA	Adolescent males 18·0	Gartrell et al. (1985)
USA	Adolescent males 16·0	Pennington et al. (1986)
Western Countries	10·0–12·0	King & Turnlund (1989)

available (Sandström, 1989). Typical zinc intakes for adults from several Western and some Third World countries are shown in Table 3.

Not surprisingly, the fact that zinc intakes in many countries habitually fall below the USA RDA has led to widespread speculation that sub-optimal zinc nutriture occurs more frequently in humans that is generally recognized, especially in groups whose increased requirement (children, pregnant women, convalescing patients) or small food intake (dieters, the elderly or the malnourished), renders them particularly vulnerable to a low level of zinc in their customary food sources (Dreosti, 1982a).

ZINC DEFICIENCY IN HUMANS

Nutritional

Although zinc deficiency in livestock had been established as a problem for several decades, it was not considered likely to occur in humans until it was demonstrated clinically in areas of Iran and Egypt (Prasad et al., 1961). Thereafter, it was recognized that inadequate zinc nutriture could exist in developing countries, and it was therefore not unexpected when zinc deficiency was noted in applicants for the Iranian Army (Halsted et al., 1972), and low zinc intakes were observed in typical diets in Turkey

(Cavdar *et al.*, 1977) and elsewhere in the Third World (Halsted *et al.*, 1974). Indeed, it has even been suggested that some of the symptoms associated with protein–energy malnutrition may arise from an accompanying zinc deficit (Golden & Golden, 1979) and from free radical-related damage associated with reduced levels of zinc and other antioxidant trace minerals (Golden & Ramdath, 1987).

Predictably, such considerations led nutritionists to question whether diets in Western countries might not also be suboptimal. Positive evidence to this effect was forthcoming in relation to delayed wound healing (Pories *et al.*, 1967), taste disorders (Henkin, 1971), and depressed growth rates in children (Hambidge *et al.*, 1972) in the USA, which drew attention to the likely existence of suboptimal zinc nutriture in North America (Mertz, 1984; Halsted, 1977). Since then, low zinc intakes have indeed been reported in the USA, the UK, Canada and Sweden (Dreosti, 1982*a*; Hambidge, 1989). Of particular interest have been the most recent reports of reduced growth rates associated with low zinc intakes in children in Beijing, China (Chen *et al.*, 1985) and Guelph, Canada (Smit-Vanderkooy & Gibson, 1987), together with indications that growth was improved by zinc supplementation. Nevertheless, while frank dietary zinc deficiency probably does exist to some extent as a nutritional problem in many countries, for most adults in the Western world, the risk of exposure to an outright zinc deficiency is relatively small. The same cannot, however, be said of a 'conditioned' zinc deficiency which may arise in the presence of an apparently adequate supply of the element, owing to modifications in its availability from the diet, or to an increased requirement following some physiological change. Various factors have been identified as conditioning agents, some of which occur naturally, but others arise as a consequence of modern technology or life-style variables (Table 4).

Special mention needs to be made of several particular groups in which zinc deficiency has emerged as a serious nutritional problem.

Acrodermatitis enteropathica
This is an inherited autosomal recessive disease, exhibiting all the symptoms of severe zinc deficiency, including death. The disease appears to arise due to a block in the absorption of zinc from the intestine, and is overcome therapeutically by high levels of zinc supplementation in the diet.

Premature infants
During the last two months of pregnancy, the human foetus accumulates

TABLE 4
Factors responsible for conditioned zinc deficiencies in man

Conditioning factor	*Mechanism of action*
Food processing	Loss or reduced availability of zinc
Dietary constituents	Antagonism between elements, complex formation.
Genetic disorders (*Acrodermatitis enteropathica*)	Impaired absorption of zinc
Medications (chelating agents, laxatives) drugs and alcohol	Reduced absorption and/or increased excretion of zinc
Disease (infection, parasitic infestation; intestinal, liver and renal disorders)	Redistribution of zinc within body compartments, decreased absorption, increased excretion and loss
Trauma (burns, haemorrhage and contusions)	Redistribution of zinc within body compartments, increased excretion and loss
Total parenteral nutrition	Inadequate zinc in infusion fluid
Dialysis	Excessive removal of zinc from blood.
Growth, pregnancy and lactation	Increased anabolic demand

about one-half of its total body zinc (Widdowson *et al.*, 1962) at a daily retention of approximately 50 μg of zinc/kg of foetal body weight (Walravens, 1980). Infants born 10–12 weeks prematurely are therefore severely compromised with respect to body zinc stores and are acutely dependent upon an external supply of the metal to provide their requirement for growth.

The predicament of the premature infant in meeting these demands is aggravated by elevated urinary zinc losses and an attendant negative zinc balance (Dauncey *et al.*, 1977). Premature infants receiving total parenteral nutrition (TPN) are especially vulnerable, due to low levels of zinc in some infusion fluids and because of a further sharp rise in urinary excretion rates (James & MacMahon, 1976; Suita *et al.*, 1984), which are generally attributed to an accompanying aminoaciduria and loss of amino acid-bound metals (James & MacMahon, 1976; Walravens, 1980).

Recent evidence suggests that the retention of zinc is directly related to the TPN intake (James *et al.*, 1979; Zlotkin & Buchanan, 1983), and estimates of the daily requirement of TPN-fed premature infants range from 30 to 500 μg/kg (James & MacMahon, 1976; American Academy of

Pediatrics, 1978; American Medical Association, 1979; James *et al.*, 1979; Zlotkin & Buchanan, 1983; Friel *et al.*, 1984), although the latest reports favour intakes around 400 µg of zinc/kg per day, which provide retention rates similar to those that occur *in utero* (Zlotkin & Buchanan, 1983).

RATE OF ONSET OF ZINC DEFICIENCY IN ANIMALS AND MAN

Early observations by Hurley *et al.* (1971) showed that relatively short periods (3–4 days) of zinc deficiency in pregnant rats rapidly affected the growth and development of the foetus. Also, growth ceases within a few days after limiting zinc intake in weanling rats (Swenerton & Hurley, 1968). The speed with which these effects occur points to the rapid onset of a physiological zinc deficiency and limited mobilization of body zinc depots—a view confirmed by studies (Dreosti *et al.*, 1968; Hurley *et al.*, 1980) which demonstrated a 40–50% decrease in plasma zinc levels in rats within one day of receiving a zinc-deficient diet. The findings are especially noteworthy in light of the fact that in serum, zinc occurs both loosely bound to albumin (60–70%) and tightly bound to α_2-macroglobulin (30–40%), with the result that most of the 50% fall in plasma zinc levels immediately following dietary deprivation occurs in the albumin-bound transport zinc fraction, leaving mainly tightly bound zinc in the plasma, which is largely unavailable for use by body tissues (Dreosti, 1982*a*).

With humans, the rapid onset of zinc deficiency following severe dietary restriction was first demonstrated in 1981 by Gordon *et al.* (1982) which indicates that in man, as in animals, a continuing intake of zinc is necessary in order to preserve a satisfactory level of the metal in plasma. It should be noted that starvation *per se* does not reduce the plasma zinc level, on the contrary due to the accompanying release of zinc arising from tissue catabolism, plasma zinc levels may rise (Dreosti *et al.*, 1985). Many manifestations of zinc deficiency are especially pronounced during periods of anabolism, when the overall food intake is adequate, but the zinc content is insufficient.

DIAGNOSIS OF ZINC DEFICIENCY

The reliability of diagnostic procedures used for the identification of zinc deficiency in man or animal has recently been perceptively reviewed by

Golden (1989), who clearly distinguishes 'Type 1' nutrients for which there is a significant body reserve and for which a deficiency leads to reduced tissue levels, from those he classes as 'Type 2', for which reserves are limited and deficiency results in cessation of growth without an accompanying loss in tissue nutrient levels. Zinc is a 'Type 2' nutrient, which itself makes the diagnosis of deficiency difficult, even without the complicating issue of the exceptionally wide involvement the metal has in most major physiological processes. Because 'Type 2' nutrients are tightly held in tissues, they tend not to be released except during tissue mobilization, which means that any situation leading to catabolism is likely to result in increased urinary zinc excretion and a negative zinc balance. Thus, normal plasma zinc levels may occur during periods of tissue wastage accompanying general starvation due to the release of bound body zinc, although the dietary zinc intake may be inadequate Golden (1989). Conversely, low plasma zinc levels are sometimes found in circumstances when the dietary intake is sufficient, due to the redistribution of zinc to other tissues as occurs during infection, trauma, pregnancy and as a result of certain medications (Dreosti, 1981).

Without doubt, the best indicator of a dietary zinc deficiency is a physiological response to zinc supplementation, for example, growth. Such therapeutic trials are however not always possible and may be complicated by secondary deficits of the 'Type 2' nutrients induced in the first place by a primary zinc deficiency (Golden, 1989). For laboratory diagnosis, use is widely made of the zinc levels in a variety of tissues or the functional activity of several zinc–containing metalloenzymes and metalloproteins (Dreosti, 1981). Plasma zinc, for all its shortcomings, can be of some value as an indicator of the current zinc status, as also is urinary zinc excretion, provided that in both cases, no complicating physiological or pathological factors are present. Zinc levels in blood cells may also be used with some effectiveness, as well as the activities of the zinc metalloenzymes serum alkaline phosphatase, pancreatic carboxypeptidase and liver alcohol dehydrogenase, the first being more readily available and the last two more sensitive (Casey & Hambidge, 1980). Hair zinc levels are frequently used in survey-type studies because of the ease with which samples may be collected and stored. Although well correlated to the past zinc status under laboratory conditions, hair zinc levels in free-living humans are so affected by contamination and cosmetic leaching of the element, that their interpretation should be treated with great caution (Buckley & Dreosti, 1984). Some limited use has been made of other body fluids and tissues including fingernails, saliva and sweat, but the questionable reliability of these indices and the risk of contamination render them unsuitable for widespread application.

Metallothionein, an intracellular zinc-binding protein, is widely considered to act as a temporary zinc buffer pool and possibly also to be involved in zinc transport. Its synthesis is induced by the presence of increased levels of zinc, with the result that some workers believe that if there is zinc bound to metallothionein-1 in the plasma, it is *prima facie* evidence that a zinc deficiency is unlikely (Bremner & Morrison, 1988; Golden, 1989). Even more indicative are metallothionein-1 levels in erythrocytes, which are sensitive to dietary zinc intakes but are not affected by endotoxins or other stresses which affect plasma zinc levels (Golden, 1989).

While the use of red cell metallothionein levels coupled with measurements of plasma zinc may well offer the best potential method for the diagnosis of zinc deficiency in the future, at present, plasma zinc levels alone provide a useful assessment of current zinc status, especially in relation to growing cells and the foetus whose only source of additional zinc must be from plasma (Hurley, 1981).

SYMPTOMS OF ZINC DEFICIENCY

The symptoms of zinc deficiency depend largely on the severity of the deficit, although some aspects of the syndrome are common to all stages of the condition. Severe zinc deficiency occurs least commonly and is usually associated with unusual circumstances (e.g. genetic disease or iatrogenically induced), which lead to a syndrome (Table 5) similar to that seen in experimental animals maintained on diets from which zinc has been almost totally removed by vigorous chemical extraction. In humans, severe zinc deficiency is always associated with untreated acrodermatitis enteropathica—an inherited defect in zinc absorption, as well as with TPN if the infusion fluid contains insufficient zinc. In addition, severe gastrointestinal/liver disease may reduce zinc absorption from the gut and its retention in the body sufficiently to precipitate the advanced syndrome (Aggett, 1989). It is also often found to accompany protein-energy malnutrition (Golden & Golden, 1981) and sometimes follows chelation therapy for Wilson's disease (Klinberg *et al.*, 1976) and treatment for thalassaemia major (Ridley, 1982).

Moderate zinc deficiency has been reported in association with malab-

TABLE 5
Reported symptoms of zinc deficiency in humans

Degree of deficiency	Symptoms
Mild	Impaired growth velocity Reduced muscle growth Diminished food intake Decreased activity of thymulin Decline in sperm count Disordered taste sensation Impaired immunocompetence, especially delayed-type hypersensitivity
Moderate	Growth retardation Male hypogonadism and impotence Depressed appetite Lethargy Thickened skin Impaired cellular immunity Night blindness Increased level of blood ammonia
Severe	Neuropsychiatric manifestations—mood lability, lethargy, memory loss, tremor, ataxia Eye abnormalities—impaired central vision, photophobia, corneal clouding and ulceration Anorexia, taste dysfunction Gastrointestinal disturbances—diarrhoea, villar atrophy Skin disorders—dermatitis around nostrils, mouth, chin, knees, elbows, heels and armpits, which may become exudative and eventually keratosed Hair is often hypopigmented or reddish in colour and may be accompanied by alopecia. Growth retardation—failure to thrive, and impaired weight gain in children. Hypogonadism in adults Poor wound healing. Birth defects. Reduced immunocompetence—thymic hypoplasia, diminished T cell, function and cellular immunity.

(Golden and Golden, 1981; Dardenne *et al.*, 1988; Aggett, 1989; Hambidge, 1989).

sorption syndrome, alcoholic liver disease, chronic renal disease, severe veganism and several chronically debilitated conditions (Prasad, 1988). Mild zinc deficiency in humans occurs sporadically in association with a low dietary zinc intake and, in many cases with a raised physiological zinc requirement, for example in growing infants and children and during convalescence and pregnancy/lactation (Prasad, 1988; Hambidge, 1989).

The symptoms associated with the full spectrum of zinc deficiency reflect the progressive sensitivity of the various zinc-dependent systems and zinc metalloenzymes, to zinc impoverishment. Foremost of all symptoms is retarded growth, a manifestation of zinc deficiency which, where applicable, must rate as the cardinal consequence of zinc insufficiency.

Ranked thereafter (Table 5) are a range of deficiency symptoms, some identifiable in relation to a particular biochemical function of zinc in the body, while others are less definable and overlap widely throughout the three arbitrary levels used to describe the extent of zinc deficiency in humans.

BIOCHEMISTRY OF ZINC

In addition to the well-recognized role of zinc as a prosthetic group in the zinc metalloenzymes, of which between 100 and 200 have been described and which collectively cover all major classes of enzyme activity (Vallee & Galdes, 1984), zinc functions also to regulate the activity of many non-metalloenzymes as well as being involved in the synthesis of proteins and the nucleic acids, and in the stabilization of biological macromolecules, polyribosomes and other cellular membranes (Clegg et al., 1989). Underlying many of these biochemical activities lies the metal's highly concentrated electrostatic charge, comparatively small ionic size and large ionization potential (Williams, 1989). Also, it is relatively easily available from the environment, and it occurs within the cell mainly in the cytoplasm. Because of its highly localized charge and electron affinity zinc is a very effective attacking group especially in a chemically non-selective, but physically constrained, manner. Its association with particular proteins ranging from mobile helical molecules (e.g. insulin), β-pleated sheet proteins (e.g. carbonic anhydrase, superoxide dismutase) and mixed proteins (e.g. carboxypeptidase, alcohol dehydrogenase), to random structures (e.g. metallothionein, transcription factor III A), confer upon the metalloprotein particular enzymic and kinetic characteristics (Williams, 1989).

In short, it can be said of zinc that it is involved enzymically in every major catalytic category. It is essential for immunocompetence and for membrane stability. It is involved in receptor modulation, in several neuroendocrine systems and plays a pivotal role in many aspects of DNA replication, transcription and translation through its association with the polymerase enzymes, certain transcription and translation factors, and because of its contribution to the structural integrity of the DNA and RNA macromolecules (Dreosti, 1984).

The recent recognition that zinc acts as a modulator substance for receptor affinity and in cell signalling now implicates the metal in the fine control of many metabolic processes (Bunce, 1989) and in neurotransmitter recognition and synaptic transmission (Dreosti, 1989). In relation to transcription, the proposed role of zinc in gene masking and unmasking (Chesters, 1978) has now been extended to include a possible involvement in mitogenic signalling through the intracellular agent diadenosine tetraphosphate (Ap4A) a putative inducer of cell division (Gummt *et al.*, 1986).

SPECIAL ROLES OF ZINC

Neurobiology and behaviour

Zinc is involved both in brain development and in brain function. In animals, maternal zinc deficiency during the critical period of embryonic organogenesis results in severe congenital malformation of the central nervous system which includes defects associated with incomplete closure of the neural tube (e.g. anencephalus, exencephalus and spina bifida) and later, distension of the ventricles, all of which are irreversible and probably occur because of disturbed cell division and cell death (Hurley & Shrader, 1972; Dreosti *et al.*, 1985).

Zinc impoverishment later in pregnancy and early postnatally, or even to some extent in adult animals, mainly affects brain function, which no doubt reflects a measure of neuronal dysmorphogenesis as well as neurophysiological dysfunctions. The accompanying behavioural abnormalities generally respond well to zinc repletion and are, to some extent reversible (Halas, 1983; Dreosti, 1989*a*). Overall, the neurochemical role of zinc in the central nervous system is complex and not well understood. The element is clearly involved in a number of zinc-containing brain

TABLE 6
Neural tube defects associated with zinc deficiency in humans

Defect	Country	Reference
Anencephalus	Middle East	Damaynov & Dutz (1971)
		Sever & Emanuel (1973)
	Turkey	Cavdar *et al.* (1980)
	USA	Stewart *et al.* (1981)
	UK	Soltan & Jenkins (1982)
Spina bifida	West Germany	Bergmann *et al.* (1980)
Myelomeningocoele	Sweden	Jameson (1976)

enzymes, with the enkephalins, in neuronal receptor binding of neurotransmitter substances and in synaptic activity (Dreosti, 1989*a*).

Generally, zinc in the brain is well protected and is not easily lost from neural tissue even under conditions of depletion leading to marked loss of zinc from other organs (Kasarskis, 1984; Wensink *et al.*, 1987). Nevertheless, postnatal and adult zinc restriction is widely reported to be associated with substantial behavioural anomalies in animals, most notably with reduced learning capacity and a marked lack of emotional control (Halas, 1983). However, the contribution made to these psychological disturbances by anorexia and the resulting energy restriction is not clear and is receiving further attention (Eberhardt & Halas, 1987).

Much attention has recently been paid to the role of zinc in the hippocampus, because of the above-average levels of the metal in the hippocampal mossy fibre pathway and because of the involvement of this brain region in emotional control and in memory processing (Crawford, 1983; Dreosti, 1983). However, it should be recognized that the metal occurs at significant levels in all brain cells and that its neurochemical role in the hippocampus probably applies more widely to include other regions of the central nervous system as well.

With humans, unlike with animals, a direct causal relationship has not yet been established between zinc deficiency and brain dysmorphogenesis and dysfunction. Nevertheless, current evidence suggests that the developing human foetus is no less vulnerable to zinc depletion than are the offspring from other species, and tentative associations have been drawn by some workers between several neural tube defects in children and gestational zinc deficiency (Table 6), as well as the identification of a

TABLE 7
Behavioural deficits associated with suspected zinc deficiency in humans

Behaviour	Cause of zinc deficiency	Reference
Mental lethargy	Dietary	Prasad *et al.* (1961)
Jitteriness, impaired concentration, depression, mood lability	Iatrogenically induced in infants and adults	Henkin *et al.* (1975) Sivasubramanian & Henkin (1978)
	Acrodermatitis enteropathica	Walravens *et al.* (1978)
Taste dysfunction, anorexia	Liver cirrhosis, nephrotic syndrome, alcoholism	Lindeman *et al.* (1978)

number of behavioural deficits in children and adults accompanying situations of apparent zinc impoverishment (Table 7).

Immunocompetence

Zinc is essential for the normal development and maintenance of immune function, and when deficient, results in a profound state of acquired immunodeficiency (Good, 1989), which may be prolonged even with repletion (Beach *et al.*, 1982). The condition is characterized by depressed T-cell mediated immunity and underdevelopment of the thymus gland. Much of the effect possibly relates to a reduced number of available leukocytes, although diminished levels of interleukin-2 and less T-lymphocyte proliferation may also be important (Fraker *et al.*, 1986).

Recently increasing attention has been drawn to the role of thymulin, a putative peptide hormone of thymic origin, which requires zinc for functional activity and appears to be involved in the production of inter-leukin-2 (Bach *et al.*, 1988; Dardenne *et al.*, 1988).

In several studies with zinc deficient children suffering from nephrotic syndrome, and subjects with sickle-cell anaemia or voluntary restricted zinc intake, all of whom had reduced zinc status, thymulin levels were significantly lowered, but responded to zinc supplementation *in vivo* or to zinc activation *in vitro*. Current data suggests that zinc may be required to render thymulin biologically active which may in part explain the depressed immune function which accompanies zinc depletion (Dardenne *et al.*, 1988).

Fertility and teratology

Severe zinc deficiency in animals affects both males and females in relation to fertility. In males, spermatogenesis is markedly reduced and libido is correspondingly diminished, a finding reported also with humans (Bunce, 1989). In female animals, severe zinc deficiency leads to disruption of the oestrus cycle and lack of mating (Keen & Hurley, 1989).

When imposed during gestation, zinc deficiency may prejudice pregnancy outcome in several ways. In rats, gestational zinc impoverishment of the preimplantation embryo leads to lack of normal development at the morula stage, and to fragmentation and necrosis of the conceptus (Hurley & Shrader, 1975). Zinc restriction later in pregnancy results in birth defects of various levels of severity, and in growth retardation (Dreosti, 1982*a*) as well as in behavioural anomalies in the surviving offspring (Halas, 1983).

With humans, the demonstration of adverse pregnancy outcome associated with maternal zinc impoverishment is less clear, although sufficient circumstantial evidence has been reported relating to reduced birth weight and to congenital anomalies to suggest that the human foetus is no less reliant on maternal zinc supplies than are other species (Dreosti, 1982*a*). This realization, together with the relatively poor dietary zinc intake of many pregnant women has stimulated considerable debate concerning the value of zinc supplementation during pregnancy as well as the possible disadvantages which may accompany high intakes of iron and folate by pregnant women leading to an attendant risk of diminished zinc bioavailability. The topic is well reviewed by Solomons (1988) and Keen & Hurley (1989).

As stated earlier, the biochemical lesion underlying zinc deficiency related teratogenesis has not been identified. The importance of zinc for DNA synthesis and cell division (Chesters, 1989; Clegg *et al.*, 1989) cannot be overlooked, but equally the recent evidence (Record *et al.*, 1985) of severe cell death associated with actively proliferating cells in zinc deficient rat foetuses has highlighted the metal's importance for membrane stability and its possible involvement as a cellular antioxidant (Dreosti, 1987, 1989*b*).

In animals, zinc deficiency towards the end of pregnancy results in delayed and prolonged labour, excessive bleeding and poor care of the newborn (Apgar, 1972; Keen & Hurley, 1989). Some analogous effects have been reported by several workers in women of apparently poor zinc status (Jameson, 1976; McMichael *et al.*, 1982). The reader is referred to the review by Keen & Hurley, (1989).

Postnatal effects of impaired zinc status during gestation in animals include behavioural defects (Halas, 1983; Golub *et al.*, 1985), retarded skeletal development, and defective immunocompetence (Haynes *et al.*, 1985), several of which symptoms have been noted to some extent in zinc-deficient children (Keen & Hurley, 1989).

Zinc as an antioxidant

The importance of antioxidants in human health is now widely recognized, as also is the role played by oxygen-derived free radicals in many degenerative diseases and in aging (Cross *et al.*, 1987). Much attention has accordingly focused on those micronutrients which act to reduce free radical damage either as primary antioxidants concerned with diminishing the free radical flux (e.g. manganese, copper and zinc in superoxide dismutase; selenium in glutathione peroxidase; iron in catalase) or as secondary antioxidants which function as free radical scavengers (vitamins A, C, E and β-carotene) (Dreosti, 1988).

As a prosthetic group of superoxide dismutase, zinc functions clearly as a primary antioxidant, a role it also fulfils by protecting vulnerable sulphydryl groups against oxidation, and by displacing loosely bound iron from sites on membranes and macromolecules where, by virtue of its redox capacity, iron may catalyse production of the highly destructive hydroxyl radical from less reactive superoxide (Dreosti, 1989*b*; Willson, 1989).

Not to be overlooked, however, is the possible role zinc may play as a secondary antioxidant due to its capacity to induce the synthesis of zinc-metallothionein which, by virtue of its many sulphydryl groups, acts effectively as a free radical scavenging agent (Dreosti, 1989). Although much of the antioxidant activity attributed to zinc is circumstantial, experimental evidence of increased lipoperoxidation in zinc-deficient rats (Dreosti & Partick, 1987) and protection by zinc against the lethal effects of X-irradiation in mice (Floersheim & Floersheim, 1986) point suggestively to an important antioxidant function of the element along with its many other biological roles.

Generally, zinc appears to be critical in the cell to protect labile sulphydryl groups on macromolecular structures, especially at the time of cell division when it acts both to defend the cell against decompartmentalized iron and also to stimulate mitosis (Willson, 1989). Much of the control of the intracellular zinc level is attributed to the plasma membrane, and to the associated enzyme protein kinase C which acts in the signal transduction of a number of substances affecting cellular function and proliferation, and which binds zinc. Also relevant is the finding that several regulatory proteins associated with gene expression also bind zinc (Willson, 1989). Both classes of compound are now known to contain zinc —cysteine or zinc–histidine domains called 'zinc fingers' which appear to play a central role in enzyme activation and DNA binding by transcription factors (Willson, 1989). The importance of zinc in all these compounds arises because, unlike copper or iron, zinc lacks redox chemistry and may therefore be used in situations in the cell where redox ions might lead to damaging radical production (Klug & Rhodes, 1987).

Therapeutic roles for zinc
Putative therapeutic roles for zinc have been exhaustively reviewed by Solomons *et al.* (1989) who stress that zinc is both a nutrient and a drug, and that while beneficial effects will invariably accompany treatment with zinc of zinc deficiency-related symptoms, the separate value of zinc therapy for conditions not related to depressed zinc status is less clear and has recently become the focus of considerable attention in medical circles. Of the 26 illnesses or conditions for which oral zinc has been used therapeutically, Solomons *et al.* (1989) conclude that the treatment appears to have some merit in relation to decoppering in Wilson's disease, in acne, and with peptic ulcers. Less certain is its role in the treatment of genital herpes, the common cold, infertility, hepatic encephalopathy and some dermatological conditions, for which there is only limited positive evidence. For the remainder, zinc behaves little better than a placebo and its use for conditions such as primary biliary cirrhosis, rheumatoid arthritis, cutaneous leg ulcers, impaired wound healing not associated with poor zinc status, chronic bacterial prostatitis etc. would appear to be ineffective (Solomons *et al.*, 1989).

ZINC TOXICITY

Generally, zinc is relatively non-toxic and non-cumulative (Dreosti, 1982*b*). Fatal zinc poisoning is rare and usually arises accidentally from ingestion of gram quantities of zinc or zinc salts, with accompanying nausea, vomiting, fever and damage to the kidneys and pancreas (Fox, 1989). Antidotal treatment of zinc toxicity involves increased urinary zinc loss following parenteral administration of chelating agents which range in effectiveness from EDTA, DTPA and CDTA through D-penicillamine, l-cysteine, sodium salicylate to glutathione and diethyldithiocarbonate (Domingo *et al.*, 1988; Llobet *et al.*, 1988).

Lower intakes of zinc (between 100 and 500 mg) may cause gastric disturbances, nausea and dizziness. Indeed weak solutions of zinc salts are widely used effectively as an emetic. Prolonged intake of sub-acute levels of zinc excess disturb several physiological functions, most notably the absorption of copper, leading to copper-responsive anaemia (Sandstead, 1982; Festa, 1985; Fox, 1989). Other reported effects include decreased levels of plasma high-density lipoprotein cholesterol, impaired *in vitro* indices of immunocompetence and adverse pregnancy outcome (Chandra, 1984; Fox, 1989). The FAO/WHO (1982) maximum tolerated zinc intake for adults is of the order of 70 mg per day, but this may be above the level at which copper absorption is disturbed (Fox, 1989).

CONCLUSIONS

The importance with which zinc is regarded in human nutrition is well reflected in the prominent position it commands in the research literature relative to other microelements. Contributing to this intense interest must be three aspects of zinc nutriture which distinguish it from most other mineral elements. Firstly, zinc is widely involved in almost every aspect of physiological function, with the result that a deficiency of the element leads to a far more complex syndrome than is associated with deficits of most other micronutrients. Secondly, the supply of zinc in the average human diet does not appear to afford a large margin of safety over the requirement, especially if associated with conditions leading to a state of induced zinc deficiency (e.g. poor bioavailability, medications, alcoholism, growth, pregnancy), or in individuals consuming very little food of poor nutrient density with respect to zinc (e.g. dieters, vegans, the elderly). Thirdly, the body appears to have very limited mobilizable zinc reserves, with the result that plasma zinc levels fall sharply if dietary zinc intake is depressed, which in turn leads to the rapid onset of a physiological zinc deficit in tissues requiring the metal for growth, and a slower reduction of zinc status in mature organs.

Together, these considerations emphasize the importance of a regular intake of zinc in human diets generally, and highlight those groups requiring particular attention because of a reduced overall zinc intake, depressed bioavailability of the element or the particular physiological requirement of the individual. At the other end of the spectrum lies the danger that the current trend towards self-medication with zinc may, if overzealous, impair the availability of other mineral nutrients and may indeed significantly depress other important physiological functions. The likelihood of nutritional zinc impoverishment in most well-fed Westerners is low. Nevertheless, it does exist in some sub-groups, and may become further exacerbated by the choice and processing of foods and by other lifestyle variables. The generally adequate zinc status enjoyed by most people should not engender complacency. Marginal zinc deficiency is hard to diagnose, but will almost certainly be accompanied by diminished health, and sub-optimal physical and mental performance. Modern nutrition must focus not only on the prevention of deficiency diseases, but must also ensure that the full contribution is made by nutrients to the development and maintenance of optimal health.

REFERENCES

Aggett, P.J. (1989). Severe zinc deficiency. In *Zinc in Human Biology*, pp. 259–80 [C.F. Mills, editor]. London: Springer-Verlag.

Aggett, P.J., Crofton, R.W., Khin, C., Gvozdanovic, S. & Gvozdanovic, D. (1983). The mutual inhibitory effects on their availability of zinc and iron. In *Zinc Deficiency in Human Subjects*, pp. 117–24 [A.S. Prasad, A.O. Cavdar, G.J. Brewer and P.J. Aggett, editors]. New York: Alan R. Liss.

American Academy of Pediatrics, Committee on Nutrition (1981). Zinc. *Pediatrics* **62**, 408–12.

American Medical Association, Nutrition Advisory Group (1979). Guidelines for essential trace element preparation for parenteral use. *Journal of the American Medical Association* **241**, 2051–4.

Apgar, J. (1972). Effect of zinc deprivation from day 12, 15 or 18 of gestation on parturition in the rat. *Journal of Nutrition* **102**, 343–8.

Bach, J.-F., Pleau, J.-M. & Savino, W. (1988). The role of zinc in the biological activity of thymulin, a thymic metallopeptide hormone. In *Essential and Toxic Trace Elements in Human Health and Disease*, pp. 319–28 [A.S. Prasad, editor]. New York: Alan R. Liss.

Baghurst, K., Worsley, A., Crawford, D., Baghurst, P., Record, S. & Syrette, J. (1987). *The Victorian Nutrition Survey (Part 2)*, Adelaide Australia: CSIRO, Division of Human Nutrition.

Beach, R.S., Gershwin, M.E. & Hurley, L.S. (1982). Gestational zinc deprivation in mice: persistence of immunodeficiency for three generations. *Science* **218**, 469–71.

Bergmann, K.E., Makosch, E. & Tews, K.H. (1980). Abnormalities of hair zinc concentration in mothers of newborn infants with spina bifida. *American Journal of Clinical Nutrition* **33**, 2145–50.

Bremner, I. & Morrison, J.N. (1988). Metallothionein as an indicator of zinc status. In *Essential and Toxic Trace Elements in Human Health and Disease*, pp. 365–79 [A.S. Prasad, editor]. New York: Alan R. Liss.

Buchet, J.P., Lauwergs, R., Vandevoorde, A. & Pycke, J.M. (1983). Oral daily intake of cadmium, lead, manganese, copper, chromium, mercury, calcium, zinc and arsenic in Belgium: a duplicate meal study. *Food and Chemical Toxicology* **21**, 19–24.

Buckley, R.A. & Dreosti, I.E. (1984). Radioisotope studies concerning the efficacy of standard washing procedures for the cleansing of hair before zinc analysis. *American Journal of Clinical Nutrition* **40**, 840–6.

Bunce, G.E. (1989). Zinc in endocrine function. In *Zinc in Human Biology*, pp. 249–58 [C.F. Mills, editor]. London: Springer-Verlag.

Casey, C.E. & Hambidge, K.M. (1980). Epidemiological aspects of human zinc deficiency. In *Zinc in the Environment*, pp. 1–27 [J.O. Nriagu, editor]. New York: John Wiley and Sons.

Cavdar, A.O., Arcasoy, A. & Cin, S. (1977). Zinc deficiency in Turkey. *American Journal of Clinical Nutrition* **30**, 833–6.

Cavdar, A.O., Arcasoy, A. & Baycu, T. (1980). Zinc deficiency and anencephaly in Turkey. *Teratology* **22**, 141.

Chandra, R.K. (1984). Excess intake of zinc impairs immune responses. *Journal of the American Medical Association* **252**, 1443–6.

Chen, Xue-Cun, Yin, Tai-An & He, Jin-Sheng. (1985). Low levels of zinc in hair and blood, pica, anorexia, and poor growth in Chinese preschool children. *American Journal of Clinical Nutrition* **42**, 694–700.

Chesters, J.K. (1978). Biochemical functions of zinc in animals. *World Review of Nutrition and Dietetics* **32**, 135–64.

Chesters, J.K. (1989). Biochemistry of zinc in cell division and tissue growth. In *Zinc in Human Biology*, pp. 109–18 [C.F. Mills, editor]. London: Springer-Verlag.

Clegg, M.S., Keen, C.L. & Hurley, L.S. (1989). Biochemical pathologies of zinc deficiency. In *Zinc in Human Biology*, pp. 129–145 [C.F. Mills, editor]. London: Springer-Verlag.

Crawford, I.L. (1983). Zinc and the hippocampus. In *Neurobiology of the Trace Elements, Vol. 1*, pp. 169–211 [I.E. Dreosti and R.M. Smith, editors]. New Jersey: Humana Press.

Cross, C.E., Halliwell, B. & Borish, E.T. (1987). Oxygen radicals and human disease. *Annals of Internal Medicine* **107**, 526–45.

Damaynov, I. & Dutz, W. (197X). Anencephaly in Shiraz, Iran. *Lancet* **i**, 82.

Dardenne, M., Wade, S., Savino, W., Nabarra, B., Prasad, A.S. & Bach, J.F. (1988). Thymulin and zinc deficiency. In *Essential and Toxic Trace Elements in Human Health and Disease*, pp. 326–36 [A.S. Prasad, editor]. New York: Alan R. Liss.

Dauncey, M.J., Shaw, J.C.L. & Urman, J. (1977). The absorption and retention of magnesium, zinc and copper by low birth weight infants fed pasteurized human breast milk. *Pediatric Research* **11**, 991–7.

Dawson-Hughes, B., Seligson, F.H. & Hughes, V.A. (1986). Effect of calcium carbonate and hydroxyapatite on zinc and iron retention in post-menopausal women. *American Journal of Clinical Nutrition* **44**, 83–8.

Domingo, T.L., Llobel, J.M., Paternain, J.L. & Corbella, J. (1988). Acute zinc intoxication: comparison of the antidote efficacy of several chelating agents. *Veterinary and Human Toxicology* **30**, 224–8.

Dreosti, I.E. (1981). Laboratory methods for mineral nutritional assessment in man. In *Transactions of the Menzies Foundation, Vol. 3, The Assessment of Nutritional Status*, pp. 123–36 [B.S. Hetzel and K.I. Baghurst, editors]. Melbourne: The Menzies Foundation.

Dreosti, I.E. (1982*a*). Zinc in prenatal development. In *Clinical Applications of Recent Advances in Zinc Metabolism*, pp. 19–38 [A.S. Prasad, I.E. Dreosti and B.S. Hetzel, editors]. New York: Alan R. Liss.

Dreosti, I.E. (1982*b*). Zinc. *Journal of Food and Nutrition* **4**, 167–73.

Dreosti, I.E. (1984). Zinc in the central nervous system: the emerging interactions. In *The Neurobiology of Zinc*, pp. 1–26 [C.J. Frederickson, G.A. Howell and E.J. Kasarskis, editors]. New York: Alan R. Liss.

Dreosti, I.E. (1987). Micronutrients, superoxide and the fetus. *Neurotoxicology* **8**, 445–50.

Dreosti, I.E. (1988). Antioxidants. Micronutrients versus free radicals. *Australian Family Physician* **17**, 684–6.

Dreosti, I.E. (1989*a*). Neurobiology of zinc. In *Zinc in Human Biology* pp. 235–48 [C.F. Mills, editor]. London: Springer-Verlag.

Dreosti, I.E. (1989*b*). Free radical pathology and the genome. In *Trace Elements, Micronutrients and Free Radicals*, pp. 149–69 [I.E. Dreosti, editor]. New Jersey: Humana Press.

Dreosti, I.E. & Partick, E.J. (1987). Zinc, ethanol and lipid peroxidation in adult and fetal rats. *Biological Trace Element Research* **14**, 179–91.

Dreosti, I.E., Tao, S. & Hurley, L.S. (1968). Plasma zinc and leukocyte changes in weanling and pregnant rats during zinc deficiency. *Proceedings of the Society of Experimental Biology and Medicine* **127**, 169–74.

Dreosti, I.E., Record, I.R. & Manuel, S.J. (1985). Zinc deficiency and the developing embryo. *Biological Trace Element Research* **7**, 103–22.

Eberhardt, M.J. & Halas, E.S. (1987). Developmental delays in offspring of rats undernourished or zinc deprived during lactation. *Physiology and Behavior* **41**, 309–14.

FAO/WHO Expert Committee on Food Additives (1982). Evaluation of certain food additives and contaminants. *WHO Technical Report Series No. 683*. Rome: FAO.

FAO (1984). *Food Balance Sheets 1979–81 Average*. Rome: FAO.

Fell, G.S. & Lyon, D.T.B. (1988). Is there need for simultaneous multielement analytical techniques in clinical chemistry? In *Essential and Toxic Elements in Human Health and Disease*, pp. 521–32 [A.S. Prasad, editor]. New York: Alan R. Liss.

Festa, M.D., Anderson, H.L., Dowdy, R.P. & Ellersieck, M.R. (1985). Effect of zinc intake on copper excretion and retention in man. *American Journal of Clinical Nutrition* **41**, 285–92.

Flanagan, P.R. & Valberg, L.S. (1988). The intestinal interaction of zinc and iron in humans: does it occurs with food? In *Essential and Toxic Trace Elements in Human Health and Disease*, pp. 501–7 [A.S. Prasad, editor]. New York: Alan R. Liss.

Floersheim, G.L. & Floersheim P. (1986). Protection against ionizing radiation and synergism with thiols by zinc aspartate. *British Journal of Radiology* **59**, 597–602.

Food and Nutrition Board (1980). *Recommended Dietary Allowances* 9th ed. Washington, D.C.: National Academy of Sciences.

Fox, M.R.S. (1989). Zinc excess. In *Zinc in Human Biology*, pp. 365–70 [C.F. Mills, editor]. London: Springer-Verlag.

Fraker, P.J., Gershwin, M.E., Good, R.A. & Prasad, A. (1986). Interrelationships between zinc and immune functions. *Federation Proceedings* **45**, 1474–9.

Friel, J.K., Gibson, R.S., Peliowski, A. & Watts, J. (1984). Serum zinc copper and selenium concentrations in preterm infants receiving enteral nutrition or parenteral nutrition supplemented with zinc and copper. *Journal of Pediatrics* **104**, 763–8.

Gartrell, M.J., Craun, J.C., Podrebarac, D.S. & Gunderson, E.L. (1985). Pesticides, selected elements and other chemicals in adult total diet samples, October 1978–September 1979. *Journal of the Association of Official Analytical Chemists* **68**, 862–75.

Golden, M.H.N. (1989). The diagnosis of zinc deficiency. In *Zinc in Human Biology*, pp. 323–34 [C.F. Mills, editor]. London: Springer-Verlag.

Golden, B.E. & Golden, M.H.N. (1979). Plasma zinc and the clinical features of malnutrition. *American Journal of Clinical Nutrition* **32**, 2490–9.

Golden, M.H.N. & Golden, B.E. (1981). Effects of zinc supplementation on the dietary intake, rate of weight gain and energy cost of tissue deposition in children recovering from severe malnutrition. *American Journal of Clinical Nutrition* **34**, 900–8.

Golden, M.H.N. & Ramdath, D. (1987). Free radicals in the pathogenesis of Kwashiorkor. *Proceedings of The Nutrition Society* **46**, 53–68.

Golub, M.S., Gershwin, M.E., Hurley, L.S. & Saito, W.Y. (1985). Studies of marginal zinc deprivation in rhesus monkeys. VII. Infant behavior. *American Journal of Clinical Nutrition* **42**, 1229–39.

Good, R.A. (1989). A note on zinc and immunocompetence. In *Zinc in Human Biology*, pp. 221–3 [C.F. Mills, editor]. London: Springer-Verlag.

Gordon, B.M. (1987). Survey of chemical speciation of trace elements using synchrotron radiation. *Biological Trace Element Research* **12**, 153–9.

Gordon, P.R., Woodruff, C.W., Anderson, H.L. & O'Dell, B.L. (1982). Effect of acute zinc deprivation on plasma zinc and platelet aggregation in adult males. *American Journal of Clinical Nutrition* **35**, 113–19.

Greger, J.L. & Snedeker, S.M. (1980). Effect of dietary protein and phosphorus levels on the utilization of zinc, copper and manganese by adult males. *Journal of Nutrition* **110**, 2243–53.

Grummt, F., Weinman-Dorsch, C., Schneider-Schanlies, J. & Lux, A. (1986). Zinc as a second messenger of mitogenic induction. Effects on diadenosine tetraphosphate (Ap4A) and DNA synthesis. *Experimental Cell Research* **163**, 191–200.

Halas, E.S. (1983). Behavioral changes accompanying zinc deficiency in animals. In *Neurobiology of the Trace Elements, Vol. 1*, pp. 213–43 [I.E. Dreosti and R.M. Smith, editors]. New Jersey: Humana Press.

Halsted, J.A. (1977). Events surrounding the original demonstration of zinc deficiency. In *Zinc Metabolism: Current Aspects in Health and Disease*, pp. 1–9 [G.J. Brewer and A.S. Prasad, editors]. New York: Alan R. Liss.

Halsted, J.A., Ronaghy, H.A. & Abadi, P. (1972). Zinc deficiency in man. *American Journal of Medicine* **53**, 277–84.

Halsted, J.A., Smith, J.C. & Irwin, M.I. (1974). A conspectus of research on zinc requirements of man. *Journal of Nutrition* **104**, 345–78.

Hambidge, K.M. (1989). Mild zinc deficiency in human subjects. In *Zinc in Human Biology*, pp. 281–96 [C.F. Mills, editor]. London: Springer-Verlag.

Hambidge, K.M., Hambidge, C., Jacobs, M. & Baum, J.D. (1972). Low levels of zinc in hair, anorexia, poor growth and hypogeusia in children. *Pediatric Research* **6**, 868–74.

Haynes, D.C., Gershwin, M.E., Golub, M.S., Cheung, A.T.W. & Hurley, L.S. (1985). Studies of marginal zinc deprivation in rhesus monkeys. VI. Influence on the immunohematology of infants in the first year. *American Journal of Clinical Nutrition* **42**, 252–62.

Hazell, T. (1985). Minerals in foods: dietary sources, chemical forms interactions, bioavailability. *World Review of Nutrition and Dietetics* **46**, 1–123.

Henkin, R.I. (1971). Newer aspects of copper and zinc metabolism. In *Newer Trace Elements in Nutrition* pp. 256–313 [W. Mertz and W.E. Cornatzer, editors]. New York: Marcel Dekker.

Henkin, R.I., Patten, B.M., Re, P.K. & Bronzert, D.A. (1975). A syndrome of acute zinc loss. *Archives of Neurology* **32**, 745–52.

Hurley, L.S. (1981). Teratogenic aspects of manganese zinc and copper in nutrition. *Physiological Reviews* **61**, 249–95.

Hurley, L.S. & Shrader, R.E. (1972). Congenital malformations of the central nervous system in zinc-deficient rats. In *Neurobiology of the Trace Metals Zinc and Copper*, pp. 7–51 [C.C. Pfeiffer, editor]. New York: Academic Press.

Hurley, L.S., Gowan, J. & Swenerton, H. (1971). Teratogenic effects of short-term and transitory zinc deficiency in rats. *Teratology* **4**, 199–204.

Hurley, L.S., Gordon, P., Keen, C.L. & Merkhofer, L. (1980). Circadian variation in rat plasma zinc and rapid effect of dietary zinc deficiency. *Federation Proceedings* **39**, 431A.

James, B.E. & MacMahon, R.A. (1976). Balance studies in nine elements during complete intravenous feeding of small premature infants. *Australian Paediatric Journal* **12**, 154–62.

James, B.E., Hendry, P.G. & MacMahon, R.A. (1979). Total parental nutrition of premature infants. 2 requirements for micronutrient elements. *Australian Paediatric Journal* **15**, 67–72.

Jameson, S. (1976). Effects of zinc deficiency on human reproduction. *Acta Medica Scandinavica* **593**, 5–89.

Janghorbani, M., Ting, B.T.G. & Zeisel, S.H. (1988). Trace element research with stable isotope tracers. In *Essential and Toxic Trace Elements in Human Health and Disease*, pp. 545–56 [A.S. Prasad, editor]. New York: Alan R. Liss.

Jones, K.W. & Pounds, J.G. (1987). Role of nuclear analytical probe technique in biological trace element research. *Biological Trace Element Research* **12**, 3–16.

Kasarskis, E.J. (1984). Zinc metabolism in normal and zinc deficient rat brain. *Experimental Neurology* **85**, 114–27.

Keen, C.L. & Hurley, L.S. (1989). Zinc and reproduction: effects of deficiency on fetal and postnatal development. In *Zinc in Human Biology*, pp. 183–220 [C.F. Mills, editor]. London: Springer-Verlag.

King, J.C. (1986). Assessment of techniques for determining human requirements. *Journal of the American Dietetic Association* **86**, 1523–8.

King, J.C. & Turnlund, J.R. (1989). Human zinc requirements. In *Zinc in Human Biology*, pp. 335–50 [C.F. Mills, editor]. London: Springer-Verlag.

Klingberg, W.G., Prasad, A.S. & Oberleas, D. (1976). Zinc deficiency following penicillamine therapy. In *Trace Elements in Human Health and Disease, Vol. 1*, pp. 51–65 [A.S. Prasad and D. Oberleas, editors]. New York: Academic Press.

Klug, A. & Rhodes, D. (1987). 'Zinc fingers': a novel protein motif for nucleic acid recognition. *Trends in Biochemical Sciences* **12**, 464–9.

Lindeman, R.D., Baxter, D.J., Yunice, A.A. & Kraikitpanitch, S. (1978). Serum concentrations and urinary excretions of zinc in cirrhosis, nephrotic syndrome and renal insufficiency. *American Journal of Medical Sciences* **275**, 17–24.

Llobet, J.M., Domingo, J.L. & Corbella, J. (1988). Antidotes for zinc intoxication in mice. *Archives of Toxicology* **61**, 321–3.

Lönnerdal, B., Stanislowski, A.G. & Hurley, L.S. (1980). Isolation of a low molecular weight zinc binding ligand from human milk. *Inorganic Biochemistry* **12**, 71–8.

McKenzie, J.M., Guthrie, B.E. & Prior, I.A.M. (1978). Zinc and copper status of Polynesian residents of the Tokelau Islands. *American Journal of Clinical Nutrition* **31**, 422–8.

McMichael, A.J., Dreosti, I.E. & Gibson, G.T. (1982). A prospective study of serial maternal zinc levels and pregnancy outcome. *Early Human Development* **7**, 59–69.

Mertz, W. (1974). The effects of zinc in man: nutritional considerations. In *Clinical Applications of Zinc Metabolism*, pp. 93–100 [W.J. Pories, W.H. Strain, J.M. Hsu and R.L. Woosley, editors]. Springfield, CT: Charles C. Thomas.

Mertz, W. (1980). Mineral elements: new perspectives. *Journal of the American Dietetic Association* **77**, 258–63.

Mills, C.F. (1989). The biological significance of zinc for man: problems and prospects. In *Zinc in Human Biology*, pp. 371–81 [C.F. Mills, editor]. London: Springer-Verlag.

Paul, A.A. & Southgate, D.H. (1978). *McCance and Widdowson's The Composition of Foods (4th edn.)*. London: H.M. Stationery Office.

Pennington, J.A.T., Young, B.E., Wilson, D.B., Johnson, R.D. & Vanderveen, J.E. (1986). Mineral contents of foods and total diets: the selected minerals in foods survey, 1982–1984. *Journal of the American Dietetic Association* **86**, 876–91.

Phillips, G.D. (1982). Zinc in total parenteral nutrition. In *Clinical Applications of Recent Advances in Zinc Metabolism*, pp. 169–80 [A.S. Prasad, I.E. Dreosti and B.S. Hetzel, editors]. New York: Alan R. Liss.

Pories, W.J., Henzel, J.H., Rob, C.E. & Strain, H.H. (1967). Promotion of wound healing in man with zinc sulphate given by mouth. *Lancet* **i**, 121–2.

Prasad, A.S. (1988). Clinical spectrum and diagnostic aspects of human zinc deficiency. In *Essential and Toxic Trace Elements in Human Health and Disease*, pp. 3–53 [A.S. Prasad, editor]. New York: Alan R. Liss.

Prasad, A.S., Halsted, J.A. & Nadimi, N. (1961). Syndrome of iron deficiency anemia, hepatosplenomegaly, hypogonadism, dwarfism and geophagia. *American Journal of Medicine* **31**, 532–46.

Record, I.R., Tulsi, R.S., Dreosti, I.E. & Fraser, F.J. (1985). Cellular necrosis in zinc-deficient rat embryos. *Teratology* **32**, 397–405.

Ridley, C.M. (1982). Zinc deficiency developing in treatment for thalassaemia. *Journal of the Royal Society of Medicine* **75**, 38-9.

Sandstead, H.H. (1973). Zinc nutrition in the United States. *American Journal of Clinical Nutrition* **26**, 1251-60.

Sandstead, H.H. (1982). Copper bioavailability and requirements. *American Journal of Clinical Nutrition* **35**, 809-14.

Sandström, B. (1989). Dietary pattern and zinc supply. In *Zinc in Human Biology*, pp. 351-64 [C.F. Mills, editor]. London: Springer-Verlag.

Sandström, B. & Lönnerdal, B. (1989). Promoters and antagonists of zinc absorption. In *Zinc in Human Biology*, pp. 57-78 [C.F. Mills, editor]. London: Springer-Verlag.

Schroeder, H.A. (1971). Losses of vitamins and trace minerals resulting from processing and preservation of foods. *American Journal of Clinical Nutrition* **24**, 562-70.

Schroeder, H.A., Nason, A.P., Tipton, I.H. & Balossa, J.J. (1967). Essential trace metals in man. Zinc. *Journal of Chronic Diseases* **20**, 179-210.

Sever, L.E. & Emanuel, I. (1973). Is there a connection between maternal zinc deficiency and congenital malformations in the central nervous system in man? *Teratology* **7**, 117-19.

Shrimpton, R. (1984). Food consumption and dietary adequacy according to income in 1200 families, Manaus, Amazonas, Brazil. *Archivos Latino-Americanas de Nutricion* **34**, 615-29.

Sivasubramanian, K.N. & Henkin, R.I. (1978). Behavioral and dermatologic changes and low serum zinc and copper concentrations in two premature infants after parenteral alimentation. *Journal of Pediatrics* **93**, 847-50.

Slorach, S., Gustafsson, I.B., Jorhem, L. & Mattsson, P. (1983). Intake of lead, cadmium and certain other metals via a typical Swedish weekly diet. *Vår Föda* **35**, Suppl. 1, 3-16.

Smith, J.C., Morris, E.R. & Ellis, R. (1983). Zinc: requirements, bioavailabilities and recommended dietary allowances. In *Zinc Deficiency in Human Subjects*, pp. 147-70 [A.S. Prasad, A.O. Cavdar, G.J. Brewer and P.J. Aggett, editors]. New York: Alan R. Liss.

Smit-Vanderkooy, P.D. & Gibson, R.S. (1987). Food consumption patterns of Canadian pre-school children in relation to zinc and growth status. *American Journal of Clinical Nutrition* **45**, 609-16.

Solomons, N.W. (1986). Competitive interaction of iron and zinc in the diet: consequences for human nutrition. *Journal of Nutrition* **116**, 927-35.

Solomons, N.W. (1988). The iron:zinc interaction in the human intestine, does it exist? An affirmative view. In *Essential and Toxic Trace Elements in Human Health and Disease*, pp. 509-18 [A.S. Prasad, editor]. New York: Alan R. Liss.

Solomons, N.W., Ruz, M. & Castillo-Duran, C. (1989). Putative therapeutic roles for zinc. In *Zinc in Human Biology*, pp. 297-322 [C.F. Mills, editor]. London: Springer-Verlag.

Soltan, M.H. & Jenkins, D.M. (1982). Maternal and fetal plasma zinc concentration and fetal abnormality. *British Journal of Obstetrics and Gynaecology* **89**, 56-8.

Soman, S.D., Panday, V.K., Joseph, K.T. & Raut, S.J. (1969). Daily intake of some major and trace elements. *Health Physics* **17**, 35-40.

Stewart, C., Katchen, B. & Collipp, P.J. (1981). Zinc and birth defects. *Pediatric Research* **15**, 515.

Suita, S., Ikeda, K. & Hayashida, Y. (1984). Zinc and copper requirements during parenteral nutrition of the newborn. *Journal of Pediatric Surgery* **19**, 126–30.

Swenerton, H. & Hurley, L.S. (1968). Severe zinc deficiency in male and female rats. *Journal of Nutrition* **95**, 8–13.

Thurnham, D.I., Zheng, S.F. & Munoz, N. (1985). Comparison of riboflavin, vitamin A and zinc status of Chinese populations at high and low risk for esophageal cancer. *Nutrition and Cancer* **7**, 131–43.

Truswell, A.S. & Chambers, T. (1983). IUNS Report on Recommended Dietary Allowances Around the World. *Nutrition Abstracts and Reviews: Series A, Clinical and Experimental* **53**, 1109–10.

Underwood, E.J. (1977). *Trace Elements in Human and Animal Nutrition*, 4th edn. New York: Academic Press.

Vallee, B.L. & Galdes, A. (1984). The metallobiochemistry of zinc enzymes. In *Advances in Enzymology*, Vol. 56, pp. 283–415 [A. Meister, editor]. New York: John Wiley & Sons.

Van Dokkum, W., De Vos, R.H., Muys, T.H. & Wesskra, J.A. (1989). Minerals and trace elements in total diets in The Netherlands. *British Journal of Nutrition* **61**, 7–15.

Varo, P. & Kovistoinen, P. (1980). Mineral element composition of Finnish foods. XII General discussion and nutritional evaluation. *Acta Agricultural Scandinavica* **22**, Suppl., 165–71.

Walravens, P.A. (1980). Nutritional importance of copper and zinc in neonates and infants. *Clinical Chemistry* **26**, 185–9.

Wensink, J., Lenglet, W.J., Vis, R.D. & Van den Hamer, C.J. (1987). The effect of dietary zinc deficiency on the mossy fiber zinc content of the rat hippocampus. *Histochemistry* **87**, 65–9.

WHO-World Health Organization (1973). Trace elements in human nutrition. WHO Tech. Ref. Series 532. pp. 9–14.

Widdowson, E.M., Dickerson, J.W.T. & McCance, R.A. (1962). Chemical composition of the body. In *Mineral Metabolism*, pp. 1–247 [C.L. Comar & F. Bromer, editors]. New York: Academic Press.

Williams, R.J.P. (1989). An introduction to the biochemistry of zinc. In *Zinc in Human Biology*, pp. 15–32 [C.F. Mills, editor]. London: Springer-Verlag.

Willson, R.L. (1989). Zinc and iron in free radical pathology and cellular control. In *Zinc in Human Biology*, pp. 147–72 [C.F. Mills, editor]. London: Springer-Verlag

Zlotkin, Z.B. & Buchanan, B.E. (1983). Meeting zinc and copper intake requirements in the parenterally-fed preterm and full-term infant. *Journal of Pediatrics* **103**, 441–6.

5

Dietary Mineral Supplementation and Bioavailability

ANDREW BEAL & ANN F. WALKER
Department of Food Science and Technology, University of Reading, UK

INTRODUCTION

Supplementation of the diet with minerals, as well as other nutrients, is becoming more widespread in the industrialized world. However, in Britain, as in other European countries, sales are still trivial in comparison with US sales, which were well in excess of $5 billion per annum in 1989.

An increasing proportion of consumers feel compelled to improve the nutritional quality of their diet. While some people take nutrient supplements for specific health reasons, e.g. iron to offset menstrual losses, for others the motivation may be to ensure the nutritional adequacy of a convenience diet. During the 1980s, people became more aware of the relationship between diet and health and all indications are that the interest is likely to continue and even increase.

The bioavailability or availability of a nutrient has been defined by Bender (1989) as 'the proportion of a nutrient capable of being absorbed and available for use or storage'. Absorption is a particularly important aspect of bioavailability, especially in the case of minerals, where it is so important that the terms absorption and availability are sometimes used synonymously. In this chapter, the current knowledge of dietary influences on mineral absorption is reviewed with emphasis given to absorptive interactions between dietary minerals. The implications of such interactions on the nutritional status of people taking mineral supplements will be examined in the light of experimental difficulties encountered in nutritional research and the bearing this has on providing reliable nutritional information to the consumer.

This chapter starts with a brief description of the absorptive mechanisms of the important mineral nutrients, calcium, iron, magnesium and zinc, which are often lacking in the diet. This overview is necessary for an understanding of mechanisms of nutrient interaction at the absorptive interface later in the Chapter.

ABSORPTIVE MECHANISMS

The intestinal mucosa has some ability to adjust mineral absorption to suit the requirements of the body: deficiency of a mineral results in increased absorption. This is well documented for iron, as well as for calcium and zinc (Pollack *et al.*, 1965). On the other hand, an excess absorption of minerals may be prevented by limiting absorption (e.g. iron) and/or by increased urinary excretion. Unfortunately, these mechanisms are not sufficient to prevent chronic toxicity in the face of prolonged overconsumption of a mineral.

The duodenum and jejunum are generally the major sites of mineral absorption, although the whole intestine is capable of absorbing most minerals. The limited ability of the colon to absorb minerals by diffusion is well known (Pike & Brown, 1983). On the other hand, James *et al.* (1978) have shown that the colon is capable of active absorption of calcium, mediated by vitamin D, but the rate of absorption is only about 10% of that of the small intestine, although, as the transit time through the colon is 20 times longer than that for the small intestine, the net capacity for colonic absorption may more than equal that of the small intestine. It is possible that other minerals may also be actively absorbed by the colon.

The large intestine hosts a microflora, whose nutritional effects are only just beginning to receive attention. In recent years, the capacity of dietary fibre to bind minerals and, therefore, to reduce their availability has been a subject of much research, although, as seen below, evidence about the effects of fibre is equivocal. One of the problems is that much of the fibre is broken down in the large intestine by microbial fermentation.

Calcium absorption
This subject is well documented though the precise sequence of events is still not clear.

Most sources are agreed that calcium is absorbed rapidly from the duodenum and jejunum, and slowly from the ileum. Absorption is against an electrochemical gradient, by a two-stage process. Sanford (1982) states that Stage 1 is probably diffusive and that Stage 2 involves the active transport of calcium from the mucosal to the serosal membrane. Indeed, Davenport (1979) suggested a mechanism involving active transport at lumen concentrations between 1 and 5 mM, at which point the mechanism becomes saturated and further absorption is by diffusion. Calcium in the lumen becomes bound to a calcium-binding protein (CaBP) in the brush border of the mucosa before transfer into the cell.

Calcium absorption is precisely regulated. Increase in plasma calcium stimulates the secretion of the thyroid hormone calcitonin, which promotes calcium deposition in bone. A decrease in plasma calcium stimulates the secretion of parathyroid hormone (PTH) from the parathyroid glands. Parathyroid hormone enhances the appropriate kidney enzyme to bring about increased hydroxylation of 25,-hydroxycholecalciferol to 1,25-dihydroxycholecalciferol (active form of vitamin D). This hormone-like vitamin acts on the cells of the intestinal epithelium, initiating the synthesis of CaBP. Together with PTH, calcitriol also increases mobilization of calcium from bone (Pike & Brown, 1983).

Increased CaBP increases the potential for uptake of calcium. There is some debate as to whether CaBP remains within the brush border or is secreted into the lumen. Most workers believe that CaBP modifies the mucosal membrane, permitting the diffusion of calcium into the cell. Transport across the cell is also a matter of speculation. One theory suggests CaBP carries the calcium to the serosal interface; in another, the mitochondria, which are known to collect calcium avidly, are thought to be the vehicle (Pike & Brown, 1983).

Iron absorption

In healthy subjects, only a small proportion of dietary iron is absorbed, although the capacity of the small intestinal mucosa (mostly duodenum and jejunum) to absorb iron increases markedly in iron deficiency. Non-haem iron is absorbed in the ferrous form, ferric iron being reduced before absorption by factors such as ascorbic acid. It is believed that iron crosses the membrane as a soluble iron ligand complex and not as free ferrous iron. In man, haem iron is absorbed intact and the iron is released into the mucosal cytosol by an enzyme, haem oxidase (Eastwood & Passmore, 1986). The initial uptake of iron by the mucosa is rapid but falls to almost zero within an hour or so. Mucosal permeability to iron appears to depend on the iron content of the mucosal cell and so depends on rate of transfer to plasma, the uptake by ferritin, and cytosolic concentration (Sanford, 1982).

Ferritin is essentially an iron storage compound and most mucosal ferritin is eventually lost when the cell desquamates (Forth, 1970). It has been suggested that the cytosol maintains a soluble iron content in complex with amino acids and these are able to transfer iron to the plasma. Transfer across the serosal membrane appears to be the rate-limiting step in the process (Barton *et al.*, 1983).

The mechanisms of mineral absorption and transfer are prone to competition between minerals (interactions) because their specificity is usually low. Mineral absorption generally relies on the formation of soluble complexes and any given ligand may operate in common with any mineral if the conditions are conducive. The iron absorption mechanism has only a limited specificity for iron. Therefore in the iron-deficient state, ferrous iron absorption is increased considerably, whereas several other metal ions also show increased absorption, but to a lesser extent. An excess of these ions, namely Co^{2+}, Mn^{2+} and Ni^{2+} (which have a similar electronic configuration to ferrous iron), are also capable of inhibiting iron absorption by competition (Pollack *et al.*, 1965).

Magnesium absorption

Much dietary magnesium is consumed as the magnesium porphyrin complex present in chlorophyll and deficiency is rarely seen in areas where green leafy vegetables constitute of significant portion of the diet (Eastwood & Passmore, 1986).

Davenport (1979), in a general text on digestive physiology, wrote that magnesium is absorbed equally well along the entire length of the intestine by passive diffusion, assisted by solvent drag. He claimed that there was little evidence to suggest facultative control of magnesium absorption in that absorption does not appear to adjust to meet requirements. A review by Tansy (1971) supports these ideas and adds that a relationship between calcium and magnesium absorption may exist and that sodium and potassium could be involved. The involvement of these monovalent cations suggests that a carrier operates. However, the carrier may act principally for calcium absorption with movement of magnesium being purely competitive. On the other hand, Briscoe & Ragan (1967) reported a correlation between serum magnesium and calcium levels indicating that perhaps magnesium responds to homeostatic mechanisms thought to act primarily for calcium. These authors made further studies on patients suffering malabsorption or depressed renal function and concluded that the transport mechanisms for the two minerals may be independent in both the intestine and in the renal tubule.

Zinc absorption

Evans & Johnson (1978) reported that zinc combines with a ligand in the intestinal lumen, possibly a prostaglandin, prior to transport into the mucosal cell. Zinc is then bound to metallothionein in the cytosol. Metallothionein modulates the uptake of zinc and copper, which compete for its sites. Incorporation of these two minerals is at a rate determined by: affinity of the thionein for the metal, cytosolic concentration, intestinal lumen concentration and plasma concentration of the competing ions. Absorption across the mucosal membrane is probably by diffusion or carrier-mediated active transport, both of which are subject to competition from similarly structured metal ions (Mills, 1985).

INTERACTIONS WITHIN FOODSTUFFS, INCLUDING THE INFLUENCE OF THE FOOD CHAIN

Foods are biological materials and will therefore vary in composition and properties depending on a wide range of factors. So far as minerals are concerned, this variability may affect both the mineral content and factors within the food that may influence the bioavailability of minerals, such as the levels of phytate (see below).

Agronomic and environmental factors

Although the use of fertilizers permits great efficiency of nitrogen and phosphate metabolism by plants, leading to high crop yields, they may also induce compositional changes. For example, protein quantity and quality may be changed, or higher levels of phytic acid may be produced, altering the potential of food derived from the plant to bind minerals. Indeed, any change in agronomic practice may have repercussions on mineral-binding potential of food, including the introduction of 'organic' farming methods. It should not be assumed that all quality changes to plant foods are desirable from a nutritional point of view.

Change in agricultural methods may not only influence composition of existing crops, but may allow the introduction of new crops with different or modified dietary components. Even climatic changes may influence food crop species grown and/or their composition. For example, acid rain is known to affect soil pH and must therefore influence mineral solubility and availability to plants. So far there has been little research on these aspects.

Food processing

Food processing commonly involves one or more of the following conditions: wet or dry heat treatment (for example, in canning or drying), freezing, change in pH (e.g. pickling), chemical or microbiological modification (e.g. the addition of additives or microbial fermentation), change in osmotic potential (e.g. brining, dry salting, addition of sugar, or evaporation) or the exclusion of air.

A number of these processes are known to affect mineral absorption, although experimental observations have not strictly followed theoretical expectations. The main problem is analogous to predicting vitamin C loss during processing, where predictive models have failed because of the number of factors involved. Similarly, many factors influence the outcome of processing on mineral bioavailability, including amounts of minerals and mineral-binding factors in raw materials, the presence of protective components in the food and pH.

Heating is, perhaps, one of the most important forms of processing. The Maillard browning reactions which occurs during heating can produce chemical species capable of forming hydrolysis-resistant metal complexes (Greger, 1987). Heat, oxidizing conditions and alkaline pH all serve to accelerate processes leading to the formation of these refractile mineral-containing compounds. In the case of iron, soluble, hydrated iron salts are able to dehydrate, becoming less soluble or forming insoluble hydroxides with time. These progress through polymerization, gelation and hardening, to form increasingly ordered refractile substances, a process described by Clydesdale (1988) as 'ageing'. As the compound becomes more ordered, it becomes more resistant to dissolution even under acidic conditions and eventually becomes irreversibly insoluble. Evidence exists that other mineral complexes, such as calcium polyphosphates, form refractile compounds in a similar way. Gastric conditions are insufficient to solubilize any but lightly complexed gels.

Fermentation is reported to increase iron bioavailability to rats from soya beans. This may occur partly by chemical changes to the fibre, resulting in the release of minerals, and partly by lowering the pH. The latter increases mineral solubility and the protonation of acidic fibre moieties, thus reducing their mineral-binding capacity.

Panary fermentations are reported to improve mineral availability, as is baking, due to the hydrolysis of phytate by yeast and wheat phytases releasing minerals from fibre (Erdman, 1981). However, toasting and boiling have been shown to decrease mineral bioavailability, again in the presence of fibre (Camire & Clydesdale, 1981). This latter point might be expected when considered in terms of the ageing effect discussed earlier. The apparently conflicting reports involving baking and toasting may be explained by the fact that leavening, in evolving carbon dioxide, creates a low oxygen tension within the bread with consequently less oxidation.

In summary, processing changes that may improve mineral solubility include: lowered pH, reducing conditions and the presence of compounds capable of forming soluble complexes. But, again, there is conflicting evidence. Sucrose, fructose and other polyols should increase iron absorption by chelation as indicated by in-vitro experimentation with the pure compounds. However, in-vitro gastrointestinal simulations with whole food materials show sugars to have little effect on iron absorption (Clydesdale, 1988). Indeed, some workers have suggested that the presence of fructose exacerbates copper deficiency in copper-depleted rats (Greger, 1987).

The formulation of a food product allows materials to be added that may improve bioavailability, although the reason for these additions is rarely primarily nutritional. Thus citric and malic acids lower pH and can form soluble mineral complexes. The role of ascorbic acid in solubilizing iron has been shown repeatedly: it does so by a combination of chelation, lowering pH and by maintaining reducing conditions. Reduced iron is much more soluble than ferric iron. Even so, at the low pH typical of the stomach, ascorbic acid can form complexes with the ferric iron which are stable to the rising pH of the intestine (Conrad & Schade, 1968).

On the negative side, the use of fibre and gums as gelling or bulking agents offers the potential for enhancing mineral binding and so reducing bioavailability.

MINERAL INTERACTION WITH OTHER FOOD COMPONENTS

Interaction of minerals with other food components can be loosely grouped into two: those involving or not involving dietary fibre.

Reactions not involving dietary fibre
Compounds within foods that inhibit mineral absorption include oxalates and tannins, which form stable insoluble mineral complexes. Tannins have a high affinity for iron. Calcium phosphates are theoretically capable of

precipitating metal ions in insoluble polymeric complexes, although this has not been satisfactorily demonstrated in a dietary context.

Iron and calcium in milk are associated with the proteins lactoferrin and casein respectively. These proteins reduce the availability of the minerals to the gut, but, by the same token, the intestinal microflora are also denied immediate access to the minerals. Protein breakdown releases the minerals for absorption and also supplies amino acids, many of which can form soluble complexes with minerals, which may assist absorption.

Haem is absorbed intact and in the gut lumen its iron component is effectively protected from sequestration by other ligands. The effect of protein in promoting the absorption of both haem and non-haem iron is well documented (e.g. Slatkavitz & Clydesdale, 1988). Indeed, absorption of iron is normally facilitated by a plentiful supply of ligands in the digesta (such as amino acids), which are capable of forming soluble complexes. These ligands are also effective in solubilizing zinc and other minerals (Sandstrom *et al.*, 1987).

Large intakes of dietary protein, typical of western diets, have been reported to increase phosphorus and calcium absorption. However, this increased absorption is offset by an increased calcium requirement due to an increase in urinary calcium (Linkswiler *et al.*, 1981). These authors noted that calcium balance in humans was achievable at low calcium intakes (500 mg/day) and low protein intakes (50 g/day) (phosphate 700–1000 mg/day), but calcium losses in urine became heavy as the protein content of the diet increased. Supplementary calcium and phosphate were successfully used to offset this loss at moderate protein intakes (95 g/day) but not at high protein intakes (142 g/day). It is thought that sulphur amino acids are responsible for the calciuretic effect by decreasing resorption of calcium at the kidney tubule. Greger (1987) suggests that the high phosphate content of many protein foods is sufficient to offset the hypercalciuric effects of protein and that the net effect on calcium balance is minimal, providing calcium intake is adequate.

A small proportion of fat normally escapes absorption in the small intestine. This fat, in the form of free fatty acids, is capable of binding calcium and magnesium to form insoluble soaps. These minerals may be absorbed from the colon after fermentation of the soaps by the indigenous microflora. However, serious losses of minerals via this route are possible in patients suffering steatorrhea (fatty diarrhoea, a symptom of severe malabsorption) or following extensive bowel resection (Tansy, 1971). The main interactions of carbohydrates with minerals are possible involvement of simple sugars as dietary chelating agents and those of the complex carbohydrates, which are dealt with in the next section.

Reactions involving dietary fibre (and phytate)

Dietary fibre components are implicated in reducing mineral bioavailability by binding minerals associated with the fibre source itself and those arising from other foodstuffs, or from gastrointestinal secretions during digestion.

The effects of dietary fibre in mineral binding are often confounded by the presence of phytic acid, with which it is usually intimately associated. Reviews of the mineral-binding effects of dietary fibre are numerous and reflect the intense research activity in this area. Much of the research has shown that an increase in dietary fibre can cause negative mineral balance for one or more minerals in man and other animals.

Some reports indicate that mineral binding is limited to particular fibre fractions, e.g. bran or phytate, but conflicing reports can always be quoted. Thus, Cook (1983) concludes in a review that bran and phytate were mainly responsible for mineral binding to dietary fibre, while Davies (1978) reviews conflicting reports on the components of fibre responsible for mineral binding and whether they are significant. He points out that in-vitro tests showing high mineral-binding capacities are often not supported *in vivo*. He claims that phytate, rather than fibre, appears to be the major determinant of zinc availability in the rat. This view is supported by Erdman (1981) who suggests that the zinc:phytate ratio is of paramount importance in zinc availability.

Dietary fibre

Dietary fibre has been defined as that material not broken down by the endogenous secretions of the human gastrointestinal tract. However, this definition must be used with care, since the material escaping such digestion includes a proportion of fat, protein and starch, which are clearly not dietary fibre. For many purposes, dietary fibre is best described in chemical terms as the sum of non-starch polysaccharides and lignin (Englyst & Cummings, 1988). Dietary fibre can be separated into heterogeneous fractions by a number of physical extraction procedures. Few of the fractions are chemically defined, though their constituent chemistry is becoming clearer (Table 1).

Other isolated fractions of plant foods are described as Acid Detergent Fibre (ADF), Neutral Detergent Fibre (NDF) and total fibre, depending on the method of extraction. Many workers regard the non-starch poly-

TABLE 1
Fractions of dietary fibre and complex carbohydrate

		Constituent	General structure
Insoluble		Lignin	Phenolic units in 3D structure
		Silica	SiO_2 residues
		Cutin	—
		Partially resistant starch	Retrograde amylopectin or highly crystalline or intimately associated with NSP
		Resistant starch	Retrograde amylose
		Inulin	Polyfructose
		Cellulose	β-1,4 polyglucose chains
		Hemicellulose	Shorter chains than cellulose and branched with monosaccharide or uronic acid units. Increased branching generally increases solubility
	Non-starch polysaccharides	Pectins	Uronic acid chains with monosaccharide sub-unit side chains
		Pectic acids	As pectins but side chains composed of uronic acid residues
Soluble		Mucilages and gums	Monosaccharide and/or uronic acid chains with monosaccharide side chains
		Oligosaccharides	e.g. raffinose and stacchyose, a trisaccharide and tetrasaccharide, respectively
		Phytic acid	Inositol hexaphosphate

NSP = Non-starch polysaccharide.
Compiled from Scheeman (1986) and Cummings & Englyst (1987).

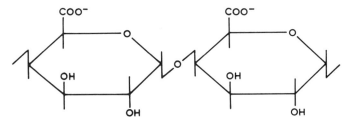

FIG. 1. Ionized uronic acid chains.

saccharide (NSP) method of Englyst as the analytical procedure for assessing dietary fibre with most relevance to digestive physiology, although it cannot be obtained as an isolated fraction for mineral-binding studies. The ability of dietary fibre to bind minerals depends on the net effect of each of its constituents. However, these do not necessarily correlate with the fractionation procedures imposed by analysts. Consequently, any proposed mechanism for mineral binding by dietary fibre must remain tentative until the subject has been more fully explored.

Fibres containing pectin, hemicellulose, mucilages and gums are rich in uronic acid groups (Fig. 1). At the pH prevalent in the small intestine, these acidic groups would be extensively ionized (James *et al.*, 1978) and capable of cation exchange. Camire & Clydesdale (1981) and Platt and Clydesdale (1984) noted high metal binding capacities of lignin, pectin and cellulose *in vitro*, the extent of which was pH dependent. Kohn (1975) suggested that, in addition to cation exchange, minerals may substitute for the bound water involved in the hydrogen bonding of polyuronic acid chains. In more neutral fibres, such as cellulose, solvation forces may attract minerals towards the hydrated fibre. However, these forces are unlikely to be strongly mineral binding since minerals are also hydrated.

There is considerable evidence that demonstrates the ability of various fibre fractions to bind minerals. These fractions have differing affinities for minerals, depending on prevailing conditions (Table 2). Dreher (1987) extensively reviews and summarizes *in vitro*, animal and human experiments on the effect of dietary fibre on mineral availability.

In summary, the effect of dietary fibre on mineral availability is a controversial subject with many apparent contradictions. Thus, Toma & Curtis (1986) review reports showing cellulose to decrease calcium retention in rats during an 8 week study. In another, baboons showed no change in calcium balance when given cellulose over a 26 week period.

Most reviewers conclude that experimental variability is responsible for

TABLE 2
Mineral binding by fibre fractions *in vitro*

Fibre	Possible binding sites	Affinity for minerals	Effect of pH[a]	Effect of heat treatment	Mineral–mineral interaction
Cellulose	Weak, ns for Fe	Weak but generally Fe > Zn > Ca		Alters extent	NI
Pectin		Ca, Zn > Mg, Fe	Uronic acid groups bind Ca ↑ with ↑ pH	NI	NI
High methoxy	s and ns for Fe				
Low methoxy	s				
Lignin	2 specific for each Fe, Cu, Zn	Fe > Cu > Zn		Alters affinity Zn > Fe > Mg > Ca	Addition of Zn, Mg, or Cu reduces bound Fe. Addition of Fe greatly reduces bound Zn or Mg or Ca in order Zn > Mg > Ca
Bran	NI	Generally Zn > Fe > Mg but depends on source	Variable. Ca binding ↑ with pH. Fibre + protein act as buffers	Extent and order varies, depending on source	Addition of Ca increases Fe binding. Presence and concentration of endogenous minerals influences binding

[a], pH alters the extent of binding in all cases; ns, non-specific; s, specific; ↑, increase. NI, no information.
Compiled from Camire & Clydesdale (1981).

TABLE 3
Reported values for digestibility of fibre fractions in humans

Fibre source	Digested (% reduction in gut)
Cellulose	0–77·6
Ileostomy patients	15·5
Hemicellulose	50–96
Ileostomy patients	72·5
Pectin	99–100
Lignin	0
NSP	69–84
Examples of fibre from specific foods:-	
Apple	57
Banana (NSP)	85–92
Carrot, celery,	63
Cabbage	63, 42
Cereal	0–6
Lettuce	25
Orange	24
Potato (NSP)	94–99

NSP, non-starch polysaccharide.
Compiled from Ali *et al.* (1981) and Cummings & Englyst (1987).

the equivocal data. A major variable in *in-vivo* experiments is the length of time of the experiment, in view of the propensity of animals to adapt to dietary change with time. Balance studies in excess of 6–8 weeks have indicated that fibre has little effect on mineral availability. Initial reductions in mineral availability may occur, but it is though that the colonic microflora adapts to the increased fibre load. Fermentation of the additional fibre may release bound minerals allowing them to be absorbed by the colon.

This theme is also pursued by Ali *et al.* (1981) who outline the variability of fibre breakdown in the colon (Table 3). Whilst hardly any lignin is broken down, all pectin, most hemicellulose and about 50% of the cellulose disappears in the human gut. They cite other studies in which hemicellulose increased zinc excretion, cellulose less so and pectin not at all. A study by Cummings *et al.* (1979) showed pectin to be fermented in the human gut with no overall effect on calcium balance. Some values for the digestibility of dietary fibre fractions in humans taken from these two publications are shown in Table 3.

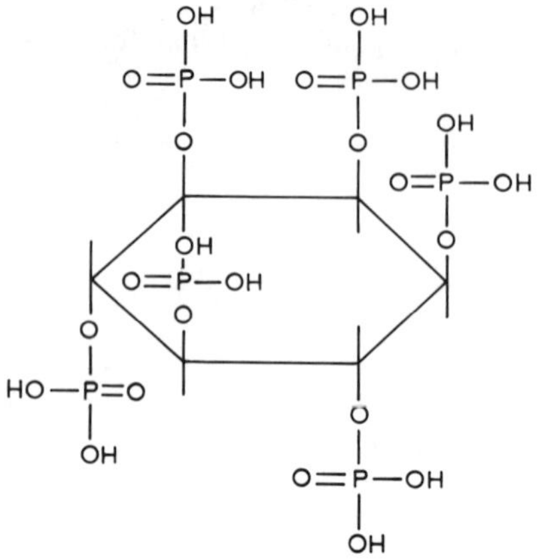

FIG. 2.   *Myo*-inositol hexaphosphate: unionized.

Phytate

Phytic acid is a term used generally to describe the phosphate esters of *myo*-inositol, but it has now become synonymous with the commonly encountered hexaphosphate (Fig. 2). Chiefly of vegetable origin, its main function appears to be as a phosphate storage for the developing seedling; consequently, it is most abundant in cereal grains, oilseeds, legumes etc. (Nolan *et al.*, 1987).

Phytic acid has 12 ionizable hydrogens of which six are quite strongly acid and three very weakly so. Ionization occurs over the range pH 2–12. The compound is extensively ionized at intestinal pH (pH 6–8). It is this property that enables it to bind minerals within the intestine and to form mineral complexes within the plants from which it originates.

A number of possible structures for metal phytate complexes have been proposed, including simple chelation by one phosphate group (Fig. 3(a)), complexation between two or more phosphate groups of the same molecule (Fig. 3(b)), or different ones to give polymeric structures (Fig. 3(c)). Increased pH increases the number of sites available for binding. The mono- and di-metal complexes are fairly soluble, but polymetal phytates are insoluble (Nolan, *et al.* (1987). The types predominating depend on pH and concentration.

According to Davies & Reid (1979), in-vitro studies show that phytate forms stable complexes with divalent ionic solutions with stability in the order Cu $>$ Zn $>$ Co $>$ Mn $>$ Fe $>$ Ca. They suggested that an insoluble calcium–zinc–phytate complex can form at around pH 6·0 in which zinc

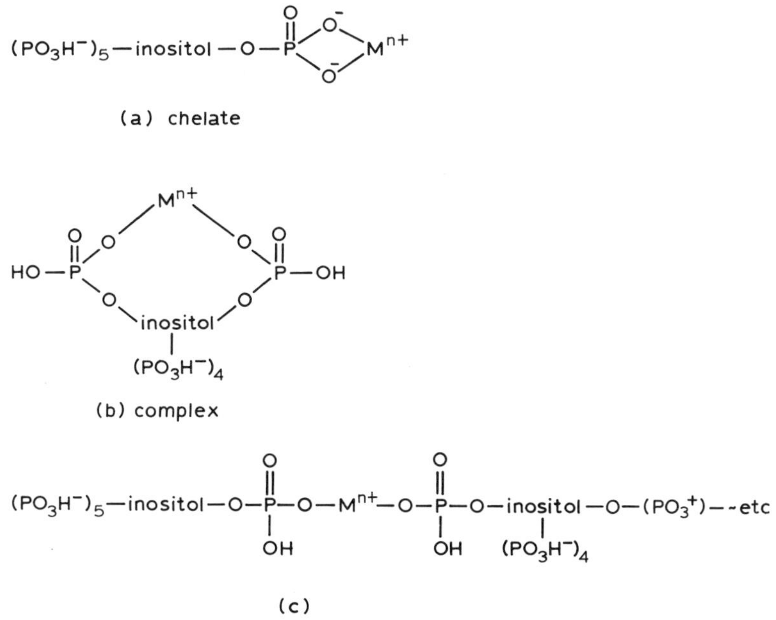

$$(PO_3H^-)_5 - \text{inositol} - O - \overset{\displaystyle O}{\underset{\displaystyle O^-}{\overset{\|}{P}}} \overset{O^-}{\underset{O^-}{<}} M^{n+}$$

(a) chelate

$$HO - \overset{\displaystyle O}{\overset{\|}{P}} \overset{O}{\diagdown} \overset{M^{n+}}{\diagup} \overset{O}{\diagdown} \overset{O}{\underset{\|}{P}} - OH$$
$$\overset{O}{\diagdown}_{\text{inositol}} \overset{O}{\diagup}$$
$$(PO_3H^-)_4$$

(b) complex

$$(PO_3H^-)_5 - \text{inositol} - O - \overset{\displaystyle O}{\underset{\displaystyle OH}{\overset{\|}{P}}} - O - M^{n+} - O - \overset{\displaystyle O}{\underset{\displaystyle OH}{\overset{\|}{P}}} - O - \text{inositol} - O - (PO_3^+) - \text{-etc}$$
$$(PO_3H^-)_4$$

(c)

FIG. 3. Postulated phytate-polycation interaction: (a) behaviour of a single phosphate group; (b) behaviour of two phosphate groups on the same molecule; and (c) behaviour of two single phosphate groups on adjacent phytate molecules (adapted from Nolan *et al.*, 1987). M^{n+}, metal.

predominates and that this accounted for a calcium-exacerbated binding of zinc by phytate. In a review of mineral–phytate interactions, Mills (1985) stresses the vulnerability of zinc and the antagonism of calcium which he concludes acts by affecting the rate of phytate hydrolysis catalysed by mucosal phytases.

On the other hand, Lyon (1984) demonstrated that phytate binds minerals in the order Zn $>$ Fe $>$ Ca $>$ Mg $>$ Cu. Copper did not readily form phytate salts. This is contrary to the earlier findings discussed above. Lyon (1984) suggests that copper is preferentially bound by solubilizing ligands within the diet. This concept is supported by Mills (1985), who quotes the ability of some amino acids to sequester minerals from phytate in the order Cu $>$ Cd $>$ Mn $>$ Zn $>$ Pb.

Lyon (1984) reports that ligands capable of removing minerals from phytate, include: citric acid (sequesters Fe $>$ Zn $>$ Ca $>$ Mg); histidine (Mg $>$ Zn $>$ Fe $>$ Ca), and ascorbic acid and lactose (in both cases,

Mg $>$ Fe $>$ Ca $>$ Zn, but not very effectively). As phytate has a greater affinity for minerals than most other fibre fractions, it follows that those ligands capable of sequestering minerals from phytate may do so with other fibre fractions. Other ligands capable of forming soluble complexes with minerals within the intestine include keto sugars, polyols, the bicarbonate ion and polypeptides.

So far as animal experiments are concerned, dietary calcium, iron and zinc requirements were found to increase with raised phytate intake in chicks and rats, and rickets has been induced in dogs fed on a high phytate diet (although the validity of using a carnivorous species for this type of study is questionable). However, more recent studies have produced conflicting reports of the role of phytate in binding dietary iron: this may be because of the high bioavailability of iron from monoferric phytate (Maga, 1982).

It has been concluded that the iron in monoferric phytate is also available in man. Wheat bran was found by Sandberg *et al.* (1982) to reduce zinc absorption and to increase apparent iron absorption in man. They presumed these effects were due to phytate in the bran being present as monoferric phytate. These results were consistent with work *in vitro* by Platt & Clydesdale (1987), who assumed a soluble iron phytate complex to be monoferric phytate. Addition of calcium and zinc decreases solubility.

Several reports indicate that adaptation to high phytate diets can occur and that poor mineral availability of such diets is a temporary phenomenon. In addition, certain processes can improve the availability of minerals from high phytate foods. Figure 4 shows the improvement of 'availability' of iron (measured by in vitro solubility) in a traditional sorghum-based weaning food by a combination treatment of milling, soaking, germination and fermentation.

MINERAL INTERACTIONS IN THE GUT

In a normal diet, although only a few food items may be involved in each meal, the number of nutritional constituents is very much larger and greatly increases as digestion breaks down complex molecules into simpler ones. This population of chemical species within the gastrointestinal tract is added to by endogenous secretions. Variation in any of these compounds must have some effect on the intestinal milieu, because all of them contribute something towards the physical and chemical environment of

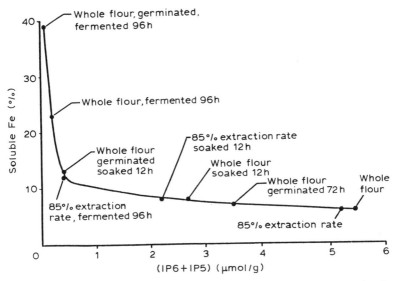

FIG. 4. The relationship of iron availability (% soluble iron after in-vitro digestion) to phytate (sum of inositol hexa- and pentaphosphates: IP6 and IP5 respectively) of a traditional African weaning-food based on sorghum, during the course of its multi-stage preparation. (From Svanberg & Sandberg (1989). Reproduced by permission from Royal Society of Chemistry, Cambridge).

the lumen of the gut. An example of this is the effect of ascorbic acid on iron absorption. Ascorbic acid greatly improves iron absorption from dietary non-haem sources, which would otherwise be poor (Cook, 1983).

With non-minerals

The presence of meat also increases the absorption of non-haem iron and of purified haem. This 'meat factor' is thought to be due to the production of solubilizing ligands during digestion (Slatkavitz & Clydesdale, 1988). Support for this theory comes from Van-Campen (1973), who found that amino acids that were structurally capable of forming tridentate ligands increased iron transfer across ligated rat intestine. The L and D forms of amino acids worked equally well, indicating that the iron complexes were not being absorbed via amino acid transport mechanisms which are specific for L-amino acids. Flynn *et al.* (1984) working *in vitro* showed that the greater the stability constant, the greater the tendency for ion–amino acid complexation to occur. However, some of these depended on high pH and may not be relevant to foods (or physiological conditions), but L-cysteine was able to complex iron within a physiological pH range.

The absorption of iron is enhanced by the presence of food constituents that form soluble complexes, such as ascorbic acid (described above) and fructose. Inhibition is caused by oxalates and tannates amongst others, which form insoluble complexes (Crosby, 1968). The loss of calcium and magnesium availability by reaction with fatty acids to form insoluble soaps has already been mentioned.

Linkswiler *et al.* (1981) reported that calcium balance at a range of intakes was maintained in young adults given a low but adequate level of protein in their diets. When calcium and phosphate were held at these levels and protein was increased, calcium losses occurred in the urine. (The calciuric effect of protein has been described earlier in this chapter.) Spencer (1986) and Linkswiler *et al.* (1981) claimed that this effect was due to using purified proteins. The latter authors suggested that the use of purified proteins allows phosphate levels to be held constant and they claimed a 'natural' protein source would have phosphate associated with it and therefore any increase in protein would increase phosphate. They found that when meat was used as a protein source no significant change in urinary calcium was seen.

With minerals

Mineral–mineral interactions of relevance to human nutrition take place at a number of levels, including: in the food prior to consumption, within the lumen of the gut, at the mucosal surface of the gut, within the mucosal cells and within the circulatory system, tissues and organs. Here, prime consideration will be given to those processes that occur from the lumen of the gut until transfer across the mucosa.

The term mineral–mineral interaction is somewhat misleading as very few minerals exert an effect directly upon another mineral. Most interactions are mediated through an organic substance. An exception perhaps is phosphate which may form insoluble precipitates with calcium in the duodenum.

Zinc and iron

Influences both of iron on zinc and zinc on iron have been reported in the literature. Dietary supplementation with iron and zinc preparations are now very common, so the repercussions of both these interactions are of consumer interest.

The interaction of zinc and iron absorption has been reported in animal studies; in particular, iron absorption was markedly reduced at high zinc levels (Davis, 1980). An example of this interaction was reported by Settlemire & Matrone, (1967), who fed rats with a high zinc diet (0·75%) and noted that blood zinc levels more than doubled, while anaemia developed. This was associated with increased faecal iron.

In another experiment with rats using similar dietary zinc levels, Coleman & Matrone (1969) reported that an iron-poor ferritin was produced. However, *de novo* ferritin synthesis was not affected by zinc toxicity as rats were able to incorporate intravenous iron into ferritin. This finding suggests that zinc interaction with iron occurs prior to transfer across the serosal membrane of the intestinal epithelium.

Solomons (1986) complains that definitive and well designed studies of this subject are yet to be conducted but he acknowledges a consensus of evidence suggesting that excess iron inhibits zinc uptake. For example, excess iron has been shown to inhibit zinc absorption in humans but at a dose much larger than any likely to be present in a normal diet (Valberg *et al.*, 1984). Effects of supplemental iron on zinc absorption and other nutrients in human diets are shown in Table 4. Similar studies of the effects of supplemental zinc are shown in Table 5.

The zinc, iron and copper triplet
The interaction of iron and zinc should not be discussed without reference to copper. The role of copper was first noted when livestock, given supplemental copper in the belief that higher doses of this essential mineral would stimulate growth, developed toxicity symptoms, including a form of anaemia (Davis, 1980). Davis extensively reviewed the zinc, iron and copper interaction, noting that excess in one or two of the triplet depresses absorption of the other(s). He suggested that competition between copper, iron and zinc for transferrin and metallothionein were probably the main sites of absorptive interaction. Other workers have shown that nutritional status with respect to these three minerals can have profound effects on the absorption, utilization and toxicity of other minerals or heavy metals.

Greger & Johnson (1981) suggested that poor iron mobilization may occur in the body due to copper-deficient caeruloplasmin (an enzyme which contains copper and is necessary for iron mobilization from stores of ferritin). This theme was explored earlier in a review by Van-Campen (1970); he cites animal studies supporting a mutual antagonism of copper, zinc and iron in rats and other animals, including:

(1) Supplementary copper alleviates the symptoms of zinc toxicity in rats.

TABLE 4

Effect of supplemental iron on mineral absorption in human studies

Subjects	Method	Details of study (effect monitored on)	Findings	Reference
9 Young women	30 day metabolic balance	22 mg Fe/day in controlled western-type diet (Ca, Mg, P, Zn, Mn, Cu)	Most minerals in positive balance, Mn and Cu in negative balance	White & Gynne (1971)
Adults	Change in plasma concentration	Fe salts or haem: pharmaceutical doses (Zn)	Zn absorption reduced but less so in the presence of haem	Solomons & Jacobs (1981)
Adults	Change in plasma concentration	Fe^{2+} or Fe^{3+} pharmaceutical doses, with or without vitamin C + Zn (Zn)	$Fe^{2+} \ggg Fe^{3+}$ in reducing Zn absorption. (Fe^{3+} + vitamin C) = Fe^{2+}	Solomons et al. (1983)
9 Adults	Whole body radioisotope count	Fe or Cu on extrinsic ^{65}Zn, 'in a turkey meal or in $ZnCl_2$ solution	Fe:Zn (10:1 and 5:1) reduced Zn absorption from Zn solution, but not from Zn incorporated into turkey meal. Cu: no effect	Valberg et al. (1984)
291, 1 year infants	Change in serum concentration over 4 months	Placebo or Fe supplement (Zn, Cu)	No effect	Yip et al. (1985)

TABLE 5
Effect of supplemental zinc on mineral absorption in human studies

Subjects	Method	Details of study (effect monitored on)	Findings	Reference
11 Adolescent girls	30 Day metabolic balance	11·5 or 14·7 mg Zn/day (Cu, Fe and Mn balance)	No effect, except, although Cu remained positive, it was lower at higher Zn level	Greger et al. (1978)
Adult women	18 Day metabolic balance	8–24 mg Zn/day (Cu)	No effect	Taper et al. (1980)
Adults	12 Weeks blood biochemistry	45–200 mg Zn/day (Fe, Mg, Ca, Zn, Cu, Pb)	No effect, except that Cu and Pb levels reduced, Zn increased	Abdulla & Svensson (1982)

(2) Excess zinc reduced the activity of the copper enzyme cytochrome oxidase in rats; this activity was restored by supplementary copper.

(3) Supplementary zinc or iron-relieved copper toxicity in pigs.

Thus it appears that in cases where diets are deficient in one mineral of the triplet, toxic symptoms were evoked by relatively low doses of another. The evidence suggests that a competitive interaction between copper and zinc occurs at the intestinal and/or absorptive level.

The situation in humans might be predicted from animals studies, although studies in humans have proved equivocal. Therefore, Taper *et al.* (1980) found no significant effect of zinc on copper uptake in women at physiological levels, while Greger *et al.* (1978) found that excess zinc depressed copper absorption in adolescent girls (Table 5).

Calcium and zinc
Using whole body counts to follow ^{65}Zn uptake in rats, Heth & Hoekstra (1965) found that calcium depressed zinc retention over a higher than normal range of calcium intakes (0·6–1·8% of diet). The effect may have operated either by decreasing zinc absorption or increasing zinc turnover. Intravenous zinc was better retained than supplemental dietary zinc at high calcium levels in the diet (i.e. body turnover of zinc was reduced). These results implied an interaction at the intestinal absorption level.

Spencer *et al.* (1965) were not able to demonstrate a calcium—zinc antagonism in man during experiments conducted at levels covering a normal dietary range. Their results were supported by Monsen & Cook (1976) at dietary levels and by Steinhardt-Bour *et al.* (1984) who found no interaction between zinc and calcium or zinc and phosphate at moderate intakes (see Table 6).

Calcium and iron
Chapman & Campbell (1957) suggested that for anaemic rats the Ca:Fe ratio in a diet needed to be large (these authors used 0·7% calcium in the diet) before iron absorption was reduced. They concluded that the interaction was due to saturation of the 'mucosal iron block' by excess calcium. However, the mucosal block theory has since been called into question. In contrast, Barton *et al.* (1983) fed phlebotomized (bled) rats diets containing calcium only slightly in excess of normal levels. Blood and tissue analyses of the cadavers suggested a dose-related inhibition of iron absorption by calcium.

The interaction of iron and calcium may be further complicated by the

TABLE 6
Effect of supplemental calcium on mineral absorption in human studies

Subjects	Method	Details of study (effect monitored on)	Findings	Reference
Adults	20–30 Day metabolic balance	268 or 1983 mg Ca/day (Zn)	No effect	Spencer et al. (1965)
34 Adults	Radio-iron tracer	Mineral salts in semisynthetic meal (Fe)	Ca and P together reduced Fe absorption: no effect separately	Monsen & Cook (1976)
Adult males	39 Day balance plasma levels	Combinations of high and low Ca and P in controlled diet with vitamin D (Zn, Fe, Cu, transferrin, ferritin)	No effect, except high Ca, high P reduced Fe and Cu absorption	Snedeker et al. (1982)
Young adult males	75 Day metabolic balance	Combinations of high and low Ca and P in controlled diet (Zn, Fe and Cu balance)	No effect, except high polyphosphate reduced Fe balance	Steinhardt–Bour et al. (1984)
13 Postmenopausal women	Whole body radioisotope count	Post-meal Ca or Ca + P supplement on extrinsic ^{65}Zn and ^{59}Fe (Zn, Fe)	Fe absorption reduced by both supplements, but not Zn absorption	Dawson–Hughes et al. (1986)
8 Adult males	18–24 day metabolic balance	Low, normal and high range doses of Ca (Cd, Cu, Mn, Zn balance)	No effect at any Ca level	Spencer et al. (1979)

action of phosphate, but here again the situation is far from clear. Mahoney & Hendricks (1978) found that phosphate salts, particularly polyphosphates, depressed iron absorption and haemoglobin concentrations in rats. They also claimed that phosphates depressed calcium absorption in growing but not in mature rats. Zemel & Bidari (1983), whilst studying the effects of phosphates on zinc absorption in weanling rats, found that zinc absorption was reduced by polyphosphates and more so if calcium was present. Orthophosphates had little effect. However, Zemel & Bidari (1983) reported only slight, insignificant effects on iron absorption by phosphates in combination with high and low calcium intakes.

An earlier experiment lends support to the results of Zemel & Bidari. Chapman & Campbell (1957), in the experiment on anaemic rats described above, showed that two levels of phosphate did not promote the effect of calcium on iron absorption. Using postmenopausal women as subjects, Dawson-Hughes *et al.* (1986) found that calcium and phosphate did not affect zinc retention, but did reduce iron retention. Their results suggested calcium, rather than phosphate, was responsible for impaired iron utilization.

Calcium and magnesium
Information on the interaction of calcium and magnesium is scarce. In an early review, Hoekstra (1964) reported that excess magnesium had a depressing effect on calcium absorption and that very high calcium and phosphate intakes (up to 2·5% and 1·7% of diet respectively) could decrease magnesium absorption in guinea pigs and in chicks. However, the data from animal experiments is equivocal. The effects of phosphate on magnesium have been reported as increasing its absorption in guinea pigs and depressing its absorption in rats (Tansy, 1971).

Possible mechanisms for competition between minerals at the gut absorptive interface
A number of researchers have attempted to explain or predict mineral absorptive interactions using known properties of the minerals involved. Both *in vitro* and *in vivo* mineral interactions have been examined with respect to pH, temperature, redox potential, concentration, solubility, electronic configuration and structure, reaction rates and stability constants. The list of physicochemical variants is almost as long as the variation in dietary composition.

From his studies *in vitro*, Clydesdale (1988) concluded that solubility and charge density are the main determinants of mineral bioavailability in the gut. He described how these change with pH and the rate of hydrolysis of soluble mineral hydrates. Hill & Matrone (1970), in a much cited piece of research, presented a hypothesis that implied that metal ions with similar electronic configurations would compete antagonistically in biological systems. Their experiments, carried out *in vivo*, supported this hypothesis and other workers have since followed it up.

The solubility of metal complexes is of paramount importance in their absorption by the intestinal mucosa and this is influenced by prevailing conditions. Solubility aids the movement of mineral complexes through the lumen contents and facilitates transport; it is essential for diffusion. Ligands present in the intestine can either enhance or inhibit absorption. Those that enhance absorption have sufficient affinity for the mineral to form soluble complexes capable of absorption (Clydesdale, 1983).

Iron and other minerals
On the subject of metal ions with similar electronic configurations competing for absorption, Flanagan *et al.* (1980) showed that mice made anaemic by dietary means had increased absorption of iron, cobalt, manganese and nickel as well as zinc, cadmium and lead. Phlebotomized mice had increased absorption of iron and cobalt only. However, in each case iron absorption increased to a greater extent than the electronically similar transition elements, indicating some absorptive specificity towards iron in anaemia, but not sufficiently so as to prevent competition from these other metals.

Calcium and other minerals
The relative complexing abilities of phosphates with calcium from *in vitro* experiments are described by Van-Wazer & Callis (1958). Chain and ring phosphates can form relatively stable soluble complexes with calcium. However, they may polymerize and become insoluble. The extent of polymerization and its onset depends on the presence of other ionic species, their concentration and the pH of the solution. Orthophosphates tend to form insoluble calcium complexes.

THE RELEVANCE OF THE EVIDENCE FOR CONSUMER NUTRITION

In a review written over 20 years ago, Hoekstra (1964) made comments which still have relevance today. He succinctly describes the problems

facing investigators of mineral interactions. He emphasized the questionable relevance of simplistic models to whole diets, but also suggested that
experimental designs that attempt to incorporate many variables, especially at limited levels of variability, would prove difficult to interpret, even
with sophisticated statistical and computing techniques. Experimental
models that manipulate only a few selected variables within a highly
variable and complex matrix can only accurately be interpreted if the
chosen variables are those that account for a significant proportion of the
variability within the model. There are 14 or so nutrient minerals, all of
which may participate in interaction. Also present in any diet are many
more trace metals, which, unless they exhibit toxicity, tend to be ignored.

These views were echoed by Mills (1985) who concluded that much of
present knowledge is based on circumstantial evidence. He expressed
satisfaction that the trend for research was now towards the examination
of interactions within a nutritional framework instead of towards demonstrating the existence of interactions regardless of nutritional consequence.

Inappropriate experimentation is also criticized by Clydesdale (1988) in
a concise review of mineral interaction from a physicochemical viewpoint.
He criticized much of the experimental methodology employed in studies
of this topic, particularly those examining mineral–fibre interactions involving two or more minerals. He reports experiments where the binding
of each mineral by fibre and to what degree has been dependent on the
order of the addition of minerals during the experiment. He also complains that the effects of pH and redox potential are too often ignored in
experiments of this type.

It is clear from the literature that mineral interactions are subject to a
huge number of variables, which make experimental design difficult and
the evaluation of results intellectually demanding. In this review circumstantial evidence is presented that, for the most part, has mineral interactions as its only common theme. The lengths of studies vary, as do the
number, sex, size, age, species and state of health of subjects. The administration of test doses varies, as do the diets containing them. This review
serves to provide information on a range of topics related to mineral
interaction in food, within the intestine and at or about the absorptive
interface and perhaps more than anything indicates our lack of knowledge
to base advice on mineral supplementation.

It would require extensive facilities to set up a model that permitted the
controlled manipulation of chosen variables whilst monitoring the effects
on consequential variables. The number of potentially reactive chemical
species appearing during digestion experiments *in vitro* is increased by

orders of magnitude *in vivo*, when the multitude of variable effects of absorptive mechanisms are included. The use of simplified experimental models only allows information to be gathered piecemeal from which a general picture may be built up. Unfortunately, there is always the danger that the simplification applied may remove all relevance to practical nutritional applications.

In a novel approach to the problem, Robb *et al.* (1986) designed a computer simulation of chemical speciation under a given set of approximate intestinal conditions. The method relied on a number of assumptions, some of major significance (e.g. no endogenous secretions and total hydrolysis of proteins and carbohydrates to amino acids and monosaccharides). Despite this, the authors concluded that the technique is applicable to the gastrointestinal condition and with sophistication could indicate useful areas of research. Such computer guided research could employ simple experimental models to explore those parameters that account for most of the variability within the model, and yet not discount the inherent variability of the global system.

In many of the studies reported in the literature, the only mention of bacterial activity was of the fermentation of indigestible material by the colonic microflora. It may be that data obtained from sterile in-vitro experiments may have little relevance to conditions within a colonized intestine: indeed, the lower ileum in health may contain a flourishing flora. Binding of minerals by bacterial slimes may occur, but the nutritional use of minerals and other dietary components by bacteria is probably in equilibrium with those released from dead cells. Nevertheless, they contribute enzymes into the gut lumen, which may assist in releasing bound minerals within the intestine.

From the literature reviewed here, it would appear that a mutual antagonism exists among copper, zinc and iron and that the intakes of these metals should be in specific proportion. It is also known that cobalt, manganese and nickel competitively interact with iron and therefore indirectly interact with copper and zinc. Calcium appears to depress iron absorption in the presence of phosphate and therefore indirectly affects all the aforementioned. This scenario is further modified when dietary fibre is included in the diet. Other modifying factors are the presence of ascorbic acid and meat. It is clear that much work needs to be done before accurate predictions can be made concerning the absorptive fates of minerals in normal diets.

As far as the consumer is concerned, the data do not contraindicate modest supplementation of the diet with single minerals (1 to 2 × the recommended daily allowance (RDA) to treat mineral deficiencies (or perceived deficiencies). However, it would seem logical, in view of the consensus views that mineral–mineral interactions have been demonstrated *in vitro* and in animal experiments under some conditions, that mineral supplements should be balanced whenever possible in the form of well formulated multi-mineral preparations. So long as the minerals are present in the formulation as complexed preparations this should prevent the formation of refractile polymineral and other soluble forms.

Bender (1988) discusses the availability of dietary supplements, popular attitudes toward them and the impact of media attention upon their sale. The range of products is enormous and increasing. Some of the reasons why consumers take mineral supplements are based on well-accepted nutritional principles. For example, slimmers might augment a low-energy diet where minerals might otherwise be low, or iron-deficiency anaemia might be treated using iron supplements. However, evidence, for example, that dietary supplements such as zinc are able to cure or alleviate the common cold is inconclusive. Real and perceived reasons for single-mineral supplementation of the diet are shown in Table 7, with the main human groups involved and minerals whose absorption may be jeopardized as a consequence. From the data reviewed, modest supplementation appears to do little harm, but when levels get excessive any effects on absorption of other minerals will be exacerbated.

CONCLUSION

This review of the literature on mineral interactions has laid particular emphasis on calcium, iron, magnesium, and zinc, which are known to be limiting in the diets of vulnerable groups of people. The inconclusive and fragmentary nature of the data appeared to be a strong feature and was acknowledged by a number of the researchers themselves. In particular, the complexity of the intestinal environment during digestion was blamed for the general lack of understanding of the interactions taking place.

The data in the literature indicates that, on the whole, single mineral supplements at modest levels (1 to 2 × RDA) do not seem to have large effects on the availability of other nutrients, but the indications from in-vitro and animal experiments indicate that the effects of large doses, as sometimes advocated by nutrition enthusiasts, may jeopardize absorption. In particular, high doses of iron may depress zinc intake and *vice versa*. High doses of calcium may limit magnesium absorption and depress iron

TABLE 7
Some consumers' reasons for dietary supplementation with certain minerals

Mineral	Reason (real or perceived)	Main human group involved	Possible inhibition of absorption by excess
Ca	High fibre diet	All	
	Low intake dairy products	All	
	Prevention osteoporosis	Postmenopausal women	Fe Zn Mg
	Prevention of Ca loss (teeth, bones)	Pregnant and lactating women	
	Prevention hypertension[a]	Middle-aged, elderly	
	Arthritis, muscle and joint pains	All	
Fe	Prevention of anaemia (or 'tiredness')	Menstruating women Pregnant and lactating women	Cu
		Vegetarians	Zn
		Children	
Mg[b]	Premenstrual tension	Women	
	Menstrual cramps		
	Toxaemia of pregnancy		
	Atherosclerosis angina	Middle aged, elderly	Ca
	Irregular heartbeat	All	
	Alcoholism	Alcoholics	
	Kidney stones	All	
	Insomnia	All	
	Hyperactivity	Children	
Zn	Colds, 'flu, viral illness	All	
	Post-viral fatigue	All	
	Prevention prostate problems	Men	Fe
	Skin complaints, e.g. eczema	All	Cu
	Loss of appetite	All	
	Anorexia nervosa	Teenage girls	

[a] High blood pressure: this use may increase in the future as more information becomes available.
[b] Widely used in the USA and parts of the EC, but not greatly in the UK.

and even, perhaps zinc absorption. Effects of high doses have not been sufficiently studied in animals and hardly any clinical trials have been reported. The public should be made aware of the gaps in our knowledge. Health conscious individuals who wish to improve their diet with supplements must choose whatever they feel suits their particular circumstance, according to information in their possession. Often the information that the consumer receives is from less well qualified sources and is misleading. There is an increasing need for nutrition scientists to take more responsibility for consumer nutrition education.

REFERENCES

Abdulla, M. & Svensson, S. (1982). Influence of oral zinc intake on other elements. In *Trace Element Metabolism in Man and Animals*, pp. 584–7 [J.M. Howell, J.M. Gawthorne and C.L. White, editors]. Heidelberg, FRG: Springer-Verlang.

Ali, R., Staub, H., Coccodrilli, G. Jr & Schanbacher, L. (1981). Nutritional significance of dietary fibre: effect on nutrient bioavailability and selected gastrointestinal function. *Journal of Agricultural and Food Chemistry* **29**, 465–72.

Barton, J.C., Conrad, M.E. & Parmley, R.T. (1983). Calcium inhibition of inorganic iron in rats. *Gastroenterology* **84**, 90–101.

Bender, A.E. (1988). Dietary supplements. *British Nutrition Foundation Nutrition Bulletin* **13**, 78–84.

Bender, A.E. (1989). Nutritional significance of bioavailability. In *Nutrient Availability: Chemical and Biological Aspects*, pp. 3–9 [D.A.T. Southgate, I.T. Johnson and G.R. Fenwick, editors]. Cambridge: Royal Society of Chemistry.

Briscoe, A.M. & Ragan, C. (1967). Relation of magnesium to calcium in human blood serum. *Nature* **214**, 1126–7.

Camire, A.L. & Clydesdale, F.M. (1981). Effect of pH and heat treatment on the binding of calcium, magnesium, zinc and iron to wheat bran and fractions of dietary fibre. *Journal of Food Science* **46**, 548–51.

Chapman, D.G. & Campbell, J.A. (1957). Effect of calcium and phosphorus salts on the utilization of iron by anaemic rats. *British Journal of Nutrition* **11**, 127–33.

Clydesdale, F.M. (1983). Physicochemical determinants of iron bioavailability. *Food Technology* **37**, 133–8.

Clydesdale, F.M. (1988). Mineral interactions in foods. In *Nutrient Interactions*, IFT Basic Symposium Series, pp. 73–113 [J. Erdman and C.E. Bodwell, editors]. New York: Marcel Dekker Inc.

Coleman, C.B. & Matrone, G. (1969). In-vivo effect of zinc on iron induced ferritin synthesis in rat liver. *Biochemica et Biophysica Acta* **177**, 106–12.

Conrad, M.E. & Schade, S.G. (1968). Ascorbic acid chelates in iron absorption: a role for hydrochloric acid and bile. *Gastroenterology* **55**, 35–45.

Cook, J.D. (1983). Determinants on non-heme iron absorption in man. *Food Technology* **37** (10), 124–6.

Dietary Mineral Supplementation and Bioavailability

Crosby, W.H. (1968). Control of iron absorption by intestinal luminal factors. *American Journal of Clinical Nutrition* **21**, 1189–93.

Cummings, J.H. & Englyst, H.N. (1987). Fermentation in the human large intestine and the available substrates. *American Journal of Clinical Nutrition* **45**, 1243–55.

Cummings, J.H., Southgate, D.A.T., Branch, W.J., Wiggins, H.S., Houston, H., Jenkins, D.J.A., Jinraj, T. & Hill, M.J. (1979). The digestion of pectin in the human gut and its effect on calcium absorption and large bowel function. *British Journal of Nutrition* **41**, 477–85.

Davenport, H.W. (1979). *Physiology of the Digestive Tract*, 4th ed. Chicago: Year Book Medical Publishers.

Davis, G.K. (1980). Microelement interactions of zinc, copper and iron in mammalian species. In *Micronutrient Interactions: Vitamins, Minerals and Hazardous Elements*, pp. 130–9 [O.A. Levander and L. Cheng, editors]. New York: New York Academy of Science.

Davies, N.T. (1978). The effects of dietary fibre on mineral availability. In *Dietary Fibre: Current Developments of Importance to Health*, pp. 113–21 [K.W. Heaton, editor]. London: John Libbey.

Davies, N.T. & Reid, H. (1979). An evaluation of the phytate, zinc, copper, iron and manganese contents of and zinc availability from soya based textured vegetable proteins, meat substitute or meat extenders. *British Journal of Nutrition* **41**, 579–89.

Dawson-Hughes, B., Seligson, F.H. & Hughes, V.A. (1986). Effects of calcium carbonate and hydroxyapatite on zinc and iron retention in post menopausal women. *American Journal of Clinical Nutrition* **44**, 83–8.

Dreher, M.L. (1987). *Handbook of Dietary Fiber: An Applied Approach*. New York: Marcel Dekker Inc.

Eastwood, M.A. & Passmore, R. (editors) (1986). *Davidson and Passmore: Human Nutrition and Dietetics*, 8th ed. Edinburgh: Churchill Livingstone.

Englyst, H.N. & Cummings, J.H. (1988). Improved method for measurement of dietary fiber as the non-starch polysaccharides in plant foods. *Journal of the Association of Official Analytical Chemists* **71**, 808–14.

Erdman, J.W. Jr (1981). Bioavailability of trace minerals from cereals and legumes. *Cereal Chemistry* **58**, 21–5.

Evans, G.W. & Johnson, P.E. (1978). Copper and zinc binding ligands in the intestinal mucosa. In *Trace Element Metabolism in Man and Animals*, 3rd ed., pp. 98–105 [M. Kirchgessner, editor]. Weihenstephan FDR: Arbeitskreig fur Tierernahrsforschung.

Flanagan, P.R., Haist, J. & Valberg, L.S. (1980). Comparative effects of iron deficiency induced bleeding and a low iron diet on the intestinal absorptive interactions of iron, cobalt, manganese, zinc, lead and cadmium. *Journal of Nutrition* **110**, 1754–63.

Flynn, S.M., Clydesdale, F.M. & Zajicek, O.T. (1984). Complexation, stability and behaviour of L-cysteine and L-lysine with different iron sources. *Journal of Food Protection* **47**, 36–40.

Forth, W. (1970). Absorption of iron and chemically related metals in vitro and in vivo; the specificity of an iron binding system in the intestinal mucosa of the rat. In *Trace Element Nutrition in Animals*, pp. 298–309 [C.F. Mills, editor]. Edinburgh: Livingstone.

Greger, J.L. (1987). Mineral bioavailability: new concepts. *Nutrition Today* **2** (4), 4–9.

Greger, J.L. & Johnson, M.A. (1981). Effect of dietary tin on zinc, copper and iron utilisation by rats. *Food and Cosmetic Toxicology* **19**, 163–6.

Greger, J.L., Zaikis, S.C., Abernathy, R.P., Bennett, O.A. & Huffman, J. (1978). Zinc, nitrogen, copper, iron and manganese balance in adolescent females fed two levels of zinc. *Journal of Nutrition* **108**, 1449–56.

Hill, C.H. & Matrone, G. (1970). Chemical parameters in the study of in vivo and in vitro interactions of transitions elements. *Federation Proceedings* **29**, 1474–81.

Heth, D.A. & Hoekstra, W.G. (1965). I. A procedure to determine zinc-65 absorption and the antagonistic effect of calcium in a practical diet. *Journal of Nutrition* **85**, 367–74.

Hoekstra, W.G. (1964). Recent observations on mineral interrelationships. *Federation Proceedings* **23**, 1068–75.

James, W.P.T., Branch, W.J. & Southgate, D.A.T. (1978). Calcium binding by dietary fibre. *Lancet* **i**, 638–9.

Kohn, S.E. (1975). Ion binding on polyuranates-alginate and pectin. *Pure and Applied Chemistry* **42**, 371. (Cited by Clydesdale, 1988).

Linkswiler, H.M., Zemel, M.B., Hegsted, M. & Schuette, S. (1981). Protein-induced hypercalciuria. *Federation Proceedings* **40**, 2429–33.

Lyon, D.B. (1984). Studies on the solubility of calcium, magnesium, zinc and copper in cereal products. *American Journal of Clinical Nutrition* **39**, 190–5.

Maga, J.A. (1982). Phytate: its chemistry, occurrence, food interactions, nutritional significance and methods of analysis. *Journal of Agricultural and Food Chemistry* **30**, 1–9.

Mahoney, A.W. & Hendricks, D.G. (1978). Some effects of different phosphate compounds on iron and calcium absorption. *Journal of Food Science* **43**, 1473–6.

Mills, C.F. (1985). Dietary interactions involving the trace elements. *Annual Review of Nutrition* **5**, 173–93.

Monsen, E.R. & Cook, J.D. (1976). Food iron absorption in human subjects. IV: The effect of calcium and phosphate salts on the absorption of non-heme iron. *American Journal of Clinical Nutrition* **29**, 1142–48.

Nolan, K.B., Duffin, P.A. & McWeeny, D.J. (1987). Effects of phytate on mineral bioavailability. In-vitro studies on Mg^{2+}, Ca^{2+}, Fe^{3+}, Cu^{2+} and Zn^{2+} (also Cd^{2+}) solubility in the presence of phytate. *Journal of the Science of Food and Agriculture* **40**, 79–85.

Pike, R.L. & Brown, M.L. (1983). *Nutrition: An Integrated Approach*, 3rd ed. New York: John Wiley & Sons.

Platt, S.R. & Clydesdale, F.M. (1984). Binding of iron by cellulose, lignin, sodium phytate and β-glucan, alone and in combination, under gastro-intestinal pH conditions. *Journal of Food Science* **49**, 531–5.

Pollack, S., George, J.N., Reba, R.C., Kaufman, R.M. & Crosby, W.H. (1965). The absorption of non-ferrous metals in iron deficiency. *Journal of Clinical Investigation* **44**, 1470–3.

Robb, P., Williams, D.R. & McWeeny, D.J. (1986). Predicted chemical speciation of essential metals in digested foods. *Inorganica Chimica Acta* **125**, 207–12.

Sandberg, A.S., Hasselblad, C., Hasselblad, K. & Hulten, L. (1982). The effect of wheat bran on the absorption of minerals in the small intestine. *British Journal of Nutrition* **48**, 185–91.

Sandstrom, B., Davidsson, L., Kivisto, B., Hasselblad, C. & Cederblad, A. (1987). The effect of vegetables and beet fibre on the absorption of zinc in humans from composite meals. *British Journal of Nutrition* **58**, 49–57.

Sanford, P.A. (1982). *Digestive System Physiology.* London: Edward Arnold.

Scheeman, B.O. (1986). Dietary fibre: physical and chemical properties; methods of analysis and physiological effects. *Food Technology* **40** (2), 104–10.

Settlemire, C.T. & Matrone, G. (1967). In-vivo effect of zinc on iron turnover and lifespan of the erythrocyte. *Journal of Nutrition* **92**, 159–64.

Slatkavitz, C.A. & Clydesdale, F.M. (1988). Solubility of inorganic iron as affected by proteolytic digestion. *American Journal of Clinical Nutrition* **47**, 487–95.

Snedeker, S.M., Smith, S.A. & Greger, J.L. (1982). Effect of dietary calcium and phosphorus levels on the utilisation of iron, copper and zinc by adult males. *Journal of Nutrition* **112**, 135–43.

Solomons, N.W. (1986). Competitive interaction of iron and zinc in the diet: consequences for human nutrition. *Journal of Nutrition* **116**, 927–35.

Solomons, N.W. & Jacobs, R.A. (1981). Studies on the bioavailability of zinc in humans: effects of heme and nonheme iron on the absorption of zinc. *American Journal of Clinical Nutrition* **34**, 475–82.

Solomons, N.W., Marchini, J.S., Duarte-Favaro, R.M., Vannuch, H. & Dutra-de Oliveira, J.E. (1983). Studies on the bioavailability of zinc in humans; intestinal interactions of tin and zin. *American Journal of Clinical Nutrition* **37**, 566–71.

Spencer, H. (1986). Minerals and mineral interactions in human beings. *Journal of the American Dietetic Association* **86**, 864–7.

Spencer, H., Vankinscott, V., Lewin, I. & Samachson, J. (1965). Zinc[65] metabolism during low and high calcium intake in man. *Journal of Nutrition* **86**, 169–77.

Spencer, H., Asmussen, C.R., Holtzman, R.B. & Kramer, L. (1979). Metabolic balances of cadmium, copper, manganese and zinc in man. *American Journal of Clinical Nutrition* **32**, 1869–875.

Steinhardt-Bour, N.S., Soullier, B.A. & Zemel, M.B. (1984). Effect of level and form of phosphorus and level of calcium intake on zinc, iron and copper bioavailability in man. *Nutrition Research* **4**, 371–9.

Svanberg, U. & Sandberg, A.-S. (1989). Improved iron availability in weaning foods using germination and fermentation. In *Nutrient Availability: Chemical and Biological Aspects*, pp. 179–84 [D.A.T. Southgate, I.T. Johnson and G.R. Fenwick, editors]. Cambridge: Royal Society of Chemistry.

Tansy, M.F. (1971). Intestinal absorption of magnesium. In *Intestinal Absorption of Metal Ions, Trace Elements and Radionuclides*, pp. 193–7 [S.C. Skoryna and D. Waldron-Edwards, editors]. Oxford: Pergamon Press.

Taper, J.L., Hinners, M.L. & Ritchey, S.J. (1980). Effect of zinc intake on copper balance in adult females. *American Journal of Clinical Nutrition* **33**, 1077–82.

Toma, R.B. & Curtis, D.J. (1986). Dietary fibre: effect on mineral bioavailability. *Food Technology* **40** (2), 111–16.

Valberg, L.S., Flanagan, P.R. & Chamberlain, M.J. (1984). Effects of iron, tin and copper on zinc absorption in humans. *American Journal of Clinical Nutrition* **40**, 536–41.

Van-Campen, D. (1970). Competition between copper and zinc during absorption. In *Trace Element Metabolism in Animals*, pp. 287–97 [C.F. Mills, editor]. Edinburgh: Livingstone.

Van-Wazer, J.R. & Callis, C.F. (1958). Metal complexing by phosphates. *Chemical Reviews* **58**, 1011–43.

White, H.S. & Gynne, T.N. (1971). Utilisation of inorganic iron by young women eating iron fortified foods. *Journal of the American Dietetic Association* **59** (7), 27–33.

Yip, R., Reeves, J.D., Lonnerdal, B., Keen, C.L. & Dallman, P.R. (1985). Does iron supplementation compromise zinc nutrition in healthy infants? *American Journal of Clinical Nutrition* **42**, 683–7.

Zemel, M.B. & Bidari, M.T. (1983). Zinc, iron and copper availability as affected by orthophosphates, polyphosphates and calcium. *Journal of Food Science* **48**, 567–69, 573.

6

Sugar Myths

Nino M. Binns
Tate & Lyle plc, Sugar Quay, Lower Thames Street,
London, EC3R 6DQ, UK

INTRODUCTION

Sugar is one of the most maligned items of our diet. Perhaps it is only because sweetness is an enjoyable taste that many people think they must feel guilty if they derive enjoyment from foods high in sugar. Certainly any such guilt has been fueled in the past by the writings of a number of fiercely anti-sugar people. The result is that the word 'sugar' provokes an unnecessarily emotional response in the minds of many, especially those of the lay public.

The aim of this paper is to present some facts that will be useful in putting into proper scientific perspective just a few of the myths about sugar. In particular, I have concentrated on providing background information on dental caries (tooth decay), the only disease with which sugar has any direct relationship. It is impossible to make judgements about the dental caries debate without understanding the mechanism of the disease process.

SUGAR-v-SUGARS

The term 'sugar' is usually taken as synonymous with 'sucrose' or indeed, 'white table sugar'. In fact sugar is a general term for a collection of

Present address: Pfizer Ltd, Sandwich, Kent, UK.

relatively low molecular mass carbohydrates and includes monosaccharides (e.g. glucose, fructose) and disaccharides (e.g. sucrose, lactose,
maltose). Trisaccharides (e.g. maltotriose) may also be considered sugars,
but in reference to dietary intake the most important dietary sugars are the
monosaccharides and disaccharides based on the hexoses (six carbon
sugars) glucose, fructose and galactose. All these sugars occur naturally in
fruits, vegetables, cereals and even animal products (except galactose
which is one of the component monosaccharides in the milk sugar lactose).

Sucrose is quantitatively the most important sugar in the western diet
and is extracted from sugar cane or sugar beet and purified to produce the
wide range of sugars available in the shops. Sucrose is generally regarded
as the best sweetener in terms of taste and in terms of technological
function.

Hydrolysed corn (or potato or wheat) starches may be used as an
alternative to sucrose. The starches are 'digested' by enzymes and acid to
produce glucose syrups (a mixture of glucose, maltose and higher sacch-
arides in varying proportions). In some cases these may be treated with
another enzyme to convert glucose to fructose, making a sweeter syrup
more equivalent to sucrose itself (the sweetness values relative to sucrose
at 100 are fructose 110–120, glucose 60–70).

DIETARY SUGAR INTAKE

The values for dietary sugar intake appearing in the scientific literature
may be derived from many sources which may give quite different values
for the same population groups. They may also represent sucrose intake
alone or total sugars intake. None of the sources of information is incor-
rect, *per se*, but a knowledge of their advantages and shortcomings is
needed to assess whether or not they are appropriate to address the issues
being considered.

Intakes of sugar and other nutrients are sometimes based on Consumption Level Estimates derived from food supply data. Whilst these data can
be useful for looking at population trends, nutritionists and others using
such information should be aware of their shortcomings.

Consumption Level Estimates of commodity foodstuffs such as sucrose,
cereal grains, potatoes, etc., are derived from data on agricultural production, import and export, corrected for stock levels. They represent the total
amount of the foodstuff supplied for food and non-food uses and are
normally quoted on a *per capita* basis. The latest (1988) figure available for

sugar consumption in the UK is 37·0 kg person per year (COMA, 1989). This value is more correctly described as a 'disappearance' value. It is the amount of available sugar that disappears per head of the population.

The disappearance figure for sucrose consumption overestimates actual intake by more than 10% because:

(1) It includes non-food uses.
(2) It includes indirect uses in brewing and pharmaceutical preparations.
(3) It does not allow for industrial and domestic wastage.

Even if corrections are made to allow for these factors, the consumption of sugar on a *per capita* basis is of limited use as it does not reflect differences known to occur by, for example, age group, sex and socio-economic class.

The *per capita* consumption of sugar (with corrections for (1)–(3) above) is about 100 g per day. However, actual intake surveys do not yield such high figures (see Table 1). The unreliability of dietary survey data is well known, but they are the best estimates we have available in most cases. Researchers using data from surveys reported in the literature should, however, always bear in mind the degree of reliability of survey data when extrapolating to conclusions of their own.

When using data on sugar intake it is also helpful to know whether it represents 'total sugars' (i.e. including glucose, fructose, lactose) or 'added sucrose'. Most recent surveys do indicate the nature of the data presented but it is not always immediately obvious in examination of tables, for example, and reference must be made to the methodological sections. The difference in values for total and added sugars that may be observed is illustrated in Table 1.

THE FACTS ABOUT DENTAL CARIES

Dental caries is a disease that has long caused controversy, not only between dentists and the food industry, but also between scientists seeking to increase our understanding of the disease. Surprisingly, now that the incidence of the disease has decreased dramatically in countries of Western Europe, North America and Australia and New Zealand, so the debate seems to have become more heated.

In order to make sense of the continuing debate on dental caries and perhaps even to offer useful advice in the course of professional work in

TABLE 1
Mean sugar consumption from recent dietary surveys

Survey	Method of data collection	Average (g/day)	Sugar consumption (kg/year)	Reference
Northumberland children, 11·5–14·5 years (n 405)	Dietary record using household measures 3 days; interview on day 4	Girls 94[a] Boys 101[a]	34·3 36·9	Hackett et al. (1984)
Cambridgeshire village, 20–79 years (n 103)	Weighed dietary record; 7 days	Girls 78[b] Boys 85[b] Women 56·7[c] Men 91·0[c]	28·5 31·0 20·7 33·2	Rugg–Gunn et al. (1986) Bingham et al. (1981)
South Wales 40–59 (n 717)	Weighed dietary record; 7 days	Women 57[d] Men 100[d]	20·8 36·5	Fehily, A.M. (pers. comm. 1984)
Dieticians 20–65 years (n 42)	Weighed dietary record; every 6th day for 1 year	Women 38[c]	13·9	Black et al. (1984)
Men (n 105) and women (n 112) in Cambridge	Weighed dietary record; 7 days	Men 150[e] Women 102[e]	— —	Nelson (1985)
Men (n 14) and women (n 14)	Weighed dietary record; 7 days	Men 76[b] Women 38[b]	27·7 13·9	Yeomans (1987)

1946 British Birth Cohort:

			Braddon F.E.M., (pers. comm. 1987)
Men			
Normal (*n* 2437)	Dietary Record	101·1[b]	—
Obese (BMI 30) (*n* 2113)	Dietary Record	70·1[b]	—
Women			
Normal (*n* 1747)		72·2[e]	—
Obese (BMI 28·6) (*n* 1409)		50·2[e]	—

[a] Total sugars less lactose and less sugars from fruit.
[b] added sugars.
[c] Reported as 'sucrose'.
[d] Total sugars less lactose.
[e] Total sugars including naturally occurring sugars.
—, No figures quoted since no correction can be made for lactose and other naturally occurring sugars.

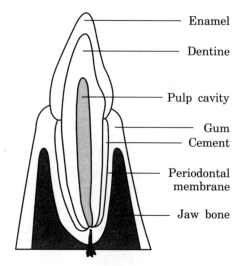

FIG. 1.   General structure of a tooth. (Reproduced by permission of the Sugar Bureau, London, UK)

the field of nutrition, it is essential to have a full *scientifically based* understanding of the causes of dental disease and the likely reasons for the changing incidence of these diseases around the world.

There are two types of dental disease commonly encountered and these are dental caries or tooth decay in which the hard tissue of the tooth is subject to decay, and periodontal disease which affects the gums and other supporting tissues. Both diseases can result in tooth loss and both diseases are influenced by diet. The emphasis is given here to dental caries which is essentially a disease of childhood and thus the most controversial. Periodontal disease is a problem for adults especially the elderly.

Firstly it is helpful to be reminded of the basic structure of the tooth (Fig. 1). A key feature of the structure of the tooth, which will be referred to again later, is the double layer of hard material which makes up the outer layer of the tooth, protecting the inner, soft pulp which contains the blood supply and the nerves.

The thin outer enamel layer is the hardest material in the body. Enamel is composed almost entirely of a highly crystalline calcium phosphate known as hydroxyapatite. Fluoride (of which more later) may become part of this crystalline structure, further increasing its resistance. The inner dentine layer is also composed of calcium phosphate but the structure is less crystalline and its hardness is equivalent to bone. It is also less resistant to decay.

The tooth is attached to the jaw from the cementum by many thousands of fibres called 'periodontal fibres'.

MECHANISM OF DENTAL DECAY

Dental caries is a disease of tooth enamel caused by bacteria. Without the bacteria dental caries scarcely occurs. In animals kept in entirely germ free conditions and fed on diets that would normally result in rampant dental caries, no caries develop. The bacterial deposit on the tooth surface is known as dental plaque, and should not be confused with food debris.

Dental plaque is composed of bacteria in a matrix of proteins sourced from saliva. Dental plaque forms in everyone regardless of tooth cleaning and diet and continues to accumulate even in people who are fasting. Plaque can be removed by toothbrushing, although not completely (try using a plaque disclosing tablet after you have brushed your teeth) but it begins to accumulate again immediately. The tooth surface is covered by a protein layer, the acquired pellicle, which, it is believed, is derived from salivary proteins. It is to this that bacteria initially adhere.

Plaque present on the teeth interacts with constituents of the diet, particularly fermentable carbohydrates. Dietary carbohydrate is used by the bacteria in two ways:

(1) It is fermented to acids and thereby used as an energy source to enable bacteria to live, grow and multiply.

(2) It is used when plentiful, to synthesize bacterial polysaccharides which form part of the matrix of the plaque. The polysaccharides (glucans) seem to change the structure of the plaque making it more 'gummy' so that the bacteria are able to adhere more firmly to the tooth surface.

Both these bacterial metabolic pathways depend on the presence of fermentable carbohydrate, which is, essentially, soluble carbohydrate that can diffuse readily into the plaque. Both sugars (glucose, fructose, maltose, sucrose, etc.) and starches, particularly cooked starches, can be fermented by oral bacteria and thus used to fuel both the pathways above.

The lactic and acetic acids produced by plaque bacteria diffuse from the bacterial cells into the plaque matrix and thus are in close contact with the surface of the tooth. The acid reacts chemically with the enamel, dissolving the hydroxyapatite structure.

If the acid is produced in sufficient quantity, and is present for long enough, the enamel continues to dissolve. However this is not a continuous process and occurs as a period of dissolution (demineralization) offset by a period of repair (remineralization). Repeated attack without sufficient repair eventually leads to cavitation until dentine is exposed. Thereafter dentine, being less resistant than enamel as mentioned above, is attacked more rapidly. At this stage the cavity must be restored by a dentist in order to preserve the tooth.

However, we do not usually eat continuously so the source of the fermentable carbohydrate is not constantly available to plaque bacteria for fermentation to acid. Furthermore, there are other 'defence mechanisms' that act to protect the tooth from acid. These are:

(1) Saliva, which is produced in quantity on eating, has a high buffering capacity and thus has the ability to neutralize acid.
(2) Saliva also helps simply to wash away food constituents.
(3) Plaque itself also contains buffering agents, which diffuse into it from saliva. Calcium, phosphate and fluoride in particular may be present as a result of exposure of the plaque to toothpaste or certain foods and these not only have buffering power but help push the balance of the chemical equation of dissolution towards remineralization.

Forgotten concepts
This introduces a concept which is often forgotten even in lengthy reviews of dental caries.

The formation of a carious lesion is *not* an irreversible process in the early stages. Enamel may dissolve, but can be redeposited until, as with many chemical reactions, a state of equilibrium is reached:

$$Ca_{10}(PO_4)_6(OH)_2 + 14H^+ \rightleftharpoons 10Ca^{2+} + 6H_2PO_4^- + 2H_2O$$

The process can be reversed by pushing the equilibrium in the direction of reforming enamel. This will occur with the help of the factors mentioned in the preceding paragraph if the pH remains above 5·5.

Equilibrium
Thus not all factors are against the preservation of our teeth. Fluoride (see below) has undoubtedly had a major role in encouraging the equilibrium to favour enamel over bacterial acid destruction.

The degree of acid produced in plaque by the actions of bacteria on food deposits can be monitored by measuring pH (the level of acidity) at the

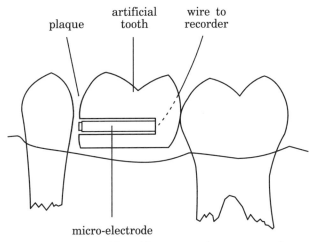

plaque   artificial tooth   wire to recorder

micro-electrode

FIG. 2. A microelectrode positioned between teeth to measure plaque pH. (From Curzon, (1989). Reproduced by permission of the British Nutrition Foundation *Nutrition Bulletin*)

tooth surface. This elegant method for measuring plaque pH was first developed in Switzerland (see Fig. 2) and is now used in that country to monitor the cariogenic potential of foodstuffs and allow, if appropriate, that they be labelled 'safe for teeth'.

If plaque pH is recorded throughout the day the type of traces shown in Fig. 3 might result. The critical pH in terms of dissolution of enamel appears to be around 5·5. If the pH at the tooth surface is maintained above this level, then the equilibrium is towards remineralization.

The pH is likely to be maintained at low levels (i.e. acidity is high) when carbohydrate food particles stick to teeth and offer a ready and prolonged supply of fermentable carbohydrate. Also it is clear from studying Fig. 3 that increasing the frequency of exposure to fermentable carbohydrate increases the likelihood of a prolonged depression of the pH below 5.5.

CARIES—A MULTIFACTORAL DISEASE

Having examined the mechanism by which dental caries occurs, it is worth studying in more detail the factors that influence outcome: that is whether or not enamel dissolves to cavitation or remineralizes.

Many authors have stated categorically that sugar is the sole cause of dental caries. However, dental caries is a disease initiated by bacterial acid

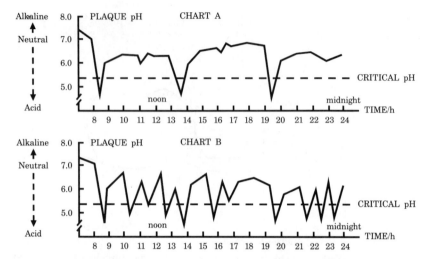

FIG. 3.   Typical traces obtained by measuring tooth plaque using a microelectrode. (Reproduced by permission of the Sugar Bureau)

dissolution. While the former statement is not true and the latter is true,
yet both are simplistic in attempting to describe completely a disease with
a multifactorial aetiology.

Even the simplest illustration of the causation of dental caries involves
four main factors (see Fig. 4) in which each factor itself may have a
number of components.

Susceptibility to dental caries

Host factors and teeth
The main host factors are:

Age
Tooth formation and composition
Immune response
Saliva
Dental plaque
Dental hygiene

Age is usually listed as a critical component of host resistance, but is
poorly understood. Children have always been considered more susceptible to caries than adults implying that resistance to decay is built up with

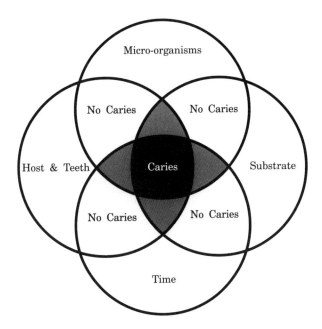

FIG. 4. The relation of aetiological factors in dental caries. For dental caries to occur, all four factors must act simultaneously. (From Kidd & Joyston-Bechal, (1987). Reproduced from John Wright and Sons Ltd, Bristol, UK)

continuing exposure to the environment. However, now the oral environment tends to include fluoride, children's teeth are more resistant to caries.

Apart from dental hygiene, which has an impact on dental plaque, other host factors influencing the development of dental caries may be genetically determined. However, tooth resistance is no doubt also radically affected by fluoride (see below). The immune response *is* important, as it should not be forgotten that dental caries is a bacterial disease.

While these factors are the major host factors affecting tooth susceptibility, it should be recognized that these may also be influenced by socioeconomic or cultural factors. For example, people of Asian extraction living in the UK traditionally do not use toothpaste and thus their teeth may not benefit from the presence of fluoride.

Bacteria

As mentioned above certain types of bacteria are essential to the disease process. The mouth is full of bacteria even in a healthy individual. This is perfectly normal! Several groups of bacteria contribute to colonization of the teeth and acid production, but those implicated in caries are streptococci and lactobacilli. In particular *S. mutans* has been implicated because it has a high capacity for the synthesis of extracellular glucans from dietary carbohydrate. The glucans help the bacteria adhere to the tooth surface.

Time
Obviously the process of dental caries is not an instantaneous one. Nor is enamel dissolution a continuous process as it occurs in waves of demineralization and remineralization (see above). Accordingly time is an important factor.

Dietary habits
The fourth factor illustrated in Fig. 4 is the diet (substrate). The influence of diet is, in itself, a very complex issue and cannot simply be considered in terms of the sugar content. Both the frequency of eating, the type of foods containing fermentable carbohydrate, the retentiveness of the foods and the presence or absence of protective factors in foodstuffs all have an influence on the outcome of caries.

Total sugars intake. On the whole, epidemiological evidence cited in the caries debate is based on very simplistic approaches which consider only one environmental (diet) variable—sugar consumption. However, when sugar consumption changes other factors also change and so it is not possible to assume such a simple correlation demonstrates a causal effect (i.e. that a high total sugar intake alone causes caries).

For example, it is often cited that during World War II the rate of dental caries in UK and Norway declined rapidly when sugar was rationed. This is true, but it is also true that food in general was in short supply and so the frequency of eating was no doubt also reduced. Conversely, the dental caries rate in some Third World countries is increasing at the same time that sugar consumption is increasing. But many other Western habits are also being introduced, which no doubt influences the outcome on dental health. Some of these factors may later prove to be beneficial, for example, increasing use of fluoride toothpaste. The current position in industrialized countries is a relatively high sugar intake yet a very low rate of dental caries (see below).

Frequency. Armed with some knowledge about the mechanism of dental caries it is not difficult to see that frequency of eating is likely to be a critical factor in any effect that diet might have. As illustrated in Fig. 3, the pH of dental plaque fluctuates throughout the day. Clearly, if fermentable carbohydrate is consumed *frequently*, there is more chance that the pH will remain below the critical value of 5·5 for longer, thus promoting demineralization.

The shape of the graph (Fig. 3) will be altered little by consuming more sugar in a meal. However if, over the course of time the individual consumes a boiled sweet every half hour, then there would be continuous presence of acid on the tooth surface. The effect on dental caries under these conditions can be dramatic.

Type of food. The consistency of food is also important. Studies have shown that carbohydrate-containing foods that stick to the teeth are more cariogenic because fermentable carbohydrate remains available to the bacteria for longer.

The classic Vipeholm dietary study conducted in the 1950s showed that frequency and type of sugar were the overwhelmingly important factors in conjunction with sugar intake. Institutionalized individuals consuming toffees between meals had a considerable increase in caries compared with individuals consuming the same amount of sucrose per day but only at meal times in baked products and beverages (Gustafsson *et al.*, 1954).

Protective foods. Some foods are regarded as protective, for example cheese. This is partly because of its high calcium and phosphate content but partly also because of its protein content. Some proteins are believed to be protective perhaps through their buffering capacity. Other minor chemical components of foods, for example cocoa, have also been implicated as protective.

The importance of dietary habits has probably been overemphasized in the past, and its contribution to caries may be much less than supposed. For example, one recent study in adolescent children (a high sugar consuming group) in northern England reported a possible correlation between the total amount of sugar consumed per day and the rate of caries increment over a two year period. However although statistically significant the correlation coefficient was only 0·143 and total sugar intake accounted for only 2·0% of the variance in caries increment. There was no relationship between frequency of intake and caries increment in this study. In practical terms, this means diet had little effect on caries and that some other factor (or other factors collectively) were far more important than diet (Rugg-Gunn *et al.*, 1984).

INVESTIGATIONS ON DIET AND DENTAL HEALTH

Previous reviews of sugar and health provide a good account of research in laboratory animals, laboratory research into the cariogenic potential of food, surveys of small groups of individuals, and large epidemiological surveys (e.g. British Nutrition Foundation, 1987). This aspect is therefore not examined further here.

Decline in dental caries
In Western Europe, North America and Australia and New Zealand there has been what can only be described as a dramatic decline in dental caries over the past 15 years (see Fig. 5; WHO, 1985). During this period there has not been a significant decrease in sugar consumption, and there has probably been an increase in the use of sugary snacks between meals.

Part of the decrease may be attributed to a number of 'host' factors, e.g. improved health and thus immune response, and improved dental hygiene. However, experts believe that the major factor is the use of fluoride, mainly in dentifrices (toothpaste) but also in water supplies, fluoride supplements, mouth rinses and preventative treatments applied by dentists. The sale of fluoride toothpaste in the UK now accounts for 95% of the market. The effect of fluoride has been so great that it is not uncommon for children to be completely free of caries both in the case of their milk teeth and in the case of their permanent teeth.

Fluoride
The use of fluoride has been the most effective weapon in the fight to improve dental health. As early as the 1930s it was shown that people who lived in areas with a naturally high fluoride content in their drinking water had a low incidence of caries. One part per million seems to be optimal in reducing caries by one half, compared with people in low fluoride areas, but higher levels can cause discolouration of the teeth so are not beneficial.

Fluoride acts in a number of ways to protect the teeth.

(1) It strengthens enamel and thus helps prevent its dissolution when acid is present.
(2) It helps remineralization of enamel following demineralization.
(3) It inhibits the production of acid by plaque bacteria.

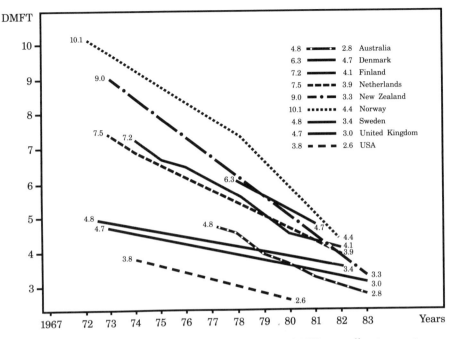

FIG. 5.   The decline in dental caries between 1967 and 1983 according to country: Decayed, Missing and Filled Teeth (DMFT) per child at 12 years. (From WHO (1985). Reproduced by permission of Butterworth–Heinemann Ltd, © *International Dental Journal*)

Fluoride present in the diet (drinking water) is reflected in fluoride in tissue fluids. Thus during growth and development fluoride ions can replace hydroxyl ions in the hydroxyapatite crystals of the enamel to form fluorapatite. Following tooth eruption fluoride continues to be taken up from the tooth's environment. Enamel from newly erupted teeth takes up more fluoride than mature enamel, hence the value to children of fluoride dentrifices and other topical preparations.

The lattice structure of hydroxyapatite crystals in enamel makes enamel a porous structure. Acid attack renders enamel more porous by damaging the structure. The more porous the enamel, the more fluoride is taken up. Hence demineralized areas of enamel will selectively take up fluoride aiding the repair process. Enamel repaired in this way is more resistant to subsequent dissolution than the original enamel.

WESTERN DISEASES

The 1989 COMA publication on Dietary Sugars and Human Diseases (COMA, 1989) reported that the Panel on Dietary Sugars found that sugars have no direct, causal link with heart disease, diabetes, cancer and other so-called Western diseases (apart from dental caries). The conclusions of the Panel are not surprising and they are not the first to conclude that sugar (sucrose) is not the arch criminal that critics such as Yudkin and his followers would have had us believe in the past.

Body weight

Everyone knows that many people maintain their ideal body weight on an incredible range of dietary habits. No single food is inherently fattening, in fact all food contributes to energy intake so it is the energy intake from the total diet that must be balanced with energy expenditure. Until recently it was generally held that carbohydrates were fattening and nutritionists recommended low carbohydrate diets for weight reduction. Carbohydrate-rich foods include potatoes, sugar, bread, cakes, biscuits, rice and pasta. Nowadays, in line with dietary guidelines, most nutritionists would recommend bread, potatoes, pasta, etc., as part of a 'healthy' diet. Sucrose has the same energy content as other carbohydrates,(i.e. 4 kcal/g compared with fat 9 kcal/g, alcohol 7 kcal/g, and protein 4 kcal/g).

In the simple energy equation:

$$\text{'energy in–energy out } = \text{ energy loss or gain'}$$

The 'energy in' component is under the control of individual but the 'energy out' component does seem to have a strong genetic component although this is still a controversial issue. There is evidence, for example, that babies born to obese parents have a lower metabolic rate (energy expenditure) than babies born to lean parents (Anon, 1988).

In terms of energy expenditure, exercise has a small quantitative effect —for example half an hour's brisk walk might burn an extra 100 kcal compared with sitting down reading a book. However, over a lifetime these small adjustments *may* be important since 100 kcal excess energy intake per day contributes 10 g adipose tissue per day or 3·65 kg adipose tissue per year. In 5 years this would be 18 kg! On a daily basis such a small variation in energy intake is very difficult to measure because of the lack of accuracy of methods of measuring dietary intake. Thus it is not possible at present to judge what scale of fluctuation is significant. Almost certainly it will vary between individuals and metabolic adaptation can probably 'absorb' such a small daily excess or deficit. In practice, for most individuals, daily fluctuations are likely to be both above and below the mean value of energy expenditure, so that the net balance sheet remains at zero in the longer term.

Carbohydrates (including sucrose) are likely to be less fattening than dietary fat because they are actually used less efficiently for conversion to body fat than is fat itself (the conversion of carbohydrate to fat is energy demanding). Calculations of the cost of the metabolic conversion of carbohydrate to adipose tissue indicates an efficiency of 72%. This compares with 93% efficiency for dietary fat.

The sugar–fat seesaw

Overeating and excess energy intake have been said to result from excessive intake of foods based on sweet–fat combinations. However, calculations based on National Food Survey data, adjusted to include soft drinks and confectionery, show that sugar–fat combinations contribute less than 11% of total energy on an average basis (McColl, 1988). Even allowing for all home-use flour to be incorporated into sweet baked products at an extreme ratio of 4:3:3 flour:fat:sugar does not increase the percentage beyond 12·3%.

There is, in fact, an *inverse* relationship between fat and carbohydrate (or sugars) intake. This has been demonstrated in a number of studies (McColl, 1988)) but is illustrated best by the extensive data from studies by Nelson and co-workers (Nelson, 1985) and presented in the COMA (1989) Report (see Tables 2 and 3).

It is impressive that at any and every level of energy intake the highest sugar consumers have a *lower* percentage of energy intake from fat. This is true even when sugar intake is expressed as g/1000 kcal energy intake. In every case illustrated the highest sugar intake group had a percentage of fat energy below 40% whereas low sugar consumers had a higher percentage fat intake—up to 44·9% in women consuming low energy intakes.

It is illuminating to consider a quote from a recent Annual Report of the National Food Survey Committee (MAFF, 1986):

The amount of fat in the diet increased in proportion to the amount of energy, so that the percentage of energy derived from fat remained at 42·6. The target recommended by the DHSS for individuals wishing to reduce their risk of cardiovascular disease is that 35 per cent of their energy intake should be derived from fat—a value not recorded in the National Food Survey since 1952, when the contribution from car-

Nino M. Binns

TABLE 2
Nutrient intake of 112 women in Cambridge according to the proportion of sugar in the diet

	Women			P
	Lowest 37 women	Middle 38 women	Highest 37 women	
	$16\cdot2^a$ (range 5·2–22·3)	$28\cdot8^a$ (range 22·4–36·5)	$49\cdot6^a$ (range 36·9–111·2)	
Total intake (per day)				
Energy (kcal)	1825	2023	1985	ns
(M$_J$)	7·67	8·50	8·34	
Protein (g)	67	68	60	*
Fat (g)	90	93	85	ns
Carbohydrate (g)	187	229	257	***
Alcohol (g)	6	8	3	*
Total sugars (g)	73	102	135	***
Non-milk extrinsic sugars (g)	30	58	99	***
Intake g/1000 kcal (4·2 M$_J$)				
Protein	36·6	33·6	30·1	***
Fat	49·3	45·7	42·6	***
Carbohydrate	102·6	113·1	129·2	***
Alcohol	3·2	3·9	1·3	ns
Total sugars	40·0	50·5	68·1	***

[a] Non-milk extrinsic sugars, grams per 1000 kcal.
***, $P < 0\cdot001$; **, $P < 0\cdot01$; *, $P < 0\cdot05$; ns, not significant.
Adapted from COMA (1989).

TABLE 3

Nutrient intake according to intake of non-milk extrinsic sugars within three levels of energy intake in Cambridge women (kcal per day)

	Cambridge women (n 112)								
	Highest (2150–3318 kcal) energy intake			Middle (1791–2134 kcal) energy intake			Lowest (794–1777 kcal) energy intake		
	Higher	P	Lower	Higher	P	Lower	Higher	P	Lower
	32·8–84·4[a] 18 women		10·9–31·8[a] 19 women	26·2–71·0[a] 19 women		12·0–25·9[a] 19 women	23·8–111·1[a] 18 women		5·2–19·9[a] 19 women
Nutrient intake									
Energy (kcal)	2507	*	2337	1934	ns	1953	1433	ns	1515
(M_J)	10·53		9·82	8·12		8·20	6·02		6·36
Protein (g)	72	ns	77	63	*	68	49	*	59
Fat (g)	110	ns	110	83	*	94	61	**	76
Total CHO (g)	318	***	253	243	***	209	177	*	149
Total sugars (g)	160	***	106	119	***	87	89	**	56
Non-milk extrinsic sugars (g)	109	***	52	80	***	43	65	***	21
Alcohol (g)	6	*	11	3	*	7	2	ns	5
Per cent of energy									
Protein	11·6	**	13·3	13·0	ns	14·0	13·6	*	15·6
Fat	39·6	*	42·5	38·7	***	43·2	38·5	***	44·9
Total carbohydrate	47·5	***	40·7	47·1	***	40·1	46·3	***	36·9
Total sugars	23·9	***	17·1	23·1	***	16·7	23·5	***	13·9
Non-milk extrinsic sugars	16·3	***	8·5	15·5	***	8·1	17·0	***	5·1

[a] Non-milk extrinsic sugars intake, grams per 1000 kcal.
*** P < 0·01; * P < 0·05; ns not significant.
Adapted from COMA (1989).

bohydrate (especially from high intakes of bread, sugar and potatoes) was much greater than now, at 52·9 per cent.

Since the relationship between fat intake and sugar intake is clearly inverse, it does seem that an increase, or at least a maintenance, of current sugar intakes will be needed to achieve the level of fat reduction recommended by COMA (1984), NACNE (1983) and others.

CONCLUSION

The scope of this review has been confined to a discussion of sugar in relation to dental caries and to some of the so-called Western diseases. It should thus be clearer to readers that sugar does not deserve the criticism levelled upon it in the past.

In order to make an adequate judgement about any controversial nutritional issues, it is necessary always to consider *scientific* information. All such scientific information should be evaluated critically in order for the individual to reach a soundly based conclusion. Hopefully the reader will now be stimulated to search for such scientific information on sugar and other similarly contentious topics.

REFERENCES AND BIBLIOGRAPHY

Anon (1988). Decreased energy expenditure as a cause of obesity in infants. *Nutrition Reviews* **46**, 255–7.

Bingham, S., McNeil, N.I. & Cummings, J.H. (1981). The diet of individuals in a study of a randomly-chosen cross section of British adults in a Cambridgeshire village. *British Journal of Nutrition* **45**, 23–35.

Black, A.E., Ravenscroft, C. & Simms, A.J. (1984). The NACNE report: are the dietary goals realistic? Comparison with the dietary patterns of dietitians. *Human Nutrition: Applied Nutrition* **38A**, 165–79.

British Nutrition Foundation (1987). *Sugars and Syrups: The Report of the British Nutrition Foundation's Task Force*. London: British Nutrition Foundation.

COMA (1984). Committee on Medical Aspects of Food Policy: Report of the Panel on Diet in Relation to Cardiovascular Disease. *Report on Health and Social Subjects* no. 28. London: H.M. Stationery Office.

COMA (1989). Committee on Medical Aspects of Food Policy: Report of the Panel on Dietary Sugars and Human Disease. *Report on Health and Social Subjects* no. 37. London: H.M. Stationery Office.

Curzon, M.E.J. (1989). Food and dental caries. *British Nutrition Foundation Nutrition Bulletin* **14**, 36–45.

Gustafsson, B.E., Quensel, C.E., Swenander Lanke, L., Lundqvist, C., Grahnen,

H., Bonow, B.E. & Krasse, B. (1954). The effect of different levels of carbohydrate intake on caries activity in 436 individuals observed for five years. (In The Vipeholm Dental Caries Study). *Acta Odontological Scandinavica* **11**, 232–365.

Hackett, A.F., Rugg-Gunn, A.J., Appleton, D.R., Allinson, M. & Eastoe, J.E. (1984). Sugar-eating habits of 405, 11 to 14 year old English children. *British Journal of Nutrition* **51**, 347–56.

Kidd, E.A.M. & Joyston-Bechal, S. (editors) (1987). *Essentials of Dental Caries.* Bristol: Wright.

McColl, K.A. (1988). The sugar–fat seesaw. *British Nutrition Foundation Nutrition Bulletin* **13**, 114–18.

MAFF (1986). *National Food Survey Committee: Household Food Consumption and Expenditure.* London: H.M. Stationery Office.

NACNE, National Advisory Committee on Nutrition Education (1983). *Proposals for Nutritional Guidelines for Health Education in Britain.* London: Health Education Council.

Nelson, M. (1985). Nutritional goals from COMA and NACNE. How can they be achieved? *Human Nutrition: Applied Nutrition* **39A**, 456–64.

Rugg-Gunn, A.J., Hackett, A.F., Appleton, D.R., Jenkins, G.N. & Eastoe, J.E. (1984). Relationship between dietary habits and caries increment assessed over two years in 405 English adolescent school children. *Archives of Oral Biology* **29**, 982–92.

Rugg-Gunn, A.J., Hackett, A.F., Appleton, D.R., Mayniham, P.J. (1986). The dietary intake of added and natural sugars in 405 English adolescents. *Human Nutrition: Applied Nutrition* **40A**, 115–24.

WHO (1985). Changing patterns of oral health and implications for oral health manpower: Part 1. *International Dental Journal* **35**, 235–51.

BIBLIOGRAPHY

Glinsmann, W.H., Irausquin, H. & Park, Y.K. (1986). Evaluation of health aspects of sugars contained in carbohydrate sweeteners: report of Sugars Task Force. *Journal of Nutrition* **116**, S1–216.

7

Nutritional Implications of Processing Fats and Oils: Products of Oxidation and Industrial Hydrogenation

MICHAEL I. GURR

The Milk Marketing Board, Thames Ditton, Surrey, UK

INTRODUCTION

Dietary guidelines as part of preventative measures against cardiovascular disease and other public health problems are now a common feature in many developed countries. Dietary fat is almost universally brought into sharp focus in these guidelines and it is quite common for many people to assume that 'processing' is inevitably detrimental to the nutritive value of food fats. Such attitudes need to be approached from a firm scientific basis.

Three-quarters of the food in the UK diet is processed in some way, and very much more than this if processing is taken to include food preparation and cooking in the home. Food fats may range from the virtually unprocessed (e.g. the fat in an avocado pear or a peanut), through various intermediate degrees of processing (e.g. bacon fat, butter, frying oil) to highly processed (e.g. margarine). The more refined the oil or fat, the more processing stages it is likely to have undergone.

Processing is necessary to remove unwanted compounds that may be too highly coloured, bad smelling or tasting, or toxic; to remove harmful organisms, thus rendering the food safe; or to change the physical properties of the food.

Present address: Maypole Scientific Services, Vale View Cottage, Maypole, St. Mary's, Isles of Scilly TR21 0NU.

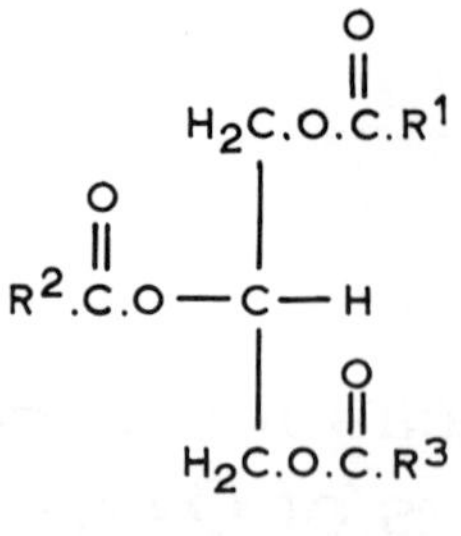

$$
\begin{array}{c}
\text{O} \\
\parallel \\
H_2C.O.C.R^1 \\
| \\
\text{O} \qquad | \\
\parallel \qquad | \\
R^2.C.O\!-\!C\!-\!H \\
| \quad \text{O} \\
| \quad \parallel \\
H_2C.O.C.R^3
\end{array}
$$

Triacylglycerols

FIG. 1.   Storage lipids. R^1, R^2 and R^3 represent different fatty acids (see Fig. 3).

THE NATURE OF FOOD FATS

Before discussing the likely influence of the various processing techniques employed, it is first necessary briefly to describe the types of fats present in foods. Fats are those foods or components of foods that are clearly fatty in nature, greasy in texture and immiscible with water. Edible fats (solid texture) and oils (liquid at ambient temperature) are all composed predominantly of esters of glycerol with fatty acids (Fig. 1). These are called 'triacylglycerols' (in older literature 'triglycerides'). Chemists use the more general term 'lipid' to describe a chemically varied group of fatty substances that have in common the property of being insoluble in water but soluble in solvents such as chloroform, hydrocarbons, alcohols or ethers. This definition includes a far wider range of chemical substances than simply the triacylglycerols. These include (Fig. 2) the phospholipids (similar to triacylglycerols except that one of the fatty acids is replaced by a phosphate ester), cholesterol and other sterols and their esters with fatty acids and the fat-soluble vitamins.

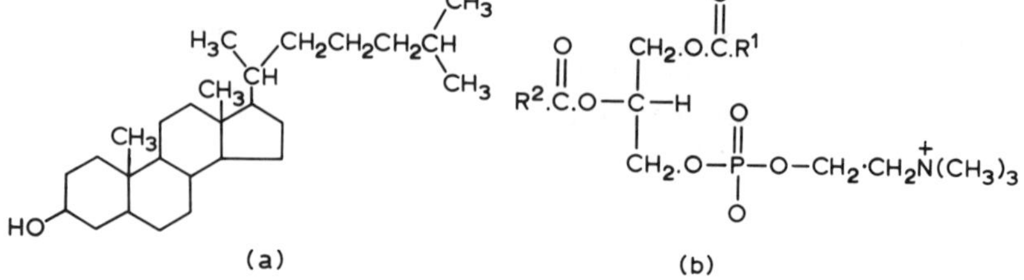

FIG. 2.   Structural lipids: (a) cholesterol; (b) phospholipid.

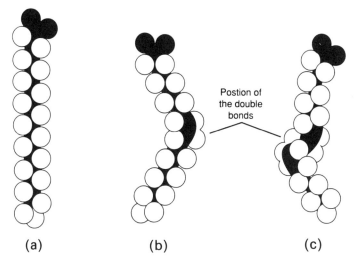

(a)   **(b)**   **(c)**

FIG. 3. Types of fatty acids: (a) saturated: $CH_3(CH_2)_{16}COOH$, stearic acid, octadecanoic; (b) monosaturated: $CH_3(CH_2)_7 CH = CH(CH_2)_7 COOH$, oleic acid, cis–9–octadecanoic; (c) polyunsaturated: $CH_3(CH_2)_4 CH = CH \cdot CH_2 \cdot CH = CH(CH_2)_7 COOH$, linoleic acid, cis,cis,9,12-octadecadienoic.

Fats in food derive from the lipids in the animals and plants that we eat. In both animals and plants, lipids fulfil two main functions: storage and structure (Gurr, 1984).

Storage fats

Fatty acids in the form of triacylglycerols constitute the major source of fuel in mammals and in the seeds of some plants. Mammals, including human beings, use triacylglycerols as a long-term supply of energy, stored in the adipose tissue. Translated into food terms, the lard of pigs and the suet of beef animals can be recognized as adipose, or storage fat. Fish, in contrast, store fat in the liver (e.g. cod) or the flesh (e.g. herring, mackerel) rather than in adipose tissue.

The fatty acids present in these lipids are of three main types: saturated, monounsaturated and polyunsaturated (Fig. 3). The fat of ruminants tends to have high concentrations of saturated and monounsaturated fatty acids, that of pigs and poultry is more dependent on the animal's diet, while the fat of fish is generally rich in polyunsaturated fatty acids (Table 1). Milk fat can also be regarded as a storage fat for the benefit of the newborn animal and also comprises mainly triacylglycerols. The storage

TABLE 1

Fatty acid composition of some food fats (g/100 g)

Fatty acid[a]	Storage fats					Structural fats	
	Beef suet	Butter	Lard[b]	Cod liver	Soya-bean oil	Beef muscle	Green leaves
4:0–12:0	—	13	—	—	—	—	—
14:0	3	12	2	6	—	3	—
16:0	28	26	27	13	10	13	13
18:0	26	11	16	3	4	16	—
16:1–18:1	36	30	44	33	25	23	10
20:1–22:1	—	—	—	18	—	—	—
16:2/3	—	—	—	—	—	—	5
18:2[c]	1	2	9	2	52	20	16
18:3[d]	—	—	—	—	7	2	56
20:4	—	—	—	—	—	19	—
Others	6	4	—	25[e]	2	—	—

[a] In this shorthand nomenclature, the number before the colon denotes the number of carbon atoms in the fatty acid hydrocarbon chain; the number after the colon refers to the numbers of double bonds, i.e. the degree of unsaturation.
[b] From pig fed on low-fat, cereal-based diet.
[c] Predominantly *cis*, *cis*-9, 12-octadecadienoic acid (linoleic acid).
[d] Predominantly *cis*, *cis*, *cis*-9, 12, 15-octadecatrienoic acid (linolenic acid).
[e] Predominantly long-chain polyunsaturated acids (20:5, 22:5, 22:6).

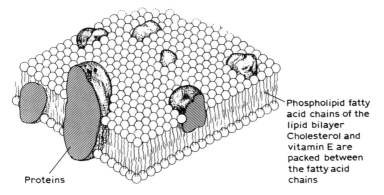

FIG. 4. Fluid mosaic model of membrane structure.

fats, however, also have small amounts of other lipids (cholesterol, fat-soluble vitamins), dissolved in them.

Structural fats

Lipids form an integral part of the structure of biological membranes, which are present in all cells to give shape to the cell and to provide a barrier against the environment (Fig. 4). They also act as sites for many biochemical reactions occurring in cells. The structural fats are not triacylglycerols but are mainly phospholipids and cholesterol. In general, the fatty acid composition of structural fats is less variable and less influenced by the animal's diet than the storage fats. They contain a relatively high proportion of polyunsaturated fatty acids (Table 1).

PROCESSES THAT INVOLVE EXTRACTION, SEPARATION AND PURIFICATION

The clear amber coloured oils or the pale cream or white fats purchased in the supermarket are obtained only after a number of processes to separate the fat from other components of the seed or the animal carcass with which they were naturally associated and to remove unwanted components that contaminate the fat (Gunstone & Norris, 1983, Table 2). In general, these processes have minimal nutritional significance.

HEATING

Heating, whether on an industrial scale or simply household cooking is

TABLE 2
Extraction separation & purification processes

Process	Description
Degumming	Heating in water at 60–90° in phosphoric acid Removes phospholipids, polysaccharides, chlorophylls No important antinutritional effects; can improve by removing sources of oxidative deterioration
Alkali refining	Removes free fatty acids—brief exposure to heat removes lipase Improves palatability; removes toxins: aflatoxins, isothiocyanates, glucosinolates (rape)—goitre
Rendering	For animal fats: steaming carcass in small amount of water No important nutritional effects; animal fats have fewer contaminants than vegetable
Churning	Butter; to create emulsion Milk fat globule membrane ruptures, releases lipase Releases free fatty acids; may be palatability problem
Bleaching	With Fuller's Earth or charcoal at 80–90°C Removes pigments, polycyclic hydrocarbons; some oxidation of PUFA
Deodorization	High pressure steam distillation to remove volatiles 240–270°C/1 hr. Improves palatability by removing unpleasant odours and tastes, also some pesticide residues; but can damage PUFA, fat-soluble vitamins

used to make the food edible and palatable and also safe by killing microorganisms. It reduces heat-labile and oxygen-senstive nutrients depending on the conditions and inevitably a balance has to be struck between acceptable palatability and safety on the one side and losses of nutrients on the other. Heating can result in chemical changes in the fats themselves, depending on the time of heating, the temperature and the degree of exposure to air. In deep fat frying, which typically occurs at 180°C, water comes out of the food, bringing volatiles with it (steam-stripping). The layer of volatiles formed above the fat acts as a barrier preventing access to too much air. Oxidation may take place during storage at room or even refrigerator temperatures but is greatly accelerated by heating. The extent to which there may be adverse nutritional implications of fat oxidation is the subject of the next section.

OXIDATION OF LIPIDS IN FOODS

Free radical mechanisms

The oxidative deterioration of lipids, leading to rancidity, has been recognized as a problem in both storage and heating of fats and oils for centuries and was studied in a scientific manner as long ago as 1820 by de Saussure. The sequence of reactions is generally known as lipid peroxidation. In this process, the chemical changes involve very reactive chemical species known as 'free radicals' (for further reading see Frankel, 1980; Logani & Davies, 1980; Halliwell & Gutteridge, 1985). The process will be described only in sufficient detail to give background to the associated nutritional and toxicological problems. Lipid peroxidation proceeds in three stages: initiation, propagation and termination (Fig. 5).

Initiation

Initiation involves the abstraction of a hydrogen atom (H·) from a methylene group (—CH_2—) in the hydrocarbon chain of a lipid. Since a hydrogen atom is itself a free radical, it leaves behind an unpaired electron on the carbon (—·CH—). Unsaturated chains are more susceptible to attack than saturated ones because the presence of a double bond weakens the C—H bonds on the adjacent carbon and so makes the removal of H· easier.

Several chemical species are known to act as initiators of lipid peroxidation. One is a particularly reactive form of oxygen known as *singlet oxygen* which itself may be formed from normal oxygen by sensitizers such as chlorophylls, bilirubin and porphyrins in the presence of light. These substances are common in foods. Another common initiating species is the reactive hydroxyl radical, which may be generated by the sequence of reactions illustrated at the top of Fig. 5.

Propagation

The first change occurring in the unsaturated lipid-free radical is the isomerization of one of the double bonds to form a *trans-cis conjugated diene*, which is a more stable structure. This radical then reacts with an oxygen molecule to form a *peroxy radical*, ROO·, which is then able to abstract a hydrogen atom from another lipid molecule to give another lipid radical and a *hydroperoxide*. Thus, once the process has been initiated, it tends to continue by a chain reaction of propagation steps.

Termination

The chain reaction may be *terminated* in a number of ways. Two lipid

1. Generation of an initiator radical

$$Fe^{3+} + O_2^- \longrightarrow Fe^{2+} + O_2$$

$$Fe^{2+} + H_2O_2 \longrightarrow Fe^{3+} + OH^\bullet + OH^-$$

2. Initiation

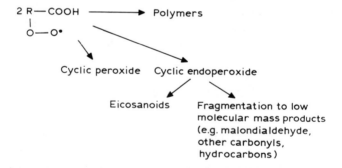

3. Propagation

4. Termination

FIG. 5. Lipid peroxidation. These are simplified examples of possible different steps. There are, of course, many other different possibilities for initiation, propagation and termination.

carbon radicals or peroxy radicals can combine to form polymeric products. Alternatively, a peroxy radical can form a cyclic peroxide, which as a free radical itself can undergo cyclization to a cyclic endoperoxide which on heating in the presence of oxygen can split into a number of end-products characteristic of lipid peroxidation: malondialdehyde, low molecular mass fatty acids, oxyacids and hydrocarbons.

The extent of peroxidation in food fats can be estimated by a number of methods. Each measures something different and none by itself is a complete guide to the degree of peroxidation that has taken place. Measurement of diene conjugation gives information about the early stages of peroxidation, as does determination of peroxides by iodometric titration. The thiobarbituric acid test is one of the oldest and most frequently used methods for measuring peroxidation of fatty acids in biological tissues and food products but its results need careful interpretation. Further discussion is beyond the scope of this chapter but a detailed account can be found in Halliwell & Gutteridge (1985) for biological tissues and Gray (1978) for foods.

Peroxidation of lipids in foods can occur very rapidly because the reaction is catalysed by other components of the foods. Catalysis may be enzymic or non-enzymic. The principal non-enzymic catalysts are iron and copper. In many reactions catalysis is effected, not by the inorganic ion as an inorganic salt, but in the form of complexes such as haem and cytochromes.

Lipid peroxidation can also be catalysed enzymically. Plant and animal tissues contain the enzyme *lipoxygenase* which catalyses the formation of hydroperoxides of unsaturated fatty acids (Halliwell & Gutteridge, 1985). The mechanism, like non-enzymic peroxidation, probably involves free radicals. The peroxy radicals generated from tissue polyunsaturated fatty acids by this enzyme may abstract hydrogen atoms from surrounding molecules. A lipid peroxidation chain reaction can then ensue, which may cause damage to surrounding tissues. A vulnerable molecule is β-carotene and, indeed, lipoxygenase is used commercially to bleach wheat flour carotenoids during bread making. Finally, in considering factors that accelerate or encourage peroxidation, the role of catalysts present in the food has been stressed. It is also worth remembering that another factor is oxygen solubility, which is 7–8 times greater in fat solvents than in water so that oxygen is readily taken up into the lipid phase of foods.

Peroxidation of cholesterol

Although emphasis is usually placed on the peroxidation of polyunsaturated fatty acids because of the ease with which they undergo free radical formation, it has been known for some time that cholesterol, generally regarded as a chemically rather stable molecule, could peroxidize in presence of oxygen. Even analytical grade cholesterol contains small quantities of oxidation products (Taylor *et al.*, 1979), but the cholesterol in dehydrated foods such as powdered eggs and powdered whole milk is highly susceptible to peroxidation when stored in air, even at room temperature. Thirty or more products have been detected. Toxic properties have been noted as described in a later section.

Protection against free radicals: antioxidants
Lipids are more susceptible to peroxidation when they are in a dispersed state than when they are highly organized and close packed as in biological membranes. Therefore, processes that tend to disrupt the lipid organization in foods are likely to increase the chances of oxidative deterioration. Because the presence of polyunsaturated fatty acids is essential to the functioning of biological tissues, it is vital that protective mechanisms exist to prevent their oxidation by free radical mechanisms, which would, if unchecked, damage the tissue and eventually cause cell death. Protection is afforded by a high degree of organization in membranes and by antioxidant mechanisms. Antioxidants either prevent the initiation of chain reactions or react with free radicals, thus preventing further propagation by terminating the reaction (Logani & Davies, 1980; Halliwell & Gutteridge, 1985).

Preventive antioxidants are substances that chelate metals involved in catalysis and enzymes, such as glutathione peroxidase, catalase and superoxide dismutase. In general, these enzymes catalyse the destruction of potential oxidants such as hydrogen peroxide and superoxide. Glutathione peroxidase is a selenium-requiring enzyme which accounts for the requirement for selenium as an essential dietary element. Chain-breaking antioxidants (Fig. 6) react with lipid-free radicals. Important naturally occurring examples are α-tocopherol (vitamin E), ubiquinone, retinol (vitamin A) and β-carotene (provitamin A). These compounds are lipid-soluble and tend to concentrate in the hydrophobic interior of membranes in close proximity to the polyunsaturated fatty acids. It is important to recognize also that water-soluble substances (e.g. ascorbic acid (vitamin C), glutathione, urate) can also function as lipid antioxidants. Vitamin C appears to interact synergistically with vitamin E *in vivo* to maintain the former in the reduced form. While many food fats (e.g. seed oils) contain high levels of natural antioxidants, it is generally necessary to use ad-

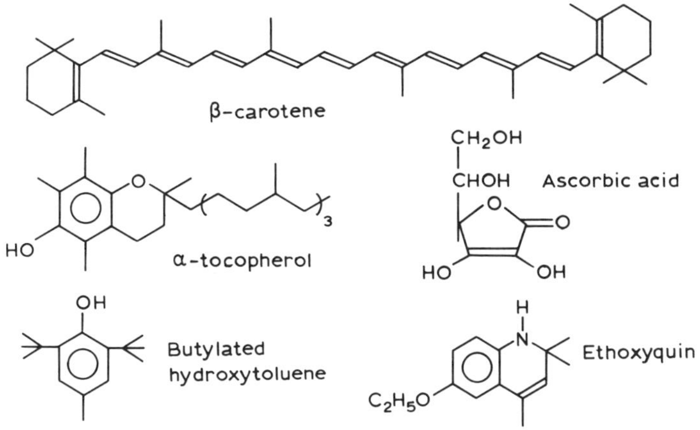

Fig. 6. Antioxidants (chain-breaking).

ditional antioxidants in processed foods to protect against damage by lipid peroxidation. Butylated hydroxyanisole and butylated hydroxytoluene are extensively used in the food industry. They act by donating a hydrogen free radical to terminate chain reactions and their addition to food fats can increase storage life from a few months to a few years.

Lipid changes in heated fats

The foregoing sections have indicated the types of chemical changes that can take place during oxidative deterioration of lipids beginning with the formation of a lipid-free radical. These reactions are accelerated by heating and the direction in which the reaction proceeds and its extent depend on several conditions including: the degree of exposure to air, the temperature achieved, the time of heating, the composition of the fat, its physical state and the presence of other components with which the free radicals can interact. The products of heating fall into several categories: volatiles, monomers, dimers and polymers.

The volatiles (e.g. hydrocarbons, alcohols, lactones, aldehydes and ketones; Reddy *et al.*, 1968) distil out of the fat at atmospheric pressure and in the frying process can form a surface layer which may hinder the access of too much oxygen into the fat. Artman and Smith (1972) identified 136 monomeric compounds in cottonseed oil heated at 182°C for six 8 h days with the fat being allowed to cool overnight and during a weekend. These compounds included unsaturated cyclic esters, hydroxyesters and ketoesters as would be expected from the free radical reaction schemes discussed earlier. The peroxides and hydroperoxides, although among the first products of oxidation even at low temperature, do not survive in heated fats and break down into the oxy- and cyclic acids as the temperature is raised. At higher temperatures and longer heating times dimeric and polymeric materials build up and under household or industrial conditions the fat may develop 10–20% of polymeric material without the functional properties of the oil becoming noticeably worse (Billek, 1985).

In assessing the contribution of heating to the dietary intake of modified fats, it is useful to consider three distinct types of cooking. Firstly, there is pan frying, which is essentially a high-temperature short-time process. The fat is generally discarded after use and the intake will be limited to a single dose of what has been absorbed into the cooked food. Secondly, there is continuous frying, such as that used for doughnuts or chips. Although the fat is absorbed into the food, the cooking fat is constantly being replaced by fresh fat and levels of end products do not have chance to accumulate. Finally, there is small volume batch frying used in catering establishments, where the fat is kept hot all day, used occasionally, cooled overnight and reused again and again. These are the type of conditions in which concentrations of modified fats build up to levels which could be potentially harmful (see later sections).

Nutritional effects
Before any nutritional effects can be observed, the first effect of oxidative changes on edible fats is the deterioration in flavour and appearance. It is probably true to say that in most cases oxidized fats are rendered unpalatable long before the changes have appreciably reduced nutritive value or created toxicity.

Because the most susceptible oils are those rich in essential fatty acids, one nutritional effect of oxidation is to reduce the essential fatty acid content of edible fats. The significance for nutrition overall, however, is likely to be minimal, since losses are usually small in relation to the total content of polyunsaturated fatty acids supplied by these susceptible oils. Perhaps more serious will be the losses of vitamin E, β-carotene and vitamin C in the cooked foods (Izaki et al., 1984; Table 3). As well as reducing the protective effect of these substances on the food itself, the overall dietary antioxidant intake will be reduced. An eloquent case has been argued for a relationship between 'antioxidant status' and cardiovascular disease (Gey, 1986).

Nutritional effects may also occur through interaction between lipid-

TABLE 3
Changes in rapeseed oil used for frying[a]

Oil characteristic	Frying time (h)				
	0	10	32	88	231
COV[b] (meq/kg)	6	44	96	159	126
POV[c] (meq/kg)	1·1	5·0	8·9	7·6	5·3
Oxidized FA[d] (%)	0	0·5	1·7	5·1	4·7
Dimers (%)	0	0·6	1·0	2·8	2·3
18:2[e] (%)	20·7	19·4	17·5	14·2	15·2
α-Tocopherol (μg/g)	136	0	0	0	0

[a] From Izaki *et al.* (1984).
[b] COV = carbonyl value.
[c] POV = peroxide value.
[d] FA = fatty acid.
[e] 18:2 = linoleic acid.

free radicals or other lipid oxidation products and other important nutrients, mainly proteins and vitamins. There can be extensive hydrophobic
and hydrogen bonding between lipid hydroperoxides or other products of
lipid peroxidation and proteins (Gardner, 1979; Table 4), but little is
known about their nutritional significance. More important are reactions
involving covalent bonds. Lipid-free radicals can interact with several
amino acids in protein molecules to induce the formation of carbon-
centred protein-free radicals. The end products of such reactions may be
polymers formed by protein–protein cross—linking and complexes involv-

TABLE 4
Reaction products of amino acids with peroxidised lipids

Amino acid	Product
Histidine	Imidazole, lactic and acetic acids, Schiff-base adducts, histamine, valine, aspartic acid, ethylamine
Cysteine	Cystine, H_2S, alanine, cystine sulphoxide
Methionine	Methionine sulphoxide
Lysine	Diaminopentane, aspartic acid, glycine, alanine, α-aminoadipic acid

From Gardner (1979).

ing lipid–protein crosslinks (Gardner, 1979). When peroxidized lipid is mixed with protein in the dehydrated state, protein scission is favoured over protein–protein crosslinking. Regardless of water activity, however, the overall effect is damage to amino acid residues, thereby reducing the nutritive value of the protein.

Finally, the secondary products of lipid peroxidation (e.g. the aldehydes, epoxides and ketones) are also capable of reacting with amino acids. One of the most extensively studied of these compounds is malondialdehyde. For example, during the storage of frozen herring the concentration of the lysine in the protein decreased in direct proportion to the increase in malondialdehyde as measured by the thiobarbituric acid test. As well as reducing the nutritive value of the proteins, these reactions lead to brown colour formation and to production of unpleasant odours and tastes.

Other nutrients particularly vulnerable to attack by peroxidation products are the vitamins that act as antioxidants (vitamins E, C and β-carotene) which are destroyed in the process of free-radical scavenging and effectively this increases the requirement for these nutrients in the diet. Those that have sensitive sulphydryl and amide groups will undergo reactions similar to those described for amino acids.

Toxicological effects
Reactive species like free radicals and peroxides are potentially damaging to cells. However, unless they are absorbed from the gut and can enter body tissue they are unlikely to be very harmful except perhaps in the gut itself (Cutler & Hayward, 1974).

There is little experimental evidence on this point, but the work of Bergan and Draper (1970) suggests that little or no linoleic acid hydroperoxide is absorbed intact and therefore cannot enter tissues and cause oxidative damage.

Nevertheless, several researchers have demonstrated effects of giving lipid peroxidation products to experimental animals that may be interpreted as due to oxidative damage. The evidence accumulated for this includes: *increases* in the relative liver weight, malondialdehyde concentrations in tissues, tissue peroxide and carbonyl values and in tissue chemiluminescence and *decreases* in α-tocopherol and linoleic acid concentrations (e.g. Miyazawa *et al.*, 1983; Izaki *et al.*, 1984). Supplementing the diet with α-tocopherol tended to protect against these induced changes (Miyazawa *et al.*, 1983; Table 5). The oxidative damage reported in these experiments may be due to low molecular mass hydroperoxyalkenals which were

TABLE 5
Effect of Methyl Linoleate Hydroperoxide (MLHPO)[a] on liver of rats[b]

Diet	Time (day)	CL[c] (cpm)	TBA[d] (abs, 532 nm)	α-Tocopherol[e] (μg/g liver)
Basal	—	225	0·168	10·1
+MLHPO	2	867*[f]	0·270*	12·9
+MLHPO + TOC	2	555*	0·190	22·2*
+MLHPO	7	471	0·170	10·2
+MLHPO + TOC	7	333	0·178	20·3*

[a] MLHPO = methyl linoleate hydroperoxide.
[b] From Miyazawa *et al.* (1983).
[c] CL = chemiluminescence.
[d] TBA = thiobarbituric acid.
[e] TOC = *alpha*-tocopherol.
[f] *, significantly different from basal value, $p < 0.05$.

apparently much more readily absorbed than linoleate hydroperoxide (Yoshioka & Kaneda, 1974; Table 6).

There is little evidence that the dimeric and polymeric materials produced by prolonged cooking of oils are absorbed by or toxic to experimental animals (Billek, 1985).

The toxicity of oxidized cholesterols has been demonstrated in several studies. For example, Taylor *et al.* (1979) studied acute and chronic toxicity for rabbits of oxidized cholesterol and impurities concentrated from USP-grade cholesterol (Table 7). The unpurified cholesterol and

TABLE 6
Effects of peroxidised lipid products on liver of mice (meq/kg)[a]

	3 h		24 h	
	POV[b]	COV[c]	POV	COV
Hydroperoxyalkenal	12·0	73·7	15·4	51·3
Linoleate hydroperoxide	2·6	5·3	2·3	1·7
Hydroxyalkenal	1·5	13·8	1·3	7·9
Alkenal	1·3	15·6	1·0	5·1
Linoleate	0·8	1·1	0·7	1·8

[a] From Yoshioka and Kaneda (1974).
[b] COV = carbonyl value.
[c] POV = peroxide value.

TABLE 7
Toxicity of oxidised cholesterol to rabbits[a]

Treatment	n	Aggregate debris (%)	Degenerated cells (%)
Control	15	0·03	0·61
Old USP[b] cholesterol (1 g/kg)	5	0·70*[c]	7·60*
New USP cholesterol (1 g/kg)	5	0·22*	4·38*
New USP cholesterol (250 mg/kg)	3	0·07	1·63*
Purified cholesterol (250 mg/kg)	4	1·20*	0·35
Concentrate (250 mg/kg)	7	5·59*	7·28*

[a] From Taylor et al. (1979).
[b] USP = United States Pharmacopoeia.
[c] *, statistically different from control values, $p < 0.05$.

especially the concentrate caused pathological changes in arteries in the rabbits 24 h after administration of 250 mg/kg. The authors suggested that studies of the induction of atherosclerosis by USP-grade cholesterol that had been stored in air at room temperature should be re-evaluated since the cholesterol used in experimental diets almost certainly contained significant quantities of oxidized sterols that could contain the atherogenic factor(s) rather than the pure cholesterol itself.

In summary, products of lipid peroxidation in foods can cause damage to tissues if those tissues are not protected by sufficient antioxidant. In practice, the most vulnerable sites of damage are in the gut, since only the smaller molecular mass products of lipid peroxidation are absorbed into the bloodstream and have access to body tissues. Even then, damage is minimal if sufficient antioxidant is also absorbed and probably one of the prime dangers from lipid oxidation in foods is not so much the oxidation products themselves as the concomitant destruction of protective substances such as tocopherols, carotenoids, ascorbic acid and folates. While every precaution should be taken to prevent lipid oxidation, it should always be borne in mind that food fats are likely to become inedible before the concentrations of lipid oxidation products have reached very toxic levels.

INDUSTRIAL HYDROGENATION

The hydrogenation process

Highly unsaturated oils, such as those found in many seeds and in fish are unsuitable for many food uses because they have very low melting points and are highly susceptible to oxidative deterioriation. The object of hydrogenation, which is one of the manufacturer's (of edible fats) most important tools, is to reduce the degree of unsaturation, thereby increasing the melting point to improve textural properties in the food and increasing oxidative stability (Gunstone & Norris, 1983). By careful choice of catalyst and temperature, the oil can be hydrogenated selectively so as to achieve a product with precisely the desired characteristics. Indeed, the process is seldom taken to completion, since fully saturated fats, especially those that would be derived from the long-chain fatty acids of fish oils, would have melting points that were too high.

Hydrogenation is carried out in an enclosed tank in the presence of 0·05–0·20% of a finely powdered catalyst (usually nickel) at temperatures up to 180°C after which all traces of catalyst are removed by filtration. Chemically, there are three main results of hydrogenation:

(1) the total number of double bonds in the fatty acid molecule is reduced;

(2) a proportion of the double bonds that are present in the original oil in the *cis* geometric configuration are isomerized to the *trans* form; and

(3) the double bonds are shifted along the hydrocarbon chain from their original positions in the natural fat (Figs. 7 & 8).

These changes may have nutritional significance that will be discussed in later sections. It is important to note that *trans* double bonds do occur in natural fats but generally much less abundantly than *cis* bonds. The most important naturally occurring isomeric fatty acids in human foods are derived from ruminant fats. Whether of natural or industrial origin, fatty acids with *trans* bonds may be monounsaturated or polyunsaturated; the latter may have *cis* and *trans* bonds within the same molecule. A characteristic of the *trans* fatty acids is that they have physical properties between those of saturated and *cis* unsaturated acids. The *trans* double bond creates a linear carbon chain that contrasts with the kinked configuration of the *cis* acids. Thus, all-*trans* fatty acids can pack together in a crystalline array and their melting points are higher than those of the corresponding *cis* acids (Gurr, 1986).

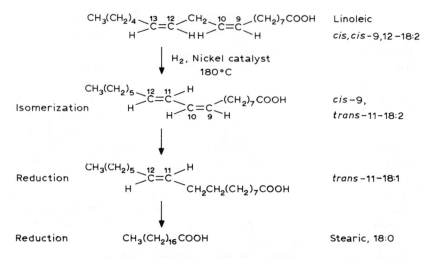

FIG. 7. Steps involved in the industrial hydrogenation of linoleic acid. This scheme is much simplified to highlight the important processes of isomerization (both geometrical and positional) and reduction of double bonds. In practice the number of different isomeric fatty acids obtained is much larger.

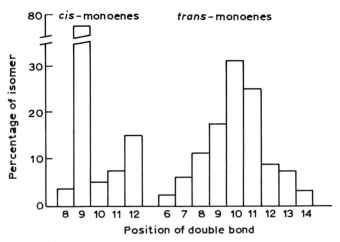

FIG. 8. Formation of positional and geometric isomers during industrial hydrogenation of a vegetable oil. (From Brisson (1981), reproduced by permission of MTP Press, New Jersey, USA).

Qualitative and quantitative information about the *trans* fatty acid content of fats can be obtained by infra-red spectrometry, by separation of the different classes of fatty acids by argentation thin-layer chromatography or by separating individual acids by capillary gas–liquid chromatography. The determination of positional isomers is more demanding and the accurate and comprehensive determination of all fatty acid isomers in a complex mixture generally requires a combination of several or all of these techniques as well as mass spectrometric analysis (Christie, 1982).

In industrially hydrogenated fats, *trans* monoenes represent the major fraction of *trans* acids, with *trans* unsaturation at positions 6-12 and a predominance of the 10-isomer. The *trans* diene fraction ranges from 0 to 25% of the total diene fraction in different margarines. *Trans* unsaturation in the dienoic acids is found in *cis*-9,*trans*-12-18:2, *trans*-9,*cis*-12-18:2 and *cis*-9,*trans*-13-18:2. Improvements in catalytic hydrogenation have reduced the amounts of *trans,trans* dienes in modern margarines, often to zero.

Dietary intake of isomeric fatty acids

Estimates of consumption of *trans* fatty acids in the UK diet vary between 5 and 7 g/person per day (Burt & Buss, 1984; Gurr, 1984; British Nutrition Foundation, 1987). Studies in some other countries have been more detailed (Brisson, 1982; Senti, 1985). The average intake in the USA in the early 1980s was thought to be 12 g head per day, 4·8% of which came from animal fat and 95·2% from partially hydrogenated vegetable oils. There, *trans* fatty acids represented about 8% of total dietary fatty acids. The corresponding figure from Canada was estimated to be 9.6 g/head per day, 94% coming from partially hydrogenated oils. National differences may be apparent because of the different sources of fats and oils used by the industry. For example, the UK margarine industry is one of the few to use marine oils in large quantities. These oils contain high proportions of polyunsaturated fatty acids with 5 or 6 double bonds. The degree of hydrogenation needed to achieve the desired physical properties is therefore more extensive and the opportunities for producing a wide variety of positional and geometric isomers are greater than in the hydrogenation of vegetable oils in which di- and tri-unsaturated fatty acids predominate.

Digestion and absorption of fats containing isomeric fatty acids

Experiments designed to investigate the metabolic effects of isomeric fatty acids have employed either semi-synthetic diets in which the lipid component contains a single isomeric fatty acid of defined structure, or in the majority of cases, an industrially produced fat containing a complex mixture of fatty acids. The former yields results that are easier to interpret and more informative in biochemical terms. The latter may be more relevant to practical human nutrition but it is frequently impossible to relate effects to a specific structural feature of the dietary lipid.

There is no scientific evidence that the lipases catalysing the digestion of fat in the gut discriminate between fatty acids according to the geometry of the double bond. However, *cis* isomers of octadecenoic acid in which the double bond occurs close to the carboxyl group are not well hydrolysed by pancreatic lipase (Holman, 1985). Very long chain fatty acids (C_{20} and above) are also more slowly hydrolysed from triacylglycerols than fatty acids of 18 carbon atoms or less (Sickinger, 1975). This is of significance for the digestion of some triacylglycerols found in fish oils and hardened fish oils, which are used as hardstock in some UK margarines, but has nothing to do with the isomeric composition of the oils or the process of hydrogenation. Likewise, there is little evidence that isomeric fatty acids differ in their absorption. In reports that claim poorer absorption of *trans* acids than *cis*, there was also a higher content of long-chain saturated fatty acids in the diet which might have accounted for the difference.

Metabolism

When isomeric fatty acids are included in the diet, they can be found in the lipids of most tissues in the body (Beare-Rogers, 1983; Senti, 1985; British Nutrition Foundation, 1987). The highest proportions of *trans* fatty acids found in human biopsy and necropsy specimens have been in the liver and adipose tissue (up to 14% of fatty acids, Johnston *et al.*, 1957). Amounts varying between 0·1 and 4·5% of total fatty acids have been found in human milk (Senti, 1985).

There is some selectivity with regard to the complex lipids into which *trans* fatty acids are incorporated. In general, a larger proportion of the *trans* fatty acids in the body is found in the triacylglycerols because of the relatively large amounts of these lipids deposited in adipose tissue (Beare-Rogers, 1983). They occur mainly in positions 1 and 3. In other tissues such as heart and brain, as much or more *trans* fatty acids may be incorporated into phospholipids (Moore *et al.*, 1980). The *trans* octadecenoic acids behave like saturated fatty acids and are preferentially incorporated into position 1 of phosphoglycerides in contrast to oleic acid which is randomly distributed. Few metabolic studies have been conducted with human subjects (e.g. see Emken *et al.*, 1980) and it is difficult to draw any conclusions about the general metabolic effects of regular ingestion of the small amounts of the isomers found in practical diets.

There is little evidence that isomeric fatty acids are broken down less readily in the body than the normal fatty acids (Anderson & Coots, 1967). Research workers in this field frequently give diets that contain partially hydrogenated marine oils or high erucic rapeseed oil, which also contain very long-chain acids as well as a mixture of isomers (e.g. Cristiansen *et al.*, 1979). The results obtained may be more related to the long-chain length of the fatty acids than to geometrical or positional isomerism.

Interactions with essential fatty acid metabolism
When young animals are fed on a diet that lacks essential fatty acids, signs of overt essential fatty acid deficiency are observed that can be reversed by feeding as little as 1% of dietary energy as linoleic acid. When the diet has only marginally sufficient linoleic acid, the addition of non-essential fatty acids can result in the appearance of deficiency signs, even though the absolute amount of linoleic acid has not been reduced. Under these conditions Hill *et al.* (1979) demonstrated that as the amount of dietary *trans* fatty acids was increased, the animals showed progressive signs of essential fatty acid deficiency. The *trans,trans* isomer of linoleic acid appeared to be more potent than the *cis,trans* isomers (Privett *et al.*, 1977).

Several reports provide evidence that one of the mechanisms by which *trans* acids influence the metabolism of essential fatty acids is to inhibit desaturases (i.e. the enzymes that introduce double bonds into fatty acid molecules to yield more highly unsaturated acids). De Schrijver and Privett (1982) showed that feeding *trans* acids to rats inhibited 6-desaturase but increased 9-desaturase. This work employed a mixture of different *trans* acids including *trans,trans*-18:2. Other research has concluded that the effects of this latter compound are far more potent than those of the *trans* monounsaturated acids (Anderson *et al.*, 1975; Shimp *et al.*, 1982). Studies with specific isomers are scientifically satisfying, but in terms of practical human nutrition the results with *trans,trans*-18:2 may not be important, since it is a very minor component of most human diets.

Certain *trans* fatty acids are themselves substrates for desaturases, so that another possible mechanism for their influence on essential fatty acid metabolism is to compete with essential fatty acids for common desaturases. *Trans* monoenes, in which the double bond is away from the 9-position, are desaturated by the 9-desaturase to form a series of *cis*-9,*trans*-x-18:2 isomers, some of which are substrates for the 6- and 5-desaturases in the further pathways of essential fatty acid metabolism (Holman 1985). The long chain polyunsaturated fatty acids formed by the alternate desaturation and elongation of dietary linoleic (n-6 family) and linolenic acids (n-3 family) have two vital functions in the tissues of the body (Fig. 9). First, their presence seems to be essential for the maintenance of stable membrane structures. Second, they are the starting points for the synthesis of a wide variety of hormone-like substances, called eicosanoids, that are important in the control of such processes as muscle contraction, the formation of blood clots and immunity. The polyunsaturated fatty acids formed from oleic acid (n-9 family) or acids containing *trans* double bonds or *cis* double bonds in unusual positions in the molecule give rise to unstable membranes and are not converted into biologically active eicosanoids.

Normally, the preferred substrates for the formation of the long-chain polyunsaturated fatty acids are linoleic and linolenic acids and so long as there are not too many *trans* acids in the diet they will compete successfully and ensure the production of sufficient long-chain polyunsaturated fatty acids to maintain functional membranes and generate the appropriate types and amounts of eicosanoids. Excessively large dietary intakes of *trans* acids may swamp these important metabolic pathways giving rise to metabolic problems akin to some aspects of essential fatty acid deficiency. Normally this does not occur but may become a problem for individuals who choose diets particularly rich in products containing large concentrations of *trans* fatty acids.

There is some uncertainty about the effects of *trans* unsaturated fatty acids on plasma lipoprotein cholesterol concentrations in man. Some studies have demonstrated an increase (e.g. see Vergroesen, 1972) and others, such as the study of Mattson *et al.* (1975) which was probably the best controlled, observed no change. Less is known about the effects on thrombus formation, although at least one author (Hornstra, 1982) has shown *trans* octadecenoate to be no more thrombogenic than *cis* octadecenoate. Recently, Mensink & Katan (1990) showed that *trans*-octadecenoate increased plasma low density lipoprotein (LDL) concentrations and reduced high density lipoprotein (HDL) concentrations when it partially replaced the *cis*-octadecenoate in the diets of human subjects. The rise in LDL-cholesterol was less than that elicited by saturated fatty acids which did not, however, affect HDL concentrations.

Recommendations for healthy eating
What are the implications of the foregoing discussion for the health of the consumer? If there are reservations about the safety of modified fats which

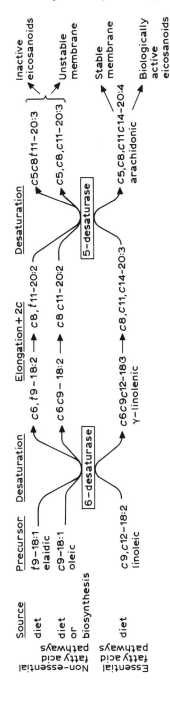

Fig. 9. Competition between essential and non-essential fatty acid pathways.

become incorporated into national dietary recommendations or into more formal legislation on food labelling, how will this affect the food manufacturer?

In the UK, the most influential document in this regard has been the report of the Department of Health's Panel on diet and cardiovascular disease (DHSS, 1984) which has been accepted by Government as official policy. Its recommendations are taken as the basis for most, if not all, the initiatives in public education programmes in healthy eating. This report made no general pronouncements about oxidized fats or antioxidants in foods. It did, however, state:

'there are no specific recommendations about the intake of oxidized cholesterol . . . in the UK diet. Further research is needed to ascertain whether dietary oxidized cholesterol is absorbed or incorporated into atherosclerotic plaques'. [It also said] 'There are no specific recommendations about the dietary intake of vitamin E which we believe will be adequate from the diet which may result from the recommendations of this report'. A more recent report from the UK Department of Health (1991) has recommended that intakes of Vitamin E should not be less than 3 mg/day for women and 4 mg/day for men.

The report did make recommendations about *trans* fatty acids. One of the report's main recommendations to the general public was to reduce the consumption of total fat and especially saturated fatty acids. For the purposes of this particular recommendation, the term saturated fatty acids was intended to include *trans* fatty acids. The panel accepted that the evidence with regard to the effects of *trans* fatty acids on cardiovascular disease were not as clear cut as for saturated fatty acids, but nevertheless they took the cautious approach to avoid the possibility of promoting, by default, dietary change (i.e. increasing the amount of *trans* fatty acids in the diet) that may have disadvantages for health until the evidence was clearer. A more recent report from the UK Department of Health (1991), clearly distinguishes *trans-* from saturated fatty acids and suggests in the text that the current population average intake of 5 g/day should not increase. However, the report is ambiguous since in Table 1.2, the quoted recommended intake is 2 g/day, implying a recommendation to reduce intake of *trans* acids substantially. If consumers are to be in a position to know which foods contain saturated, *trans*-unsaturated and polyunsaturated fatty acids and in what quantities, this information must be available to them, preferably on product labels. In a later section of the report, therefore, the panel make recommendations that information on these categories of fats should be printed on product labels. This clearly has important implications for food manufacturers, especially in terms of the cost of conforming to these regulations. There is also the danger in such cases that such foods automatically become associated as 'bad' in the consumer's mind. It is therefore a subject of continuing discussion between the Ministry of Agriculture Fisheries and Food, the Health Department, manufacturers and food scientists.

One effect of the necessity to declare *trans* fatty acids on food labels could be to influence the source of raw materials for the UK edible oils' industry. The UK industry is one of the few that uses fish oils as raw materials on a large scale. Because of the large proportion of unsaturated fatty acids with 5 and 6 double bonds in fish oils, the products of hydrogenation are more complex and the content of *trans* fatty acids in the final product likely to be higher than in the products of hydrogenation of most vegetable oils. UK manufacturers could be encouraged to switch more to vegetable oils as sources of raw materials and there is evidence that this is happening anyway. Another unknown factor is the way in which UK legislation will be required to harmonize with that of the EC. This, too, is a subject of current discussion after recent publication by the EC of draft guidelines for nutrition labelling. These did not include a requirement to label for *trans* acids.

In terms of influencing public health, the provision of information on labels is in itself insufficient. It must be accompanied by programmes designed to increase the awareness of consumers about nutritional principles, preferably at school age, so that they are educated to be able to make their own decisions on food choice. Consumers can avoid potential problems discussed in this article by choosing a varied diet, which should ensure adequate intakes of antioxidants and which should enable them to avoid an imbalance with respect to any particular type of fat: saturated, *trans* or polyunsaturated. By avoiding overcooking and the re-use of deteriorated oils, which destroys antioxidants and essential nutrients, they can adequately reduce the risks of oxidative damage, and nutrient and antioxidant depletion.

REFERENCES

Anderson, R.L. & Coots, R.H. (1967). The catabolism of the geometric isomers of uniformly ^{14}C-labelled 9-octadecenoic and uniformly ^{14}C-labelled, 9,12-octadecadienoic acid by the fasting rat. *Biochimica et Biophysica Acta* **144**, 525–31.
Anderson, R.L., Fullmer, C.S. & Hollenbach, E.J. (1975). Effect of the *trans*

isomers of linoleic acid on the metabolism of linoleic acid in rats. *Journal of Nutrition* **105**, 303–400.

Artman, N.R. & Smith, D.E. (1972). Systematic isolation and identification of minor components in heated and unheated fat. *Journal of the American Oil Chemists' Society* **49**, 318–26.

Beare-Rogers, J.L. (1983). *Trans* and positional isomers of common fatty acids. *Advances in Nutrition Research* **5**, 171–200.

Bergan, J.G. & Draper, H.H. (1970). Absorption and metabolism of 1-^{14}C-methyl linoleate hydroperoxide. *Lipids* **5**, 976–82.

Billek, G. (1985). Heated fats in the diet. In *The Role of Fats in Human Nutrition*, pp. 163–72 [F.B. Padley and J. Podmore, editors]. Chichester: Ellis Horwood/ Society of Chemical Industry.

Brisson, G.D. (1982). *Lipids in Human Nutrition*, pp. 48–50 Lancaster, UK: MTP Press.

British Nutrition Foundation (1987). *Report of a Task Force on* Trans *Fatty Acids.* London: British Nutrition Foundation.

Burt, R. & Buss, D.H. (1984). Dietary fatty acids in the UK. *British Journal of Clinical Practice* **3**, Suppl. 51, 20–1.

Christiansen, E.N., Thomassen, M.S., Christiansen, R.Z., Osmundsen, H. & Norum, K.R. (1979). Metabolism of erucic acid in the perfused rat liver. Increased chain shortening after feeding partially hydrogenated marine oil and rapeseed oil. *Lipids* **14**, 829–35.

Christie, W.W. (1982). *Lipid Analysis.* Oxford: Pergamon Press.

Cutler, M.G. & Hayward, M.A. (1974). Effect of lipid peroxides on fat absorption and folic acid status in the rat. *Nutrition and Metabolism* **16**, 87–93.

De Schrijver, R. & Privett, O.S. (1982). Interrelationships between dietary *trans* fatty acids and the 6- and 9-desaturases in the rat. *Lipids* **17**, 27–34.

DHSS (1984). Committee on Medical Aspects of Food Policy (COMA). *Diet and cardiovascular disease.* Reports on health and social subjects no. 28. London: H.M. Stationery Office.

DH (1991). *Dietary Reference Values for Food Energy and Nutrients for the United Kingdom.* Report on Health and Social Subjects no. 41. London: H.M. Stationery Office.

Emken, E.A., Dutton, H.J., Rohwedder, W.K., Rakoff, H., Adlof, R.O., Gulley, R.M. & Canary, J.J. (1980). Distribution of deuterium labelled *cis* and *trans*-12-octadecenoic acids in human plasma and lipoprotein lipids. *Lipids* **15**, 864–71.

Frankel, E.N. (1980). Lipid oxidation. *Progress in Lipid Research* **19**, 1–22.

Gardner, H.W. (1979). Lipid hydroperoxide reactivity with proteins and amino acids: a review. *Journal of Agricultural and Food Chemistry* **27**, 220–9.

Gey, K.F. (1986). On the antioxidant hypothesis with regard to arteriosclerosis. *Bibliotheca Nutritia Dieta* **37**, 53–91.

Gray, J.I. (1978). Measurement of lipid oxidation: a review. *Journal of the American Oil Chemists' Society* **55**, 539–46.

Gunstone, F.D. & Norris, F.A. (1983). *Lipids in Food: Chemistry, Biochemistry and Technology.* Oxford: Pergamon Press.

Gurr, M.I. (1984). *The Role of Fats in Food and Nutrition*, p. 127. London: Elsevier Applied Science Publishers.

Gurr, M.I. (1986). *Trans* fatty acids—metabolic and nutritional significance. *British Nutrition Foundation Nutrition Bulletin* **11**, 105–22.

Halliwell, B. & Gutteridge, J.M.C. (1985). *Free Radicals in Biology and Medicine.* Oxford: Clarendon Press.

Hill, E.G., Johnson, S.B. & Holman, R.T. (1979). Intensification of essential fatty acid deficiency in the rat by dietary *trans* fatty acids. *Journal of Nutrition* **109**, 1759–66.

Holman, R.T. (1985). Influence of hydrogenated fats on the metabolism of polyunsaturated fatty acids. In *The Role of Fats in Human Nutrition*, pp. 48–61 [F.B. Padley and J. Podmore, editors]. Chichester: Ellis Horwood/Society of Chemical Industry.

Hornstra, G. (1982). *Developments in Haematology & Immunology*, vol. 4. London: Martinus Nijhoff.

Izaki, Y., Yoshikawa, S. & Uchiyama, M. (1984). Effect of ingestion of thermally oxidized frying oil on peroxidative criteria in rats. *Lipids* **19**, 324–31.

Johnston, P.V., Johnson, O.C. & Kummerow, F.A. (1957). Occurrence of *trans* fatty acids in human tissue. *Science* **126**, 698–9.

Logani, M.K. & Davies, R.E. (1980). Lipid oxidation: biologic effects and antioxidants: a review. *Lipids* **15**, 485–95.

Mattson, F.H., Hollenback, E.J. & Kligman, A.M. (1975). Effect of hydrogenated fat on the plasma cholesterol and triglyceride levels of man. *American Journal of Clinical Nutrition* **28**, 726–31.

Mensink, R.P. & Katan, M.B. (1990). Effect of dietary *trans* fatty acids on high density and low density lipoprotein cholesterol levels in healthy subjects. *New England Journal of Medicine* **323**, 439–45.

Miyazawa, T., Nagaoka, A. & Kaneda, T. (1983). Tissue lipid peroxidation and ultraweak chemiluminescence in rats dosed with methyl linoleate hydroperoxide. *Agricultural and Biological Chemistry* **47**, 1333–9.

Moore, C.E., Alfin-Slater, R.B. & Aftergood, L. (1980). Incorporation and disappearance of *trans* fatty acids in rat tissues. *American Journal of Clinical Nutrition* **33**, 2318–23.

Privett, O.S., Phillips, F., Shimasaki, H., Nozawa, T. & Nickell, E.C. (1977). Studies of effects of *trans* fatty acids in the diet on lipid metabolism in essential fatty acid deficient rats. *American Journal of Clinical Nutrition* **30**, 1009–17.

Reddy, B.R., Yasuda, K., Krishnamurthy, R.G. & Chang, S.S. (1968). Chemical reactions involved in deep fat frying of foods. V. Identification of nonacidic volatile decomposition products of hydrogenated cottonseed oil. *Journal of the American Oil Chemists' Society* **45**, 629–31.

Senti, F.R. (1985). *Health Aspects of Dietary* Trans *Fatty Acids.* Bethesda, MD: Federation of American Societies of Experimental Biology.

Sickinger, K. (1975). Clinical aspects and therapy of fat malassimilation with particular reference to the use of medium-chain triglycerides. In *The Role of Fats in Human Nutrition* , pp. 115–209 [A.J. Vergroesen, editor]. London: Academic Press.

Shimp, J.L., Bruckner, G. & Kinsella, J.E. (1982). The effects of dietary trilinolaidin on fatty acid and acyl desaturases in rat liver. *Journal of Nutrition* **112**, 722–35.

Taylor, C.B., Peng, S.K., Werthesen, N.T., Tham, P. & Lee, K.T. (1979).

Spontaneously occurring angiotoxic derivatives of cholesterol. *American Journal of Clinical Nutrition* **32**, 40–57.

Vergroesen, A.J. (1972). Dietary fat and cardiovascular disease: possible modes of action of linoleic acid. *Proceedings of the Nutrition Society* **31**, 323–9.

Yoshioka, M. & Kaneda, T. (1974). Toxicity of hydroperoxyalkenals in autoxidized oils. *Proceedings of the IV International Congress of Food Science and Technology* **1**, 276–82.

8

Vegetarianism: The Healthy Alternative?

Tracy J. Hallas & Ann F. Walker
Department of Food Science and Technology, University of Reading, UK

INTRODUCTION

The Oxford Dictionary defines a vegetarian as 'one who abstains from the use of flesh, fish and fowl as food'. However, the degree of abstinence from animal products varies among vegetarians. At the lower end of the spectrum pescovegetarians exclude only flesh and fowl from the diet, whilst lactovegetarians and ovo-vegetarians both exclude fish, but consume milk and eggs, respectively. Lacto-ovovegetarians, as their name suggests, will eat both eggs and milk. It should be noted, however, that many researchers regard the terms lacto-ovovegetarian and lactovegetarian as interchangeable and do not attempt to distinguish between the two. At the opposite end of the spectrum, strict vegetarians (vegans) consume no food of animal origin whatsoever.

A largely vegetarian diet is practiced over the centuries by many in the Third World through necessity. In the West, until recently, it has been dismissed by many as 'faddist' (Carlson *et al.*, 1985). Not surprisingly, the food industry took little account for what was considered a minority and possibly eccentric eating pattern. However, the recent upsurge in interest in the vegetarian diet and its growing number of adherents has provided the impetus for the food industry in general, and the meat industry in particular, to accommodate vegetarians in their marketing policies. Indeed, its popularity has produced an opening in the market that many have sought to exploit.

While it is generally believed that vegetarian diets provide a healthy alternative to an omnivorous Western diet, concerns have been raised about the nutritional adequacy of such diets, particularly those that are vegan. The nutritional issues raised by vegetarianism are whether the diet is adequate for requirements and to what extent it complies with the current views on the association between diet and good health.

REASONS FOR BECOMING VEGETARIAN

As a form of dietary practice, vegetarianism is an ancient as mankind. However, the underlying motivations dictating adherence to such a diet have indeed become multifarious in the West. Many people are vegetarian due to cultural and religious reasons. Asian, Indian and East African immigrants into the UK account for a large proportion of these (Sanders, 1983).

Early in this century the advocacy by influential individuals of a simple life in harmony with nature converted many people to vegetarianism. Further concerns over adulteration of foodstuffs, instigated by prominent food reformers, prompted a move away from foods considered as unnatural. However, the vast majority of people continued to view vegetarianism with derision. Inadequate incomes and poor availability of animal produce were predominant reasons for becoming vegetarian at this time, rather than concerns over health and animal welfare (Dwyer *et al.*, 1974).

The second half of this century has seen the emergence of new reasons for becoming vegetarian. Moral objections to the treatment of animals in addition to aversion at the deliberate taking of life to sustain humanity causes many people to become vegetarian. Increased awareness of ecological and health-related issues has furthered the interest. Concerns over Third World famine and environmental or 'Green' issues accounts for a comparatively large number of vegetarians in the UK. Other factors involved are dislike of the taste and look of meat, the relative cheapness of vegetarian diets in comparison with meat diets, concerns over food poisoning and political reasons (MSI, 1989). In addition, links have been established between vegetarianism, peace movements opposed to the cruelty inflicted on animals other than in meat production and the use of alternative medicines (Dwyer *et al.*, 1974).

The primary reasons submitted for changing to a vegetarian diet these days are concerns over health and an abhorrence of animal suffering (Carlson *et al.*, 1985). Recent data suggest that health concerns are now the major impetus for avoiding meat (MSI, 1989). Usually, however, individuals will change to a vegetarian diet for a number of reasons, rather than one alone (Woodward, 1988).

The most frequent explanations given by those expressing health concerns in the seventies were the beliefs that diets devoid of meat would lead to reduced 'grogginess' and improved mental functioning (Dwyer *et al.*, 1974). Although not perceiving meat as hazardous to health, many consumers believed certain components of meat such as saturated fat, hormones and chemicals, to be deleterious. In the UK, increased public awareness of the potential risks of a meat diet in relation to chronic disease incidence such as coronary heart disease (CHD) followed the publication of dietary guidelines by NACNA (1983) and the COMA Report (DHSS, 1984), persuading many people to turn to a vegetarian diet as a preventative measure (Bender, 1985).

There can be no doubt that vegetarianism has become more fashionable in recent years in the UK, particularly among young people. However, such a motive lacks commitment: people who become vegetarian for the sake of image are liable to tire quickly of the initial attraction.

TRENDS IN VEGETARIANISM

How many vegetarians are there?
There is considerable difficulty in estimating the numbers of vegetarians in Britain at the present time. Figures representing membership of vegetarian and vegan societies show substantial increases in the number of subscribers but, of course, these figures do not accurately reflect the full scale of vegetarianism in the UK.

Gallop (1988; see MSI, 1989) indicated that 4·3 million people in the UK in 1987 were either vegetarian or had reduced their intake of red meat. This corresponds to an approximately 43% increase in those turning to vegetarian diets and an 89% increase in the number of people avoiding red meat since 1984 or an increase of 129 000 and 221 000 individuals respectively.

Estimates of the size of the UK vegetarian population in 1988 suggest almost 5 million people or 8·6% of the entire population are vegan, vegetarian or avoiders of red meat (MSI, 1989). In contrast, the Vegetarian Society UK Ltd. (Parkdale, Dunham Road, Altrincham, Cheshire) has proposed that almost 8·5% of the population are vegetarian, exclusive of those who avoid red meat (MSI, 1989). Such a discrepancy is difficult to justify. However, the partiality of organisations committed to the

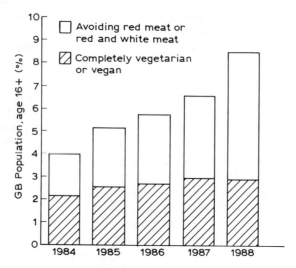

FIG. 1.   Percentage of the UK population who were non-meat eaters in the 1980s.
Compiled from Anon. (1987) and MSI (1989).

promotion of their ideals cannot be totally dismissed in influencing reported figures. Similarly, claims by the meat trade suggesting that only 3% of
the total UK population do not eat meat, a value which has remained
'largely unchanged for several years' (Anon., 1989), can be viewed with
some scepticism.

The growth of vegetarianism amongst members of the population aged
16 and above, between 1984 and 1988 is represented in Fig. 1. Most recent
estimates indicate that 3% of the adult population or 1·3 million adults are
vegetarian. The greatest rate of growth occurred between 1984 and 1985,
suggesting a considerable stimulation of public interest in diet-related
health issues following the release of the COMA (DHSS, 1984) dietary
guidelines. However, these estimated do not account for people below 16
years of age. Estimates for 1988 proposed that 9·3% of the child population or 1·2 million children in the UK were vegetarian (Gallup; MSI,
1988). Additionally, women are becoming increasingly more important in
making up the UK vegetarian population, being almost twice as likely to
avoid red meat as men. In particular, young women (16–24 years) constitute a large group of non-meat eaters (12·5%). Between 1984 and 1987
the number of vegetarians in this sector almost doubled (MSI, 1989).

The emergence of regional differences in the prevalence of vegetarianism
is also becoming evident. Although non-meat eating is increasing through-

out the UK, the trend towards vegetarianism is most prominent in the South (7·7%) (MSI, 1989). Financial considerations and the presence of societies in universities dedicated to the abolition of animal cruelty have encouraged many students to turn to vegetarianism (MSI, 1989).

Response of the food industry and food retailer

The potential to exploit an expanding vegetarian market has now been recognized by many manufacturers and retailers, who have responded to this opportunity by developing a wide range of vegetarian products. The persistence of the demand has provided the incentive for a number of non-specialist companies to reformulate their existing product ranges to suit vegetarians so as not to limit the market potential. The most common example involves the replacement of animal fat by vegetable fat in bakery products (MSI, 1989). Such changes are of little consequence to meat eaters, but refusal to make these changes would have lost the custom of a significant proportion of the non-meat eating population.

Large supermarket chains are all involved in increasing potential sales of their vegetarian product ranges by continually formulating ready-meal products with new and exciting flavours, textures and colours. Considerable effort is being put into promoting the 'healthfulness' and diversity of vegetarian products, not only to appeal more widely to existing vegetarians, but also in an attempt to attract the interest of meat eaters. In this way, manufacturers of innovative ready-meals can expect to increase their market. It is also anticipated that supplementation of meat diets with vegetarian meals will become more widespread as these products become more widely available (MSI, 1989).

Possibly most indicative of the growth in importance of vegetarianism within the food industry is the wide availability of vegetarian products among food retailing outlets. The demand for these products has had such an impact that the vast majority now stock at least some products. In the UK catering for vegetarians was traditionally the role of specialist health-food outlets. Between 1982 and 1986 the number of these outlets increased by 100, on average, each year, such that by 1986 there were approximately 1600 specialist health-food outlets in the UK. However, estimated figures for 1987 showed that the growth rate of these outlets had decreased substantially, with the establishment of only 50 new ones.

The most significant threat to the specialist outlets is the rapidly growing dominance of the multiple grocers in providing vegetarian food. Furthermore, the highly competitive position of the multiples, in addition to changes in lifestyle that favour shopping at these outlets, has conferred

TABLE 1
The value of the UK vegetarian foods
market 1988

Description	Value (£ millions)
Specialist retailers	250
Other	250
Total	500

^a Wholesalers, cash and carry, independent
grocers, excluding supermarkets.
Source: MSI (1989).

considerable advantage upon them. Multiple grocers are now believed to account for the largest share of the total UK vegetarian market (MSI, 1989). The mere presence of vegetarian foods in multiples indicates their market potential, since only by reaching sales expectations can new products justify their place on the shelf. It can be reasonably suggested that the multiples are greatly responsible for increasing demand for vegetarian foods to its current level.

The provision of ready-meal vegetarian alternatives to popular meat dishes by the multiples has resulted partly in the move away from specialist outlets, which tend to concentrate more on vegetarian meal ingredients such as tofu and soya (MSI, 1989). The specialized outlets are beginning to review their retailing strategies rather than taking a competitive stance. Thus, the UK's largest health food chain is now placing greater emphasis on providing choice of products for the consumer and is tending to concentrate on those products that are more closely connected with health, such as dietary supplements, rather than vegetarian products *per se* (MSI, 1989). Another recognition of the market potential is that retail chemists now stock some vegetarian products.

The value of the vegetarian market
Estimates of the total value of the vegetarian foods market in the UK in 1988 are around £1000 million. However, some foods and ingredients were included in these figures that cannot strictly be classified as pertaining to a vegetarian diet. Another estimate, excluding the value of vegetarian foods sold through multiples, indicate the value to exceed £500 million in 1988 (Table 1). It is believed that inclusion of the multiples will almost double the value. Therefore, estimates imply a value approaching £1000

million (MSI, 1989). Sales of chilled and frozen vegetarian ready-meals account for 21% of the total sales in ready-meals (MSI, 1989) which indicates that many meat eaters are consuming these products.

The caterer's response
Vegetarianism has undoubtedly made less impression on the UK catering sector. The need to provide some vegetarian meals as alternatives has now been widely acknowledged by restaurants, hotels and to some extent, fast-food outlets. However, perhaps indicative of the fear that vegetarianism was just another 'passing phase', there are very few all-vegetarian catering establishments (MSI, 1989).

In 1985 more than 25% of restaurants claimed that they were offering a vegetarian alternative to the main course (Carewell & Penn, 1986). Earlier, little effort was made in producing innovative meals, in the belief that a salad or omelette would suffice, but the realization that this is no longer acceptable (if indeed it ever was), has led to serious attempts to improve the selection of meals on offer to vegetarians.

The area in catering most reluctant to respond to demand for vegetarian meals has been the fast-food sector. In 1988, 19% of the fast-food market provided what they considered to be a vegetarian alternative (MSI, 1989). However, the extent to which some of these so-called 'alternatives' were suitable for dedicated vegetarians is highly questionable—vegeburgers cooked in animal fat were frequently found. Clearly, the question of authenticity of vegetarian foods in catering is of importance if vegetarians are not to be deterred from sampling them.

It is apparent, therefore, that some progress has been made in catering to improve vegetarian foods on offer, but minimal concern has been shown for the needs of vegans. Considerable potential may exist in the vegan market for manufacturers and retailers of ready-meals.

The reaction of the meat industry
Approximately 86% of people in the UK claim to have made at least one change towards a 'healthier' diet. Red meats and meat products have, in particular, been singled out by dietary advisors as products that should be reduced in the diet. Although other factors such as the increasing cost of meat will adversely affect meat purchasing, evidence implicates the role of advice on health and diet in this downward trend (Woodward, 1988). These changes have been accompanied by an increasing demand for white meat since 1984 (MAFF, 1988).

Such developments have placed the meat industry in the difficult position of having to promote the positive aspects of meat over non-meat products to recapture the market or arrest any further decline. Other responses have included producing a range of reduced-fat sausages, leaner cuts of meat and many other meat products containing 'low' contents of fat (Slattery, 1986). However, these improved quality products are commanding premium prices, which may prevent a substantial proportion of the population purchasing them (Woodward, 1988).

THE NUTRITIONAL ADEQUACY OF A VEGETARIAN DIET

The adequacy of vegetarian diets in terms of providing sufficient intakes of all nutrients compatible with good nutritional health is not always recognized. Nutritional adequacy is associated with the consumption of a wide variety of foodstuffs and although it remains widely held that vegetarian diets are restricted, the diets of British vegetarians often include more variety than those of non-vegetarians (Sanders, 1983). If sufficient care is taken in planning such a diet, especially when the diet becomes more restrictive with the exclusion of all animals produce (veganism), then most nutritionists agree that nutritionally adequate diets are perfectly feasible.

Inevitably, ignorance and misinformation will dictate the existence of some poor vegetarian diets, particularly if no attempt has been made to compensate for the withdrawal of meat and fish from the diet, which can make significant contributions to the intakes of protein, vitamin B_{12}, retinol, vitamin D and iron (Lawrie, 1979). Milk, other dairy products and eggs (all of which are excluded in vegan diets) will provide calcium, protein, fat and many vitamins and trace minerals in substantial quantities (Porter, 1975). Thus, in order to assess the adequacy and potential risk involved in the adoption of vegetarian diets, the ability of plant foods to provide these nutrients deserves consideration.

Generalization concerning the adequacy of a 'vegetarian diet' should be treated with caution. Vegetarianism includes such a broad spectrum of diets that to classify all vegetarian diets as 'good' or 'bad' would be pointless (Sanders, 1983). Distinct nutritional differences exist between the consumption of milk and eggs by lacto-ovovegetarians at one extreme and the total exclusion of all animal products by vegans at the other. Obviously, the more restrictive the diet, the greater the risk of nutrient deficiency.

Energy
While it is a commonly held view that vegans are lighter in weight than

TABLE 2
The sources of energy (% of total energy intake) compared in three different diets

	Fat	*Animal fat*	*Carbohydrate*	*Protein*	*Alcohol*
NACNE (1983) guidelines	30	—	55	11·0	4·0
Vegans	32·6	—	54·4	11·4	2·0
Lacto-ovovegetarians	38·5	15·6	45·1	14·1	2·8
Omnivores	41·0	21·5	38·5	14·0	7·0

Source: Carlson *et al.* (1985).

omnivores and lacto-ovovegetarians, supporting data on this point is difficult to find and that which exists is equivocal. The majority of studies assessing energy intakes of vegetarians have shown that they are marginal with respect to Recommended Daily Amounts (RDA) (DHSS, 1979) when considerations for age, sex and weight have been made. However, values obtained by some workers are similar to those for omnivores (Bull & Barber, 1984; Carlson *et al.*, 1985; Shultz & Leklem, 1987). Indeed, Carlson *et al.* (1985) considered that it was the high consumption of energy-dense foods by many vegans that accounted for energy intakes typically higher than lacto-ovovegetarians. On the other hand, Shultz and Leklem (1987) demonstrated the mean energy intake of vegetarian women to be exceptionally low (7·2 MJ). In contrast, another study has reported mean energy intakes of vegetarian women of 9·3 MJ and men of 10·7 MJ, which would be regarded as adequate (Roshanai & Sanders, 1984). However, in the latter study a wide range of values was noted. The importance of an adequate intake of energy cannot be over-emphasized, since it is widely acknowledged that diets low in energy can restrict intakes of other nutrients.

The relative importance of sources of energy in the diet has been highlighted in dietary guidelines (Table 2). Energy from fat in the vegan diet is significantly lower than the others and the only one to approximate dietary goals (NACNE, 1983; COMA: DHSS, 1984) in all energy sources.

The sources of energy in the diet

Quantity and quality of protein. There has been a tendency for lay people faced with the problem of ensuring nutritional adequacy of a vegetarian diet to over-focus on protein (Mutch, 1988). Only about one third of protein is supplied by meat in traditional omnivorous diets (Bender, 1985). When it is recognized that the quality of some plant proteins when eaten as the sole protein source is generally lower than single animal sources, concern over protein adequacy seemed to be reasonably founded. However, protein obtained from several vegetable sources such as soya can be of as high a quality as protein from animal sources. In addition, the complementary effect of different proteins of vegetable origin allows a better overall quality compared with a single source. In any case, requirements for protein of humans, even infants, are relatively modest compared with most species.

Protein quality is dependent upon the amounts and utilization of eight essential amino acids. Animal sources provide all eight in near optimum amounts, hence they are high quality proteins. Conversely, individual plant sources may have amino acid profiles deficient in one or two essential amino acids. By consuming a variety of vegetable protein sources, any amino acid deficiencies in one plant source can be signicantly improved by the presence of the specific amino acids in another. In this way, all eight essential amino acids, can be provided by a vegetable diet. For example, cereal grain proteins are low in lysine, an essential amino acid, while pulses contain ample lysine, but are themselves low in methionine. Thus, when consumed together the balance of amino acid supply improves and a high quality protein ensues (Winick, 1980). Since the complementary effect of one plant protein with another has been recognized, the differentiation in nutritional value of plant compared with animal protein has now largely been discarded.

Cereals, pulses and nuts, which often form the mainstay of vegan diets and may also form a substantial proportion of lactovegetarian diets, are rich sources of protein. Together, these typically provide about 10% of energy as protein (Sanders, 1983). Dairy products and eggs in lacto-ovovegetarian diets are also rich providers of protein. If consumption of these foods is frequent, there should be no difficulties in meeting requirements.

Carlson *et al.* (1985) found that the protein content of vegan diets easily met dietary recommendations. As a percentage of RDA (DHSS, 1979), a mean figure of 110·2% was obtained. A value of 123·7% was obtained from analysis of the dietary intakes of lacto-ovovegetarians. This higher value can be attributed to the lacto-ovovegetarians' frequent consumption of dairy produce and eggs. A wide variety of foods was consumed and thus it is unlikely that the diets were deficient in essential amino acids.

A further study (Shultz & Leklem, 1987) on dietary intakes of 13 vegans and lacto-ovovegetarians, assessed as a single group, also indicated adequate protein intakes: a mean intake of 59 g was calculated. Considering that all subjects were aged 56 years and above, this figure relates approximately to 131% of the RDA (DHSS, 1979). It would perhaps have been of more dietetic use if the vegans and lacto-ovovegetarians had been assessed separately since milk products and eggs would make substantial contributions to protein intake. Indeed, a high standard deviation supports this view.

These studies have that currently approved dietary recommendations for protein can be easily met by vegetarians. However, this may not always be the case for vegans. Roshanai & Sanders (1984) calculated the mean protein intakes of male and female vegans to be 70 g and 69 g per day respectively. Thus, it would seem that the female vegan diet, in particular, is more than adequate. However, further analysis of the individual values obtained showed some exceptionally poor intakes below the RDA: the lowest being 54% of RDA (DHSS, 1979) exhibited by one female. It can be concluded that for some individuals, advice concerning the nutritional planning of diet should be promoted.

It has been proposed (Acosta, 1988) that a high dietary fibre intake may adversely affect the availability of essential amino acids. This may be of significance to vegans where fibre intakes are high, and protein intakes are low, although only small effects of high-fibre diets on protein availability have been shown. Indeed, Acosta (1988) suggested that such an effect would be unlikely to pose a problem to adults but may be more important for children.

Carbohydrate. Assimilable carbohydrate intakes have been shown to be similar (Bull & Barber, 1984) or slightly higher (Carlson *et al.*, 1985; Davies *et al.*, 1985) in lacto-ovovegetarian diets compared with omnivores. However, vegan diets contain significantly greater quantities compared with both groups (Roshanai & Sanders, 1984; Davies *et al.*, 1985). Dietary guidelines currently recommend that approximately 55% of total energy intake should be derived from carbohydrate (NACNE, 1983). The likelihood of achieving this figure has been shown to be greater in lactovegetarian and particularly vegan diets than omnivore diets (Carlson *et al.*, 1985—see Table 2; Bull & Barber, 1984).

Fat. In comparison with omnivore diets, vegetarian diets commonly contribute lower levels of fat (Carlson *et al.*, 1985; Shultz & Leklem, 1987).

Indeed, the fat content of most plant sources is comparatively low (Truesdell *et al.*, 1984). It needs to be acknowledged, however, that dairy products and eggs collectively provide approximately 40% of total fat intake in traditional diets (Hazell & Southgate, 1985) and, as such, the fat intakes of lacto-ovovegetarians, whose diet incorporates substantial quantities of these foods, may approximate those of omnivores. Conversely, it has been shown that the fat intakes of vegans are significantly lower (Carlson *et al.*, 1985) due to their abstinence from animal foodstuffs.

The preferential intake of fat from plant foods by vegans modifies fatty acid intakes. Roshanai & Sanders (1984) reported the absence of the long-chain derivatives of the essential fatty acids (particularly arachidonic acid) among vegans in addition to comparatively low intakes of myristic, palmitic, margaric and stearic fatty acids. Long-chain fatty acids may be required in diets because the capacity to synthesize them is low (Sanders, 1983). However, the ability to synthesize arachidonic acid (a fatty acid found in lean meat) from linoleic acid was demonstrated by its presence in the plasma of vegans. The implications of these findings are undetermined, but the absence of any abnormalities in vegans due to their fatty acid intakes suggests there is no problem.

Vitamins

Vitamin B_{12}. The requirement for B_{12} is still subject to debate. In the UK there is no RDA set for it (Bender, 1985) on the grounds that ample B_{12} is supplied by the average diet and adequate information on requirements is not available. Herbert (1988) suggests that no more than 1 μg/day is necessary since this amount would be used therapeutically in the deficiency state to achieve health. Even amounts as minimal as 0·2–0·5 μg/day he considers as sufficient, since there is a lack of evidence suggesting that any more would be beneficial.

The absence of vitamin B_{12} from all plant foods necessitates the vegan ensuring an adequate intake through supplementation or the consumption of fortified foods. Contamination of plant foods by micro-organisms may, however, produce minute quantities. All meat substitutes in the UK are fortified by law. However, many vegetarians consider these to be unacceptable, hence fortification may not necessarily act as an absolute safeguard against deficiency (Sanders, 1983). Spirolina, a blue–green algae, has been credited with containing a rich source of vitamin B_{12}, although Herbert (1988) suggests from analysis that Spirolina and many fortified soy products, in fact, contain very little B_{12} in an active form.

Lactovegetarians should have no problems in meeting requirements since all animal sources provide this vitamin.

Deficiency of B_{12} results in megaloblastic anaemia. However, because it takes approximately 4–5 years to deplete the liver stores, any deficiency through an inadequate intake may take a long time to develop. High folate intakes characteristic of vegetarian diets can mask the clinical signs of B_{12} deficiency (Bender, 1985). The problem, therefore, of overlooking a deficiency in B_{12} is apparent.

Helman & Darnton-Hill (1987) found that 16% of lacto-ovovegetarians observed had a vitamin B_{12} status below the specified lower limit (< 200 pg/ml blood plasma) and of these, a few values fell below 150 pg/ mg. However, none of the subjects demonstrated abnormalities characteristic of B_{12} deficiency. Such findings may indicate that lower limits of adequacy have been set too high, or, absence of deficiency may reflect a 'hidden' intake of vitamin B_{12} on unwashed vegetables. Indeed, some people have the ability to obtain small amounts from the activity of the microflora in the bowel (Lockie *et al.*, 1985). Conversely, folate intakes reported as high in the study may have influenced the outcome. Racial variations may exist also where seemingly high vitamin B_{12} levels are maintained despite low intakes. Thus, in determining vitamin B_{12} status of individuals, it may be important to consider racial origin (Sheppard & Shehade, 1988). Further evidence (Carlson *et al.*, 1985) has indicated that lactovegetarian diets provided sufficient B_{12}. Mean values obtained for the lacto-ovovegetarian and vegan diets studied were 2·36 µg/day and 1·4 µg/ day respectively (in this study the RDA used was 2·0 µg/day).

The frequency of consumption of milk and dairy products is perhaps the most readily attributable feature determining the discrepancy in results between studies investigating B_{12} adequacy of lactovegetarian diets. It has been suggested that vegetarians who consume only small amounts of dairy produce should take some precautions with regard to vitamin B_{12} (Davies *et al.*, 1985).

Herbert (1988) postulated that high intakes of dietary fibre may lead to increased faecal B_{12} excretion. Therefore, the analysis of dietary intake alone may not be sufficient in assessing the adequacy of a vegetarian diet in meeting B_{12} requirements. A more useful indication would be the analysis of nutritional status by biochemical methods on body tissues.

Vitamin D. Provided almost exclusively by foods of animal origin, vitamin D would seem to be a nutrient of some concern, particularly with regard to vegan diets. It is believed that a few plants do contain the vitamin

TABLE 3
Comparison of the vitamin adequacy of vegan and lacto-ovovegetarian diets, expressed as a percentage of the RDA (DHSS, 1979)

Vitamin	Vegans		Lacto-ovovegetarians	
	%	SD	%	SD
Thiamin	176	41·8	160	60·5
Riboflavin	75	24·9	139	60·4
Niacin	197	63·3	203	97·5
A	165	36·5	208	85·0
C	704	383	639	506

Modified from Carlson *et al.* (1985).

in a water-soluble form, however, these are obscure and not readily available (Sanders, 1983). It appears that regardless of their origin, few foods provide vitamin D. Milk, eggs, dairy produce, fish, meat and fortified foods remain the only available foods sources. The action of ultraviolet light from the sun on the skin is thought to be the major source for humans.

In a study by Bull & Barber (1984), results showed that most people obtain vitamin D through sunlight, irrespective of their diet. Indeed, the average vitamin D content of the vegetarian diet ($2·5 \mu g$/day) did not differ significantly from that of omnivore diets ($2·8 \mu g$/day), suggesting an external source of vitamin D. Similar findings reporting lactovegetarian, vegan *and* omnivore diets to be low in vitamin D (about 33% of the estimated requirement) were reported by Carlson *et al.* (1985). It is noted that dietary sources of vitamin D may not be necessary for children over six years and adults, when exposure to sunlight is sufficient (DHSS, 1979).

It is important to recognize that further supplementation is required for pregnant and lactating vegetarian women and by Asian vegetarians who may not be sufficiently exposed to the rays of the sun.

Other vitamins. With the possible exception of riboflavin, obtaining adequate intakes of the B-complex vitamins and vitamins, A, B_6, C, E and folate, should pose no difficulties to all vegetarians. Their predilection for fruits, salads, and unrefined cereals ensures ample quantities (Truesdell *et al.*, 1984). Milk consumed on a frequent basis will, in addition, provide the lactovegetarian with an adequate supply. Results expressed as a percentage of RDA from the analysis of vitamin intakes of vegans and lacto-ovovegetarians are presented in Table 3. Although riboflavin is widely distributed in plant foods, the mean value of the vegan diet was low. However, no signs of deficiency were detected. In contrast, with regard to lacto-ovovegetarian diets, recommended riboflavin intakes were amply met. This significant difference can be attributed to intakes of milk and eggs by the lacto-ovovegetarians. These foods are also major sources of riboflavin in omnivore diets (Hazell & Southgate, 1985).

Further studies have reported the adequacy of vegetarian diets in the provision of vitamins (Bull & Barber, 1984; Shultz & Leklem, 1987). However, in these studies no distinction was made between vegans and lactovegetarians. Thus, all vegetarian diets analysed were reflected in the mean values recorded as being substantially greater than the RDA for riboflavin intakes.

Helman and Darnton-Hill's study (1987) assessing the vitamin and iron status of lacto-ovovegetarians, found that 9% of the sample (approximately 11 people) had thiamin blood levels below the stated lower limit. It is probable that this reflects poor food choice rather than a deficiency in vegetarian foods, since the adequacy of thiamin intake in vegetarian diets is well documented (Bull & Barber, 1984; Carlson *et al.*, 1985).

Research concerning vitamin E intakes of vegetarians is minimal. Nonetheless, adequate intakes have been reported (Helman & Darnton-Hill, 1987) and compare favourably with those obtained from omnivore diets.

One of the positive aspects associated with a vegetarian diet is the potentially very high vitamin C content which is believed to improve the absorption of inorganic iron present in plant diets, (see below). A number of investigators have reported mean vitamin C intakes of vegetarians in excess of 150 mg/day (Carlson *et al.*, 1985; Davies *et al.*, 1985, Shultz & Leklem, 1987). Recommended intakes for adults (DHSS, 1979) are 30 mg/day in the UK. Thus, some vegetarian diets provide at least five times this amount. Values are, however, often accompanied by large standard deviations, implying that wide variations in intake frequently exist. Nonetheless, it can be assumed that almost all vegetarian diets receive ample vitamin C. Vegans may tend to compensate for the withdrawal of milk products from the diet by consuming foods that happen to contain high levels of vitamin C.

Vitamin A and folate are amply supplied by all vegetarian diets (Bull & Barber, 1984; Carlson *et al.*, 1985). Furthermore, vitamin B_6 status is similar for vegetarians and omnivores, providing 85% of the RDA (Shultz & Leklem, 1987).

Dietary fibre and minerals

An abundance of unrefined foods, commonly characteristic of vegetarian diets, undoubtedly accounts for recorded intakes of dietary fibre in vegetarians, which exceed the recommendation of 30 g/day (Carlson *et al.*, 1985; Davies *et al.*, 1985) proposed by NACNE (1983). Whole-grain cereals, nuts, pulses and fruit represent the major source of fibre in all diets.

Davies *et al.* (1985) studied the dietary intakes of vegans, lacto-vegetarians and omnivores. Substantial variations in mean fibre intake existed among the three groups; vegans consuming twice that of omnivores (47 g/day vs 23 g/day). However, large variations also existed among individuals in the same group and were attributed mainly to differences in cereal fibre intake. Similarly, considerably greater quantities of cereal fibre consumed by the vegans can partly account for the large differences in absolute intakes among groups. Other sources of fibre were also prevalent in the vegan diets, in particular legumes (beans and peas), which are a rich source of fibre. Lacto-ovovegetarians consumed intermediate amounts (37 g/day). Similar data have been reported by Carlson *et al.* (1985).

Alongside the literature acknowledging the advantages of fibre is a growth in evidence suggesting its deleterious effects. Most prominent among these is the ability of fibre to bind minerals in the gut, hence rendering them unavailable (Treuhuertz, 1982). It is relevant, therefore, to discuss the mineral adequacy of vegetarian diets in relation to fibre intakes.

Iron. On the basis of food values, the iron content of a balanced vegetarian diet should be adequate (Truesdell *et al.*, 1984). Indeed, several studies have reported the mean iron intakes of vegetarians to approximate (Shultz & Leklem, 1987) or more frequently, exceed (Latta & Liebman, 1984; Carlson *et al.*, 1985) current dietary recommendations. However, adoption of such diets with respect to iron status has provoked some concern. This would seem especially true for premenopausal women, who have a high susceptibility to iron deficiency.

Evidence suggests that plant sources of iron, solely available in an inorganic form, are less readily absorbed than haem iron derived purely from animal sources (Hazell & Southgate, 1985; Fig. 2). In addition, the absorptive efficiency of inorganic (non-haem) iron may be further reduced by the presence of dietary fibre, phytate and oxalate (Davies *et al.*, 1985). It has been suggested that high intakes of vitamin C and the presence of haem iron sources in the diet may counteract or promote absorption of non-haem iron (Brune *et al.*, 1989). Therefore, it would be more indicative

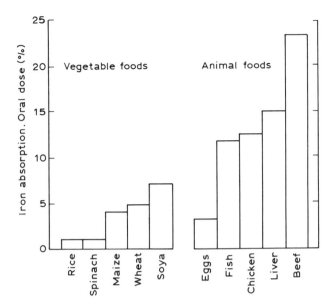

FIG. 2.   Iron absorption from a range of vegetable and animal foods. Source: Hazell and Southgate (1985).

of the adequacy, in terms of iron provision, of a vegetarian diet to consider iron status rather than iron intakes, since many factors may alter iron availability.

Worthington-Roberts *et al.* (1988) reported that despite similar iron intakes, iron status was significantly lower in the vegetarians analyses (11·8 vs 12·7 ng/ml blood). Although all values did fall within an acceptable range, these results do support the concept that a higher iron status is maintained with animal protein (haem sources of iron). This is further supported by research showing the iron status of lacto-ovovegetarians to be lower than omnivores despite the mean intake of the latter being significantly lower. However, no clinical signs of anaemia were apparent (McEndree *et al.*, 1983).

Helman & Darnton-Hill (1987) also showed iron status to be lower in lactovegetarians. It is important to note, however, that although mean iron status of the females was within a normal range (45 ng/ml blood), 27% of the population observed had an iron status below 'low' limits (< 15 ng/ml blood) and of these, 10% fell below 10 ng/ml. Conversely, Latta & Liebman (1984) have reported no significant difference between lactovegetarians and omnivores in iron status, despite similar iron intakes and a much higher fibre intake by the lactovegetarians. However, the vegetarians did occasionally consume meat and fish, in addition to milk, which may have influenced the findings.

It is probable that vegans are at a potentially greater risk from developing iron deficiency. High fibre intakes characteristic of vegan diets may adversely affect their iron status. Indeed, research has shown that irrespective of very high intakes (186% of RDA) (DHSS, 1979), vegans have low iron stores. Vitamin C intakes were particularly high, providing evidence of poor non-haem iron absorption (Carlson *et al.*, 1985). Brune *et al.* (1989) showed that a high-fibre diet marginally decreases iron availability for both vegetarians and omnivores; however, high vitamin C intakes may account for acceptable iron stores in both groups despite high fibre intakes.

Calcium. Calcium is principally provided in most western diets by milk and its derivatives: only 3% of calcium intake is obtained from meat (Hazell & Southgate, 1985). It might, therefore, be expected that the diets of lacto-ovovegetarians would not be too dissimilar to those of omnivores. While all mean values have been reported as adequate, a number of studies have shown calcium intakes in lacto-ovovegetarians to exceed significantly that of omnivores (Nnakwe *et al.*, 1984; Carlson *et al.*, 1985). However, others have reported similar (Davies *et al.*, 1985) or considerably lower results (Shultz & Leklem, 1987). Variations in milk intake will account for these seemingly contradictory data.

In contrast, calcium intakes may be markedly lower in vegans, since plant sources, in general, are poor sources of calcium. Thus Carlson *et al.*, (1985) showed calcium intakes to be marginal in vegan diets (98·5% RDA). Cooking and drinking water can provide fairly substantial quantities (15% of RDA) but wide ranges exist among individuals (Carlson *et al.*, 1985). Furthermore, the presence of fibre, phytate and oxalate in high amounts may exacerbate effects of a low intake by reducing calcium bioavailability (Treuhertz, 1982).

Calcium absorption and excretion may be profoundly affected by the level and amino acid content of protein in the diet. Indeed high protein intakes increase calcium excretion. More specifically, it may be the sulphur-amino acids in the protein that increase calcium excretion. Phosphorus which accompanies protein intake may exert independent effects, counteracting the effects of the protein (Zemel, 1988). Dietary source of protein may be significant particularly with respect to vegans, whose calcium intakes are limited. However, enhanced calcium excretion is unlikely, as soyaprotein, commonly consumed by vegans, is low in sulphur-amino acids and the phosphorus content is high (Zemel, 1988). In addition, protein intakes are also unlikely to be excessive.

Fat and cholesterol contents of the diet have also been implicated in affecting calcium availability. Higher intakes of both may be beneficial towards improving calcium absorption (Kies, 1988). This may be of relevance to vegans who may be well advised to avoid excessively lowering their fat intake when calcium intakes are very low.

Mineral absorption may vary with physiological status and calcium is no exception. Nnakwe & Kies (1985) found that with similar calcium intakes (200% of RDA), lacto-ovovegetarians showed a superior mean calcium absorption (49%), compared with omnivores (35%) suggesting adaption of some kind. However, Nnakwe *et al.* (1984) queried the role of body status in accounting for this difference. They found no difference in calcium status (as assessed by serum levels) between lacto-ovovegetarians and omnivores (Table 4) despite calcium intake being significantly higher in the vegetarians, implying the presence of factors within the vegetarian diet that inhibited absorption. However, calcium status is notoriously difficult to assess: blood levels are held constant by homeostatic mechanisms despite loss or accretion. Nevertheless, these reports show that large differences in calcium intake occur among individuals eating vegetarian diets, emphasizing widely varying dairy produce consumption.

Calcium status of vegans may be substantially lower than lacto-ovovegetarians. Lactating and pregnant women require high calcium intakes (1200 mg/day; DHSS, 1979). Thus, it is essential for pregnant vegetarians to ensure an ample intake, by supplementation if necessary.

Zinc. Vegetarian diets have the potential to be limited in zinc since the richest food sources are of animal origin. Furthermore, zinc bioavailability may be profoundly altered by the high fibre content and presence of other components that inhibit absorption in vegetarian diets. The effect of phytate, for example, may be particularly important for zinc. Indeed, plant sources richest in zinc, such as whole-grains, nuts and legumes (Truesdell *et al.*, 1984), are also those characteristically abundant in fibre and phytate. Thus zinc availability may be poor from plant foods, despite adequate intakes.

Latta & Liebman (1984) found no significant difference in zinc status between lacto-ovovegetarian and omnivore men, despite the mean fibre intake of the vegetarians being significantly higher (Table 5). It was

TABLE 4

Calcium intakes and blood serum levels of lacto-ovovegetarians and omnivores

Subject no.	Omnivores		Lacto-ovovegetarians	
	Mean intake (mg/day)	Serum levels (mg/dl)	Mean intake (mg/day)	Serum levels (mg/dl)
1	684	9·6	639	—
2	976	9·9	1416	9·9
3	778	9·7	902	9·6
4	815	9·6	1285	10·3
5	296	10·0	721	10·3
6	652	10·1	497	9·7
7	925	9·5	809	9·7
8	706	9·7	1473	9·3
9	692	10·0	1448	10·1
10			741	9·7
11			1176	10·4
12			576	10·2
13			803	9·3
14			836	9·3
15			944	—
Mean for group	725	9·7	951	9·8

RDA for calcium, 500 mg/day (DHSS, 1979).
Modified from Nnakwe et al. (1984).

ascertained that 33% of the vegetarians, as compared with 22% of the omnivores, had plasma zinc levels below 65 µg/day, a value considered to be low. The study could have been improved by the assessment of zinc intakes since it would have been useful to determine whether low intakes could have been partly responsible for the higher percentage of vegetarians exhibiting low plasma zinc levels. Nevertheless, it was reported that liberal amounts of wholegrains, legumes and cheeses were eaten, all of which are good sources.

The negative correlation found between fibre and plasma zinc in the vegetarian population is consistent with the assertion that dietary fibre and/or phytate are important determinants in zinc bioavailability. However, support has been given to the concept that adaptation may occur to a high-fibre diet. Omnivores who abruptly switched to a vegetarian diet for 22 days showed an enhanced response to a zinc plasma

TABLE 5
The relationship between fibre intake and zinc status in vegetarians and omnivores

	Crude fibre intake (g)	Status		Correlation with crude fibre	
		Plasma zinc	RBC zinc	Plasma zinc	RBC zinc
Vegetarian	7·1 ± 2·4	68 ± 14	12 ± 1·2	− 0·30**	− 0·27
Omnivore	4·6 ± 2·0*	73 ± 13	12·7 ± 1·5	− 0·13	− 0·28

*, Significant difference between groups ($p < 0.001$); **, significant difference between groups ($p < 0.05$).
Source: Latta & Liebman (1984).

tolerance test, illustrating adaptation to increased zinc absorption (Free-land-Graves, 1988).

LONG-TERM HEALTH IMPLICATIONS FOR VEGETARIAN DIETS

Inevitably, mounting evidence linking the characteristic diseases of afflu-ence such as coronary heart disease (CHD), obesity and hypertension with Western diets has alerted attention towards the potential benefits of a vegetarian diet. Growing numbers of people are adopting such a diet with the expectation that it will provide a 'healthier' option. The impetus for this movement in the UK was undoubtedly the publication of NACNE (1983) and COMA (DHSS, 1984) reports. Vegetarianism is perceived by many as an alternative to a Western diet, conducive to optimum health. The following discussion is centred on whether a vegetarian diet can indeed provide a truly 'healthy' alternative.

The COMA and NACNE reports and diets of vegetarians
Second only to Finland, Britain in the late 1980s had one of the highest death rates from cardiovascular disease in the world. It has been esta-blished by epidemiological studies that the risk of having a heart attack can be increased by several factors, of which diet is an important one. In the UK the evidence for the link with diet has been evaluated by the

Committee on Medical Aspects of Food Policy (COMA) of the DHSS (Department of Health and Social Security; DHSS, 1984). Their report, like NACNE (1983) before it, makes a number of specific recommendations on changes which it considers should be made in the UK diet, and have been termed the 'dietary guidelines'.

The very nature of CHD calls for preventative rather than curative measures. Just how effective such advice is in reducing incidences of diet-related diseases such as CHD remains to be seen, particularly in the light of new evidence indicating the merits of (for example) antioxidant nutrients, which were not addressed in these reports. Nevertheless the guidelines provide the yardstick of authoritative advice against which the diet and health of vegetarians can be evaluated.

The most significant recommendation in both the NACNE and COMA reports is concerned with the reduction of dietary total and saturated fat. The impetus for such changes is an abundance of epidemiological evidence relating high intakes of saturated fatty acids (SFAs) to the incidence of CHD. Other studies have suggested alternatively that linoleic acid, a polyunsaturated fatty acid (PUFA) is negatively correlated with mortality from CHD (COMA: DHSS, 1984). COMA acknowledged that decreasing the intake of SFAs will increase the ratio. However, some scientific authorities, writing after the publication of the COMA Report contend that increasing the P/S ratio (that is, the ratio of the contents of polyunsaturated fatty acids to saturated fatty acids in a fat or food) of the diet would be more important than decreasing total fat intake (Vergroesen & Crawford, 1989).

While a weak relationship between CHD and total plasma cholesterol has also been identified, (COMA: DHSS, 1984), the extent to which cholesterol in the diet can be correlated with CHD is questionable since increasing dietary cholesterol has only marginal effects on increasing plasma cholesterol. It is for this reason that there are no specific recommendations concerning intake of dietary cholesterol in the UK dietary guidelines.

COMA recommendations concerning fat in the UK diet are summarized in Table 6. Similar recommendations have been proposed by NACNE (1983). These figures represent an approximate decrease of 17% in fat and 25% in SFAs. An increase in PUFAs would also be desirable.

In terms of approximating to these recommendations, the diets of vegetarians and those of vegans in particular are superior to those of omnivores. The study of Roshanai & Sanders (1984) of the fatty acid intakes of vegans and omnivores reported significantly lower SFA intakes

TABLE 6
Recommended average daily intakes of total fat, saturated and polyunsaturated fatty acids

Category	1981 average	Recommended average
Total fat		
g/day	104	77–87[a]
% Energy	42	31–35
Saturates		
g/day	49	37
% Energy	20	15
Polyunsaturates		
g/day	11·4	8·6–16·7
% Energy	4·7	3·5–6·8
P/S ratio	0·23	0·23–0·45

[a] Depends on the P/S ratio, the upper limit corresponds to the recommended ratio of approximately 0·45.
Source: COMA (DHSS, 1984).

by the vegans. In addition, intakes of linolenic and linoleic acids (PUFAs) were substantially greater (Table 7). It was noted that values calculated using composition of foods tables were greater for all intakes determined when compared with analytical values.

Comparison of plasma cholesterol concentrations showed the mean low density lipoprotein (LDL) cholesterol level in vegans (1·97 mmol/litre) to

TABLE 7
Calculated compared with analysed fatty acid intakes of vegans and omnivores for 3-day intakes

	Calculated (g/day)		Analysed (g/day)	
	Vegan	Omnivore	Vegan	Omnivore
Total fat	84 ± 6·5	91 ± 5·6	78 ± 7·7	75 ± 6·9
Saturates	21 ± 1·7	40 ± 2·2	18 ± 2·0	31 ± 2·9
Mono-unsaturates	34 ± 2·1	37 ± 2·3	33 ± 2·7	33 ± 2·9
Linoleic acid	27 ± 2·5	11 ± 1·0	26 ± 2·8	10 ± 1·0
Linolenic acid	1·9 ± 0·22	1·4 ± 0·12	1·5 ± 0·19	1·0 ± 0·11
P/S ratio	1·4	0·3	1·5	0·4

Adapted from Roshanai & Sanders (1984).

be significantly lower than omnivores (2·61 mmol/litre) which correlated with their lower intakes of SFAs. High density lipoprotein (HDL) cholesterol concentrations were found to be similar among the groups.

Burslem *et al.* (1978) found that the mean dietary cholesterol intake of vegans was less than 10 mg/day, which would be expected as cholesterol is not found in plant food sources. Furthermore, the P/S ratio was considerably larger in the vegan diet compared with that of meat eaters. The vegans had lower total cholesterol levels and considerably larger HDL/ LDL cholesterol ratios than meat eaters. (A high HDL/LDL cholesterol ratio is considered to be protective against CHD, as HDL take part in 'reverse cholesterol transport', i.e. 'scavenges' cholesterol from tissues, including the linings of arteries and return it to the liver where it is metabolized.)

The ability of lacto-ovovegetarians to comply with dietary guidelines is very much dependent on the frequency of consumption of milk, dairy products and eggs, the latter providing abundant quantities of cholesterol. Indeed, lacto-ovovegetarian diets rich in milk products and eggs may contain similar amounts of cholesterol and SFAs contained in an omnivorous diet.

Epidemiological data suggest that cereal fibre is protective against CHD (COMA: DHSS, 1984), although it is not possible to establish conclusively whether this effect is independent of all other dietary variables. COMA recognized the advantages of compensating for a decreased fat intake by increasing the intake of fibre-rich carbohydrates but there are no specific recommendations concerning dietary fibre intake. NACNE, in contrast, recommends intakes of greater than 25 g/day, taking a stronger view that dietary fibre is instrumental in the lowering of serum cholesterol levels. The diets of vegetarians have been shown to exceed recommendations significantly (see above) and mean intakes of those on omnivore diets.

Other recommendations include decreasing salt, sugar and alcohol consumption, in addition to avoiding obesity. High salt intakes have been associated with high blood pressure, which may be a contributory factor to CHD and strokes. Excess intakes of alcohol may adversely affect the incidence of cardiovascular disease; obesity may partly account for an increased risk of CHD (COMA: DHSS, 1984). In general vegetarians exhibit lower body weights than non-vegetarians, but the intakes of salt, sugar and alcohol amongst vegetarians will depend largely on the individual food choice. Carlson *et al.* (1985) reported lower intakes of salt from the consumption of vegetarian diets as compared with omnivore diets. However, values obtained between groups were not statistically significant. The considerably greater potassium content of vegan diets found by Carlson *et al.* (1985) may possibly contribute to the prevention of hypertension when coupled with a low sodium intake. Alcohol intake is subject to substantial variation in vegetarians (Carlson *et al.*, 1985).

CHD in vegetarians

Two studies are of particular relevance here. The first was conducted on vegetarian and non-vegetarian Seventh-Day Adventists in the USA (Snowden *et al.*, 1984). This prospective study showed that those who ate meat had a higher risk of death from CHD. (A prospective study is one in which people are taken into the study before the development of disease and their health monitored: a method regarded as far more rigorous than retrospective studies in which patients developing a disease are asked to give details of past diet and lifestyle.)

The second study was a comparative 12 year investigation of all-cause mortality amongst vegetarians and omnivores who were customers of health-food shops or belonged to vegetarian societies. This showed that CHD accounted for the deaths of fewer vegetarians than omnivores (Burr & Butland, 1988). The number of observed deaths in both groups from CHD was lower than expected, but this observation was found to be particularly apparent in the vegetarians when standardized mortality rates (SMR) were calculated. (SMR is the number of actual deaths as a percentage of those expected.) Values obtained were 42·8 and 60·1 for the vegetarians and omnivores respectively.

However, the extent to which findings such as these can be solely attributed to the differences in dietary intake is questionable. Indeed, even if vegetarian diets are positively identified in preventing CHD, ascertaining whether the avoidance of meat or the extra intake of vegetables is responsible for the lower incidence of CHD has proved difficult.

Despite the agreement between these two discussed above, it should not be just assumed that it was the vegetarian diet that reduced risk of CHD. Lifestyle is an unknown variable. In the study by Burr & Butland (1988) the vegetarians were lighter in weight than omnivores. Therefore, a further explanation of the reduced risk could have been that the vegetarians had a greater preoccupation with health.

Neither should decreased risk of CHD necessarily be equated with increased longevity. Indeed, Burr & Butland (1988) showed that all-cause mortality was similar in both groups studied. On the other hand, Snowdon (1988) showed that for men who were Seventh-Day Adventists all-cause mortality was higher in those eating meat.

If a vegetarian diet reduces risk of CHD, the question of mechanism will have to be addressed. Measurement of plasma cholesterol levels (Burr & Butland, 1988) showed the vegetarians to have significantly lower levels (5·47 mmol/litre) in comparison with the omnivores (5·95 mmol/litre). However, the cause of the lower values was not entirely clear since a series of controlled trials in which meat was replaced by other foodstuffs did not produce interpretable or entirely consistent results. Burr & Sweetnam (1982) also tested the hypothesis that dietary fibre is protective against CHD. However the higher consumption of wholemeal bread by the vegetarians was not associated with any significant differences between vegetarians and omnivores in mortality, although the former did demonstrate a lower mean SMR.

In summary, it would seem that a vegetarian diet may protect against CHD, although the precise mechanism involved is not understood; low SFA intakes may be but one factor. The fact that some studies and not others have reported dietary fibre as being protective against CHD may reflect the differential role of dietary fibre components in the lowering of serum cholesterol. It is possible that both avoidance of meat and high fibre intakes characteristic of vegetarian diets are involved in the lowering of serum cholesterol levels.

Blood pressure in vegetarians

Blood pressure (BP) trials with vegetarians have yielded conflicting results. Melby *et al.* (1985) found mean systolic and diastolic BPs of male and female vegetarians to be lower than matched omnivores. However, on adjustment for differences in age, sex and body mass index (BMI), statistically significant differences were eliminated. Extensive analyses revealed that the lower BP in vegetarians appeared best explained by their lower BMI. It is relevant to note, however, that the omnivore and vegetarian diets in this study were not too dissimilar: this might explain the lack of an independent relationship between diet and BP. Perhaps the major influence of a vegetarian diet on BP operates via its effect on body weight, thus suggesting an indirect relationship.

In contrast to the study by Melby *et al.* (1985), the BPs of two religious groups, dissimilar in their dietary intakes only, have been shown to be significantly different; the vegetarians demonstrating a considerably lower BP than omnivores (Rouse *et al.*, 1983a). Perhaps a more conclusive study, in terms of providing evidence on the cause-and-effect relationship of vegetarian diets on BP, involved the introduction of a vegetarian diet to a group of omnivores (Rouse *et al.*, 1983b). Mean systolic and diastolic

BPs reduced substantially when the vegetarian diet was consumed but increased again on resumption of the meat diet. A control group consuming an omnivore diet throughout showed no change. The possible role of sodium was discounted since urinary sodium excretion was similar in both groups.

It is very difficult to isolate any one component of a vegetarian diet that might be responsible for lowering BP since the diets of omnivores and vegetarians differ in so many respects, other than in animal produce consumption. Indeed, not all studies comparing vegetarians and omnivores have shown differences in BP. Burr *et al.* (1981) investigated the relationship between cholesterol status and BP in vegetarians and omnivores. Mean systolic and diastolic BP showed no consistent or significant differences between the two groups, although the vegetarians had considerably lower total plasma cholesterol concentrations.

Contradictory data on the effects of fatty acid profile on the diet and BP have also been published. Rouse *et al.* (1983b) were not able to provide evidence supporting the view that BP is lowered solely by an increase in the P/S ratio. However, they indicated that P/S ratio may affect BP when total fat intake is also reduced. Partly in support of this work, Sacks & Kass (1988) showed that changes in the amount or type of fat in the diet did not directly affect BP. Conversely, Margetts *et al.* (1988) concluded that most trials have tended to show a decrease in BP associated with either a reduction in total fat intake or elevation of the P/S ratio.

The effect of dietary fibre intakes on BP has also been reviewed by Margetts *et al.* (1988). Although some studies were reported to show a decrease in BP when fibre intakes were increased, other studies found no association. The difficulty of isolating dietary fibre from other possible confounding variables was acknowledged by these authors.

Prevalence of osteoporosis in vegetarians
Although it is still widely believed that diets deficient in calcium are the primary cause of osteoporosis, the low prevalence of the disease among vegans whose intake of calcium is low would imply the potential role of other factors. A multitude of life-style factors including smoking, malabsorption, early menopause, being underweight and a family history of osteoporosis have been proposed as contributory factors, in addition to numerous diet-related causes, including excessive alcohol intake. In many of these respects, vegetarians may be less prone to osteoporosis than omnivores. However, the tendency for vegetarians, particularly vegans, to be underweight may increase the risk (Dwyer, 1988).

TABLE 8
The relationship between bone density and age in vegetarians and omnivores
(mean ± SD)

Age (years)	Density of proximal phalanx of 3rd finger		Density of 3rd metacarpal	
	Vegetarians	Controls	Vegetarians	Controls
59–69	1·50 ± 0·22	1·02 ± 0·19	1·14 ± 0·18	0·71 ± 0·17
60–69	1·27 ± 0·27	0·88 ± 0·27	1·01 ± 0·19	0·68 ± 0·19
70–79	1·32 ± 0·40	0·73 ± 0·17	1·03 ± 0·36	0·55 ± 0·14

Source: Ellis *et al.* (1972).

It has been hypothesized that omnivore diets, a primary source of acid ash, may greatly increase the degree of bone dissolution since the release of calcium ions from bone tissue will act as buffering agents against residual acid following metabolism (Ellis *et al.*, 1972). Average bone density in the vegetarians was found to be significantly greater than matched omnivores, thus supporting the hypothesis. However, whether this effect was due to acid ash or another dietary difference was inconclusive.

Subsequent examination showed bone density to decrease with age, but the extent of this decrease was considerably less in the vegetarians (Table 8). Furthermore, no reduction was demonstrated by the vegetarians after 69 years, which contrasts significantly with the omnivores. Despite a higher intake of calcium by the vegetarians, serum levels were significantly lower compared with controls. Ellis *et al.* (1972) proposed that this difference may reflect a greater dissolution of bone tissue in the omnivores, resulting in higher serum calcium levels.

Unpublished observations (Marsh *et al.*, (1983) further implicate the role of high acid ash diets in the aetiology of osteoporosis. These workers found that a lacto-ovovegetarian diet had a mean value of 26·1 mmol excess NaOH/100 g whereas the omnivore diet had a mean value of 9·8 mmol excess HCl/100 g. Other nutrient intakes were similar between the groups. Marsh *et al.* (1980), on matching vegetarian and omnivore females, discovered no significant differences in bone mineral density under the age of 50. However, increasing differences in bone mass between the ages of 50 and 87 became apparent. By their 80th year the vegetarians had more bone mineral (18% less compared with 35% less). Again, nutrient intakes were not dissimilar.

These studies provide support for the postulation that the lacto-ovovegetarian diet may be a protective factor in preventing osteoporosis. However, the exact mechanism is unknown and, again, lifestyle factors are liable to affect results.

Disease prevalence in general in vegetarians

Although the evidence for enhanced longevity of vegetarians compared with omnivores is equivocal, studies are not reported for life-long vegetarians. Despite lack of evidence of clearly extended lifetimes many vegetarians would argue that morbidity is reduced, so that the quality of life is enhanced.

The difficulty of diagnosing diseases that do not manifest themselves in the form of detectable symptoms suggests that actual disease prevalence among populations may not be accurately represented (Dickerson *et al.*, 1985). Nevertheless, studies assessing disease patterns in individuals who consume different diets may provide some indication of the 'healthfulness' of the respective diets if the same stringent diagnostic methods are employed.

Examination of vegetarians and matched omnivores reported significantly fewer cases of disease incidence in the former group (Dickerson *et al.*, 1985). No cases of diabetes mellitus or coronary thrombosis were reported by the life-long vegetarians and instances of constipation, appendicitis, irritable bowel syndrome and varicose veins were also markedly lower. Further analysis showed a downward trend in disease prevalence on the adoption of a vegetarian diet in addition to differences between the two groups in the age at which the disease was first diagnosed. The conditions investigated also tended to occur at an earlier age in the omnivores.

While Dickerson *et al.* (1985) found little difference in the occurrence of other disorders investigated between the groups, notably diverticular disease and gallstones, other groups have reported differently. Pixley *et al.* (1985) found that 25% of omnivore women compared with 12% of vegetarian women had gallstones, concluding that a vegetarian diet is preventive against gallstones. These results imply that a potentially greater benefit may ensue in terms of preventing disease and delaying its onset in the adoption of a vegetarian diet early in life. Furthermore, there may be advantages in changing to a vegetarian diet at any stage in life, in terms of reducing disease incidence. There is too little data to assess the role played in this by dietary fibre, which is currently being investigated for its therapeutic and protective effects against a range of diseases of affluence.

VEGETARIANISM AND CHILDREN

Considerable concern has centred upon the ability of vegetarian diets to provide children with adequate nutrient intakes. Vegetarian diets that sustain adults in good health may not necessarily be appropriate for children (Jacobs & Dwyer, 1988). When it is taken into account that, relative to body weight, the requirements of children are greater than those of adults and the average intake by vegetarian adults is marginal with respect to RDA for some nutrients, problems of dietary inadequacy in children seem more likely to occur. In addition, limited stomach capacity in very young children will dictate the need for diets containing greater amounts of energy-dense foods (Jacobs & Dwyer, 1988). Bulky diets characterized by large amounts of dietary fibre, complex carbohydrates and water may jeopardize growth in children since calorific and nutrient density will be low (Sanders, 1988).

Dietary deficiency in lacto-ovovegetarian children is unlikely to occur. However, vegan diets frequently acknowledged to be marginal with regard to energy content, vitamin B_{12}, vitamin D, calcium, zinc and iron may pose health risks to children. Young infants may require certain long-chain polyunsaturated fatty acids absent in all plant diets. If they are breast fed, however, this should not pose a problem since breast milk will provide sufficient amounts. In general, vegan mothers recognize the need to supplement their diets with vitamin B_{12}.

Instances of vitamin D deficiency rickets have been reported in vegan children (Ward et al., 1982). Indeed, risk of developing rickets will exist if vitamin D supplements, fortified soya milk and ample exposure to sunlight are not readily available. On some diets, vegan children may have inadequate intakes of protein particularly when energy intake is low. However, complementing protein sources or, alternatively, incorporating substantial variety into the diet should provide ample quantities. The importance of restricting high fibre intakes in very young children is not only important with respect to energy intake, but also for mineral nutrition. The bioavailability of minerals may be adversely affected by high intakes.

A longitudinal study assessing the nutrient intakes and growth of vegan children found the majority had energy intakes below recommended amounts (Sanders, 1988). Protein intakes were satisfactory but there were wide variations in fat intake (16–39%). It is probable, therefore, that the major contributory factor in low energy intakes in vegan children is their low fat intake. Calcium and vitamin D intakes were below recommendations, but many parents were aware of the need to provide vitamin D supplements, particularly in winter. Furthermore, vitamin B_{12} and iron intakes were adequate on average, but again, wide ranges existed in the former nutrient.

The majority of children exhibited 'normal' growth and development. However, they did tend to be smaller in stature and lighter in weight than omnivore children. This difference may be the result of variations in energy intake or quality of the diet, although cereals, pulses and nuts were consumed in abundance, in addition to fortified soya milks, peanut butter and ample quantities of fruit and vegetables. It is, therefore, unlikely that a poor quality diet was the reason for the difference.

Dwyer (1988) reported inadequate intakes of several micro-nutrients in lacto-ovovegetarian pre-school children. However, adequacy was gauged in relation to approximating to USA RDAs which generally exceed those currently recommended in the UK (DHSS, 1979). However, nutritional and health status was found to be satisfactory in all participants, indeed, the amounts of fat, carbohydrate, protein and cholesterol provided by the vegetarian diets was seen to resemble proposed dietary guidelines more closely than omnivore diets.

Vegan parents need to be aware of potentially hazardous areas with respect to a total plant diet. Carefully planned vegan diets which avoid the known pitfalls will not impair normal functioning; indeed, nutritionally adequate vegan diets, characteristically low in fat and cholesterol may be beneficial in establishing good health as a basis for a future healthy adult life.

THE FUTURE FOR VEGETARIANISM

The vegetarian population is set to expand in the future as the major factors influencing the trend towards vegetarianism seem likely to continue to have a significant bearing on food choice. Environmental issues, which have become notably important in the latter half of this decade and which look to provoke much concern in the next, may account for increasing numbers of people adopting vegetarian or near-vegetarian diets. The current trend in concern over diet and its relationship with health is gathering momentum too. Additionally, recent discussions on the effects of radiation, food chemicals and hormones on meat have aroused a greater consumer awareness of these controversial issues. Emotive reasons for becoming vegetarian are set to increase further.

A large proportion of the current vegetarian population comprises children and young women, and this has important implications for the future of vegetarianism. Vegetarian mothers influence their spouses and encourage their children to adopt such diets.

There is little doubt that the market for vegetarian foods is still at a very early stage of development. Considerable potential exists for manufacturers to appeal to a wider range of consumers interested in health, but not necessary vegetarian or avoiders of red meat, by providing a variety of nutritious, diverse, and convenient wholesome vegetarian products. Vegetarian foods that simulate meat are likely to be a major feature within the ready-meal sector in the 1990s. 'Quorn'® mycoprotein (Marlow Foods plc, Buckinghamshire) is illustrative of the efforts being made in this sector to attract a wide range of consumer. Versatile, 'healthy' and surprisingly similar to meat, Quorn, along with many new, innovative products, may dispel the notion that vegetarian diets are monotonous and bland.

Future market potential in the UK may include the provision of vegan ready-meals, and growth in the vegetarian catering sector. Growth in the market is likely to be most closely associated with the increasing dominance of the multiple retailers in the future, who will account for much of the vegetarian ready-meals market. In all probability the multiples will continue to threaten the role of the specialists in this market but the latter will remain important through their provision of diverse and obscure health products (MSI, 1989). Specialist outlets have attracted much loyalty over the years and it can be argued that they will continue to do so. The growing importance of health as a marketing asset is inevitable in the future. However, the health-conscious consumer may face a dilemma in deciding which products are genuinely beneficial. Vegetarian foods, widely acknowledged as 'healthy' may become increasingly viewed as an 'easy option' in health food choice.

CONCLUSION

Evidence reviewed here suggests that, if properly devised, both lactovegetarian and vegan diets provide adequate amounts of nutrients. The diets of vegans may, however, pose a greater risk of deficiency. However, the fact that some mean nutrient intakes have been shown to be marginal with respect to RDA is of concern since 50% of those studied will be consuming less than the RDA. However, lack of gross clinical signs of deficiency suggests that RDAs may overestimate requirements for the many individuals.

Although study numbers are often small thus reducing statistical significance, the frequent finding that vegetarian diets provide nutrients in excess of RDA does imply that they can be nutritionally adequate. Poor food choices and lack of planning account for inadequate vegetarian diets as it does for inadequate omnivore ones. However, the need for vegans to ensure an adequate intake of B_{12} and perhaps calcium through supplementation is evident.

Consumption of a wide variety of foods is the most effective safeguard for adequate nutrition. However, during pregnancy and lactation, vegetarian and especially vegan mothers should be extremely vigilant over intakes of energy, protein, minerals and vitamins, and some supplementation may be prudent. The absence of gross nutritional deficiencies in vegetarian children suggests that the diets are adequate. However, the importance of ensuring sufficient nutrient intakes, considering the possible detrimental effects of high dietary fibre consumption in children, is paramount. For example, small stature in the majority of vegan children may be indicative of nutrient deficiency, perhaps zinc.

Evidence reviewed here suggests that vegetarian diets, particularly those of vegans, are more beneficial to health than those of omnivores. Indeed, it appears that vegetarian diets more closely approximate to dietary guidelines than omnivore diets. While there is some evidence implicating vegetarian diets in lowering BP and protecting against CHD, osteoporosis and some other disorders, major problems can exist in the interpretation of health data. Even in studies minimizing potential confounding effects, life-style factors cannot be entirely discarded. Small study numbers and the variable lengths of time to which the subjects have followed their diets may also distort results.

In view of the findings reviewed here which suggest health benefits of vegetarian diets over those of omnivores, it would appear that those who consume vegetarian diets are indeed adopting a 'healthy' alternative. This would seem especially true for vegan diets, a point which emphasizes the importance of distinguishing between the different degrees of vegetarianism. However, whether any benefit is due to the absence of animal products from the diet, replacement of animal products by additional plant foods or other life-style factors is uncertain.

While the potential for strict vegetarian diets to be nutritionally inadequate is apparent, poor nutritional health is associated with ignorance and a lack of planning rather than the inability of plant foods to provide sufficient nutrients. Vegan diets are deficient in vitamin B_{12}, vitamin D and commonly calcium, but a wide variety of supplements is available. If the known pitfalls of vegan diets are recognized, as they frequently are, nutritional problems should not occur.

It is clear that vegetarianism in the UK is set to expand with the growing number of adherents under 16 years of age. The food industry in general has been swift to exploit this opening in the market. The provision of a varied and highly nutritious range of vegetarian ready, convenience meals by the food industry in response to the upsurge in demand will ensure plenty of choice for the vegetarian of the future.

REFERENCES

Anon (1987). Veggies on the increase. *Caterer and Housekeeper* December, p. 3.

Anon (1989). Vegetarianism not as rife as claimed. *The Grocer* November, p. 4.

Acosta, P.B. (1988). Availability of essential amino acids and nitrogen in vegan diets. *American Journal of Clinical Nutrition* **48**, 868–74.

Bender, A.E. (1985). Nutritional requirements. *The Journal of the Royal Society of Health* **105** (1), 1–4.

Brune, M., Rossander, L. & Hallberg, L.(1989). Iron absorption: No intestinal adaption to a high-phytate diet. *American Journal of Clinical Nutrition* **49**, 542–5.

Bull, N.L. & Barber, S.A. (1984). Food and nutrient intakes of vegetarians in Britain. *Human Nutrition: Applied Nutrition* **38A**, 288–93.

Burr, M.L. & Butland, B.K. (1988). Heart disease in British vegetarians. *American Journal of Clinical Nutrition* **48**, 380–2.

Burr, M.L. & Sweetnam, P.M. (1982). Vegetarianism, dietary fiber and mortality. *American Journal of Clinical Nutrition* **36**, 873–7.

Burr, M.L., Bates, C.J., Fehily, A.M. & Leger, A.S.S.T. (1981). Plasma cholesterol and blood pressure in vegetarians. *Journal of Human Nutrition* **35**, 437–41.

Burslem, J., Schonfeld, G., Howald, M.A., Weidman, S.W. & Miller, J.P. (1978). Plasma apoprotein and lipoprotein levels in vegetarians. *Metabolism* **27**, 711–17.

Carewell, A. & Penn, J. (1986). Health food marketing: The impact of changes in consumer awareness and preference on production policy. *Food Marketing* **2** (3), 45–54.

Carlson, E., Kepps, M., Lockie, A. & Thompson, J. (1985). A comparative evaluation of vegan, vegetarian and omnivore diets. *Journal of Plant Foods* **6**, 89–100.

Davies, G.J., Crowder, M. & Dickerson, J.W.T. (1985). Dietary fibre intakes of individuals with different eating patterns. *Human Nutrition: Applied Nutrition* **39A**, 139–48.

DHSS (Department of Health and Social Security) (1984). *Diet and Cardiovascular Disease* (The COMA report). Report on Health and Social Subjects no. 28. London: H.M. Stationery Office.

DHSS (Department of Health and Social Security) (1979) *Recommended Daily Amounts of Food Energy and Nutrients for Groups of People in the United*

Kingdom. Report on Health and Social Subjects no. 15. London: H.M. Stationery Office.

Dickerson, J.W.T., Davies, G.J. & Crowder, M. (1985). Disease patterns in individuals with different eating patterns. *The Journal of the Royal Society of Health* **105**, 191–4.

Dwyer, J.T. (1988). Health aspects of vegetarian diets. *American Journal of Clinical Nutrition* **48**, 712–38.

Dwyer, J.T., Mayer, L.D.V.H., Dowd, K., Candell, R.F. & Mayer, J. (1974). The new vegetarians: The natural high. *Journal of the American Dietetic Association* **65**, 529–36.

Ellis, F.R., Holesh, S. & Ellis, J.W. (1972). Incidence of osteoporosis in vegetarians and omnivores. *American Journal of Clinical Nutrition* **25**, 555–8.

Freeland-Graves, J. (1988). Mineral adequacy of vegetarian diets. *American Journal of Clinical Nutrition* **48**, 859–62.

Hazell, T. & Southgate, D.A.T. (1985). Trends in the consumption of red meat and poultry—nutritional implications. *British Nutrition Foundation Nutrition Bulletin* **10**, 104–17.

Helman, A.D. & Darnton-Hill, I. (1987). Vitamin and iron status in new vegetarians. *American Journal of Clinical Nutrition* **48**, 852–8.

Herbert, V. (1988). Vitamin B_{12}: plant sources, requirements and assay. *American Journal of Clinical Nutrition* **48**, 852–8.

Jacobs, C. & Dwyer, T. (1988). Vegetarian children: appropriate and inappropriate diets. *American Journal of Clinical Nutrition* **48**, 811–18.

Kies, C.V. (1988). Mineral utilization of vegetarians: Impact of variation in fat intake. *American Journal of Clinical Nutrition* **48**, 884–7.

Latta, D. & Liebman, M. (1984). Iron and zinc status of vegetarian and non-vegetarian males. *Nutrition Reports International* **30**, 141–9.

Lawrie, R.A. (1979). *Meat Science,* 2nd ed. Oxford: Pergamon Press.

Lockie, A.H., Carlson, E., Kipps, M. & Thompson, J. (1985). Comparison of four types of diet using clinical, laboratory and psychological studies. *Journal of the Royal College of General Practitioners* **35**, 333–6.

MAFF (Ministry of Agriculture Fisheries and Food). (1988). *Household Food Consumption and Expenditure.* Annual report of the National Food Survey Committee. London: H.M. Stationery Office.

Margetts, B.M., Beilen, L.J., Armstrong, B.K. & Vandongen, R. (1988). Vegetarian diet in mild hypertension: effects of fat and fiber. *American Journal of Clinical Nutrition* **48**, 801–5.

Marsh, A.G., Sanchez, T.V., Mickelson, O., Keiser, J. & Mayer, G. (1980). Cortical bone density of adult lacto-ovo-vegetarian and omnivorous women. *Journal of the American Dietetic Association* **76**, 148–51.

Marsh, A.G., Sanchez, T.V., Chaffee, F.L., Mayer, G.H. & Mickelson, O. (1983). Bone mineral mass in adult lacto-ovo-vegetarian and omnivorous males. *American Journal of Clinical Nutrition* **37**, 453–6.

McEndree, L.S., Kies, C.V. & Fox, H.M. (1983). Iron intake and iron nutritional status of lacto-ovo-vegetarian and omnivore students eating in a lacto-ovo-vegetarian food service. *Nutrition Reports International* **27**, 199–205.

Melby, C.L., Hyner, G.C. & Zoog, B. (1985). Blood pressure in vegetarians and non-vegetarians: A cross-sectional analysis. *Nutrition Research* **5**, 1077–82.

MSI (Marketing Strategies for Industry, UK Ltd) (1989). *Databrief Report on Vegetarian Foods UK.* June. London: MSI.

Mutch, P.B. (1988). Food guides for the vegetarian. *American Journal of Clinical Nutrition* **48**, 913–19.

NACNE (National Advisory Committee for Nutrition Education) (1983). *Proposals for Nutritional Guidelines for Health Education.* London: Health Education Council.

Nnakwe, N. & Kies, C. (1985). Calcium and phosphorus utilization by omnivores and lacto-ovo-vegetarians fed laboratory-controlled lacto-vegetarian diets. *Nutrition Reports International* **31**, 1009–14.

Nnakwe, N., Kies, C. & McEndree, L. (1984). Calcium and phosphorus nutritional status of lacto-ovo-vegetarian and omnivore students consuming meals in a lacto-ovo-vegetarian food service. *Nutrition Reports International* **29**, 365–9.

Pixley, F., Wilson, D., McPherson, K. & Mann, J. (1985). Effect of vegetarianism on development of gallstones in women. *British Medical Journal* **291**, 11–12.

Porter, J.W.G. (1975). *Milk and Dairy Foods.* Oxford: Oxford University Press.

Roshanai, F. & Sanders, T.A.B. (1984). Assessment of fatty acid intakes in vegans and omnivores. *Human Nutrition: Applied Nutrition* **38A**, 345–354.

Rouse, I.L., Armstrong, B.K. & Beilin, L.J. (1983*a*). The relationship of blood pressure to diet and lifestyle in two religious populations. *Journal of Hypertension* **1**, 65–71.

Rouse, I.L., Beilin, L.J., Armstrong, B.K. & Vandongen, R. (1983*b*). Blood pressure lowering effect of a vegetarian diet: a controlled trial in normotensive subjects. *Lancet* **i**, 5–10.

Sacks, F.M. & Kass, E.H. (1988). Low blood pressure in vegetarians: effects of specific foods and nutrients. *American Journal of Clinical Nutrition* **48**, 795–800.

Sanders, T.A.B. (1983). Vegetarianism: Dietetic and medical aspects. *Journal of Plant Foods* **5**, 3–14.

Sanders, T.A. (1988). Growth and development of British vegan children. *American Journal of Clinical Nutrition* **48**, 822–5.

Shultz, T.D. & Leklem, J.E. (1987). Vitamin B_6 status and bioavailability in vegetarian women. *American Journal of Clinical Nutrition* **46**, 647–51.

Sheppard, K. & Shehade, S.A. (1988). Vitamin B_{12} levels in non-Caucasian vegetarians. *European Journal of Clinical Nutrition* **42**, 539–40.

Slattery, J. (1986). *Diet and Health: Food Industry Initiatives.* Briefing Paper, Food Policy Research Unit Report. Bradford (UK): Horton Publishing Ltd.

Snowden, D.A. (1988). Animal product consumption and mortality because of all causes combined, coronary heart disease, stroke, diabetes, and cancer in Seventh-Day Adventists. *American Journal of Clinical Nutrition* **48**, 739–48.

Snowden, D.A., Phillips, R.L. & Fraser, G.E. (1984). Meat consumption and fatal ischemic heart disease. *Preventive Medicine* **13**, 490–500.

Treuhertz, J. (1982). Possible inter-relationship between zinc and dietary fibre in a group of lacto-ovo-vegetarian adolescents. *Journal of Plant Foods* **4**, 89–93.

Truesdell, D., Whitney, E.N. & Acosta, P.B. (1984). Nutrients in vegetarian foods. *Journal of the American Dietetic Association* **84**, 28–35.

Vergroesen, A.J. & Crawford, M. (1989). *The Role of Fats in Human Nutrition.* London: Academic Press.

Ward, P.S., Drakeford, J.P., Milton, J. & James, A. (1982). Nutritional rickets in Rastafarian children. *British Medical Journal* **285**, 1242–3.

Winick, M.D. (1980). *Nutrition in Health and Disease*. New York: John Wiley and Sons.

Woodward, J. (1988). Consumer attitudes towards meat and meat products. *British Food Journal* **90**, 101–4.

Worthington-Roberts, B.S., Breskin, M.W. & Monsen, E.R. (1988). Iron status of premenopausal women in a university community and its relationship to habitual dietary sources of protein. *American Journal of Clinical Nutrition* **47**, 275–9.

Zemel, M.B. (1988). Calcium utilization: effect of varying level and source of dietary protein. *American Journal of Clinical Nutrition* **48**, 880–3.

9

Nutrition for Specific Disease Conditions

Royal Berkshire Hospital, Reading, UK

INTRODUCTION

In recent years a substantial market has been created for food products and supplements that meet specialized dietary requirements. The target groups for such products are people with specific medical conditions, but as most of these foods are not available on the supermarket shelves, manufacturers direct their marketing at doctors and dietitians who prescribe the products for their patients.

When a person is ill and the indications are that nutritional manipulation of the diet could be of benefit, a therapeutic diet may be indicated. The diet, usually formulated by a dietitian, can be designed to control the blood concentration of some specific constituent, e.g. blood cholesterol, or it may have an influence at the physiological level, e.g. dietary fibre. Some diets involve restricting particular dietary substances (e.g. controlling blood cholesterol level) whilst other diets involve the addition of certain components as with fibre. Restrictions and additions may be directed at the macronutrients, protein, fat, carbohydrate and fibre, in which case they are general in nature, or they may be directed at micronutrients in which case they are quite specific and may involve control at the molecular level. The latter diets are usually quite complex.

In addition to a consideration of the biochemical and physiological factors, the diet must be acceptable to the individual for whom it is intended. Therefore the diet must also be palatable and convenient as without these characteristics dietary compliance will be compromised.

Specialized products that have been manufactured with the objectives of a particular diet in mind are available and are very helpful as they can make the diet easier to follow.

Within this chapter specialized and prescribable dietary products are discussed in general terms and then in the context of four different disease states to illustrate how they can be used in the treatment of a particular condition. Each of these is just one example of the many dietary manipulations available in diet therapy for different disease conditions (Thomas, 1988). For each of the four conditions, a brief background to the condition will be followed by a discussion of the dietary objectives and the type of specialized products available.

DIETARY PRODUCTS

A dietary product is any manufactured food product that has been altered to make it more suitable for use in a dietary regimen. Thus in its widest sense low-fat spreads, which offer slimmers low-calorie alternatives to ordinary spreading fats, or low-sugar fruit squashes, which offer diabetics alternatives to ordinary fruit squashes, are dietary products. Both these foods and many more like them are available to the discerning consumer through the usual retail outlets.

Specialized dietary products
A specialized dietary product works along similar principles but as the product is intended for a minority group of the population it is unlikely to be found in the local supermarket. Moreover, because of low demand the product will almost certainly be more expensive than its non-therapeutic equivalent. A proportion of specialized therapeutic products are considered to be essential for the maintenance of the diet and can therefore be obtained on a doctor's prescription in much the same way as a drug.

Prescribable dietary products
A prescribable dietary product is a specialized product which may be obtained on a doctor's prescription. The conditions for which an item can be prescribed are clearly defined in the Borderline Substances Section of the British National Formulary (BNF). Doctors who prescribe outside these criteria are likely to incur financial penalties.

Additional products are continually being developed to meet new requirements or to add to existing ranges. When a manufacturer introduces

TABLE 1
Function of the kidney

Several important functions of the kidney
1) The production of urine
2) The excretion of the toxic products of metabolism
3) The control of fluid and electrolyte balance
4) The maintenance of the normal acid-base equilibrium of the blood
5) The retention of vital substances essential to the body
6) The production of the hormones erythropoietin and renin

a new product there is considerable incentive to get it recognized as a prescribable product. To achieve this the product must be submitted to the Advisory Committee for Borderline Substances (ACBS). There are different criteria for each type of product but trial data demonstrating that the new product is both safe and efficacious is a prerequisite for all products (see for example Lee *et al.*, 1987; Parkinson *et al.*, 1987; Wardley & Taitz, 1988). Some products fail to gain recognition on the grounds that they are luxury items or are superfluous.

CHRONIC RENAL FAILURE

The kidney has several important functions which are listed in Table 1. In chronic renal failure, these vital functions begin to fail. Accordingly, waste products accumulate in the blood and the normal water and electrolyte balances are upset. Accumulation of acid waste products in the circulating blood results in acidosis. Accumulation of waste products, particularly urea, a protein breakdown product, causes uraemia, a clinical condition which features headache, nausea, drowsiness and mental confusion.

The objectives of dietary treatment
Dietary manipulation in chronic renal failure serves two functions. In the early, asymptomatic stage of the disease a modest protein restriction can help to preserve the remaining kidney function (Bennett *et al.* 1983). In the later stages of the disease diet helps to control uraemia and fluid retention thus maintaining optimal nutritional status. This latter point is of paramount importance as chronic renal failure is a wasting disease and usually sufferers have little or no interest in food.

The parameters of the diet that need to be considered in chronic renal failure are protein, energy, electrolytes and fluids.

Protein restriction

In health, the Western diet contains on average about 70 g of protein daily (Gregory *et al.* 1990). The DHSS Recommended Dietary Allowances (RDA) for most adults lie between 42 and 84 g protein/day depending on sex and activity, DHSS (1979). Thus, many of us eat more protein than our bodies actually require. There is no evidence to suggest that excess dietary protein has any deleterious effect on the healthy adult kidney. In fact, the body is able to use the surplus protein as an energy source and the kidneys readily eliminate the additional urea which is produced.

In chronic renal failure the excretory function of the kidney is impaired so there is good reason to restrict dietary protein as this will reduce the kidney's work and offset the symptoms of uraemia. However, it is impossible to prevent protein metabolism simply by eliminating dietary protein, since there is an obligatory protein loss of 20–40 g protein/day. This protein must be replaced by the diet if optimal nutrition is to be maintained. The amount of protein actually given on a low-protein diet can, however, be minimized by using protein foods of high biological value, e.g. proteins that come from animal sources such as meat, fish, cheese, eggs and milk and restricting the protein which comes from cereals and pulse vegetables. The actual amount of protein allowed on a low-protein diet will be a function of the individual's weight and renal condition. Typically 0·6 g protein/kg of ideal body weight is given (Thomas 1988). This usually amounts to between 30 and 50 g of protein daily and is achieved by strictly limiting all animal and cereal protein and virtually eliminating vegetable protein.

Table 2 illustrates how a normal diet containing about 90 g protein and 9·24 MJ (2 200 kcal) could be made low protein. It should be noted that this modification seriously affects the energy level of the diet, which must be corrected by the introduction of high energy supplements (see next section) and specialized low-protein products.

Specialized low-protein products that are available on prescription include low-protein flour, and foods such as bread, pasta and biscuits made from low-protein flour (Fig. 1). When the protein is extracted from flour the properties of the residual product are somewhat modified. The elasticity typical of wheat dough is particularly affected as this property is conferred by gluten, one of the principal proteins in wheat flour. The end product is much finer in texture and to handle is more like corn than wheat

TABLE 2
The effect on energy of reducing dietary protein

Meal	Normal protein intake	Reduced protein intake
Breakfast	Porridge with milk and sugar Boiled egg 1 Slice of toast with butter Coffee with milk	Porridge with sugar 1 Slice of toast with butter Coffee with a dash of milk
Mid-morning	Coffee with milk 2 Digestive biscuits	Coffee with a dash of milk
Lunch	Sandwich (with 45 g cheese) Fruit yoghurt Orange	Sandwich (with 30 g cheese) Orange
Mid-afternoon	Tea with milk	Tea with a dash of milk
Evening meal	Roast beef (75 g) Carrots Peas Roast potatoes Yorkshire pudding Apple pie Ice cream	Roast beef (50 g) Carrots Roast potatoes Stewed apples
Bedtime	Drinking chocolate 1 Slice of toast with butter	Drinking chocolate (no milk)
	Protein = 93 g MJ = 9·24 kcal = 2200	Protein = 43 g MJ = 4·83 kcal = 1150

Compiled from Paul & Southgate (1978).

flour. Not surprisingly foods made from low-protein flour have a different texture: bread tends to be more crumbly and pastry can be rather hard. Nevertheless many renal patients find these substitutes very helpful as they offer a convenient source of low-protein food and the patients adjust to the altered taste and texture.

Energy
Energy is a very important component of a low-protein diet, for if the energy content is not high enough to meet the body's needs dietary and muscle protein will be 'burnt' as an energy source to correct the deficit. The main sources of low-protein energy are pure fat (butter, margarine, cooking oil and cream) and pure sugar (sucrose, glucose, fructose, etc.).

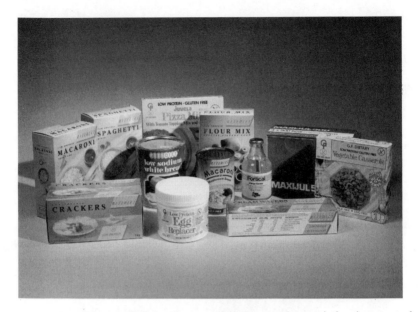

FIG. 1.   For patients with chronic renal failure, protein restriction is a central feature of the diet. This reduces the load on the kidneys, but it is essential that an adequate energy level be maintained. Patients in latter stages of chronic renal failure may also require low sodium products to achieve electrolyte balance.

However, pure fats and sugars can be very nauseating and they are tolerated better when they are 'carried' by starch. Thus low-protein flour and its products serve a dual role in that they are an energy source in their own right yet also convey fats and sugars, e.g. butter and jam on bread.

Another way of introducing energy is through the use of glucose polymers. These are high molecular weight chains of glucose that are very energy dense yet without the sweet taste of glucose. Glucose polymers are also very soluble in water and viscous solutions can be made and offered in a variety of flavours. Some freeze very well and make acceptable 'ice lollies'. Again, these products are available on prescription for renal patients. Table 3 illustrates how a low-protein, high-energy diet can be built up using suitable low-protein and high-energy products.

Electrolytes and fluid
In the terminal stages of renal failure the kidney loses control over the fluid and electrolyte balance of the body. At this stage, it is necessary to control the diet further as sodium, potassium and fluid intake will need to be

TABLE 3
The effect on energy of adding specialized and high-energy products to a low-protein diet

Meal	Low-protein high-energy diet
Breakfast	Porridge with cream and sugar 2 Slices of low protein bread, toasted (with butter and marmalade) Coffee with cream
Mid-morning	Coffee with a dash of milk 2 Low-protein biscuits
Lunch	2 Slices of ordinary bread as a salad sandwich 4 Low-protein crackers with butter and cheese (30 g) Orange
Mid-afternoon	Tea with a dash of milk Low-protein jam tart
Evening meal	Roast beef (50 g) Carrots Roast potatoes Low-protein apple pie Cream and water custard
Bedtime	Drinking chocolate (no milk) 2 Low-protein biscuits
	Protein = 45 g MJ = 11·09 kcal = 2640

Compiled from Paul & Southgate (1978).

limited. For this reason, it is possible to get low-protein products that are also restricted in their sodium (salt) content, e.g. low-protein, low-salt bread and crackers. One low-sodium product that is quite unsuitable in the treatment of chronic renal failure is salt substitute. Although it has a similar taste to common table salt, this product (potassium chloride), is actually dangerous as the potassium component can be even more harmful than sodium.

Fluid restriction is contraindicated until the production of urine virtually ceases. Under these circumstances the fluid intake is limited to 500 ml plus the volume of the previous day's urinary output. Such strict fluid control poses a further challenge to the manufacturers of dietetic foods. One of the reasons why glucose polymer solutions are perceived as thick and syrupy is that they contain a high solid content in an attempt to achieve a high energy density so that fluid may be spared.

CANCER CACHEXIA

Cancer cachexia is the term given to the generalized wasting of body tissues often observed in individuals suffering from cancer. It is a complex syndrome and the symptoms include significant biochemical disturbances in addition to severe anorexia and organ wasting (Kern & Norton, 1988). Originally it was thought that these symptoms could be attributed to the direct action of the tumour on host tissues but it is now believed to be a host-mediated response to tumour invasion (Beutler, 1988).

Further complicating the situation is the fact that cancer treatments such as surgery, radiation and chemotherapy can also have adverse nutritional effects by contributing to the anorexia (Fig. 2) and interfering with nutrient absorption (Fig. 3) (Holmes, 1987). The interplay of these factors results in an accelerating downward spiral and eventually death, often from malnutrition.

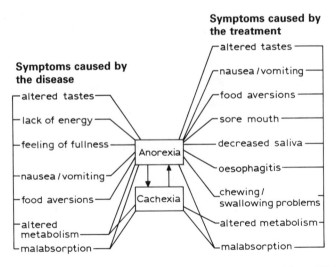

FIG. 2. How cancer and cancer therapy affect appetite (adapted from Whitney & Cataldo, 1983).

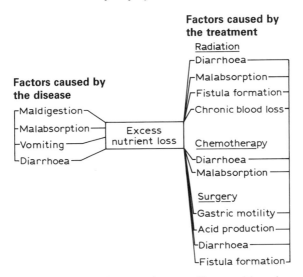

FIG. 3.   How cancer and cancer therapy affect nutrition absorption.

The objectives of dietary treatment

The objective of diet therapy in the treatment of cancer is to arrest some of the nutritional problems thereby preserving nutritional status which in turn will improve the quality of life, reduce susceptibility to infections and increase tolerance to cancer therapy. In designing a diet the dietitian will need to take into account the type and location of the tumour, in addition to all the problems associated with cachexia and cancer treatment previously described. The diet will need to contain a high level of nutrients in a small volume, i.e. it will need to be nutrient dense but as high-fat diets tend to be nauseating and difficult to digest the overall fat content should be kept low.

Other factors that may need to be given special consideration in the development of a suitable product include familiarity with the food, the flavour intensity and the food temperature, all of which can help when taste perception is altered (Stubbs, 1989).

Maintaining a highly nutritious diet in the minimum volume can be achieved through enrichment, supplementation, tube feeding or a combination of these methods.

Enrichment

Enrichment ensures that the small volumes of foods that are eaten contain the maximum levels of energy, protein, vitamins and minerals. Prescrib-

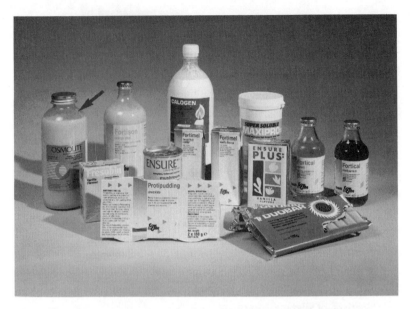

FIG. 4.   In cancer cachexia, the aim of therapy is to preserve nutritional status to improve the quality of life. As patients often find fatty foods nauseating, these are kept to a minimum. Poor appetite means low intake, so foods need to be of high energy and nutrient density. For some patients tube (enteral) feeding may be necessary with products specially formulated to meet nutrient requirements (such as that shown with the arrow).

able products for protein enrichment are usually based on dried milk proteins with additional vitamin and mineral supplementation. Energy enrichment is achieved using the glucose polymers described in the previous section. These are available in liquid and powder form (Fig. 4). The protein and energy-rich liquids and powders are added to normally prepared home-made foods to increase their nutrient density. Soups and milk-based puddings are particularly useful carriers of these products.

Some manufacturers offer supersoluble glucose polymer powders in 100 g sachets. These are useful, for when dissolved into a litre of water the powder is virtually tasteless and can provide a further 1680 KJ (400 kcal) when taken as drinking water throughout the day.

Supplementation
Prescribable nutritional supplements are also available for cancer patients. These are usually presented in the form of ready-made drinks carrying a

complete nutritional analysis. They come in a wide variety of sweet flavours. Some savoury flavours have also been developed and offer a welcomed change. However, savoury flavours are more difficult to perfect and the range is more limited.

Supplements can be used as complete meal replacements when food is rejected or as drinks offered in between meals for patients to 'sip feed'. Some manufacturers have developed their own range of ready made high-protein, high-energy soups and puddings. These are convenient to use and, like the drinks, guarantee a defined level of nutrient intake per unit consumed. However, the flavour and texture variations are limited and the diet will become monotonous unless they are used in conjunction with enriched home made foods. Table 4 illustrates how enrichment and supplementation can enhance the energy and protein levels above the basic diet.

Tube feeding
Tube feeding takes away the responsibility of the individual for feeding himself or herself. This procedure is particularly useful when the patient is unable to swallow or unable to manage the large volume of food required. To tube feed it is necessary to pass a fine bore tube through the nose, down the oesophagus and into the stomach. A reservoir which is filled with a defined liquid feed is then connected to the tube via a giving set and the feed passes by gravity through the tube and into the stomach, (Fig. 5).

There is a wide range of prescribable tube feeds (Fig. 4). Most are based on milk protein but some offer alternative protein sources, e.g. soya for individuals who are milk or lactose intolerant. Similarly, different concentrations of protein and energy can be selected so that it is possible to design a feed that very closely matches the individual's requirements. There is also great variation in the presentation. Most are supplied in liquid form but some are available as a powder which has to be reconstituted with water. Some liquid feeds are marketed as a 'closed system'; this reduces the possibility of contamination as compared with those feeds that have to be decanted into a reservoir.

Tube feeding can completely replace oral feeding or can be used as a form of supplementation when some food is being taken orally. It is also possible to use the procedure at night while the patient is asleep (MacIntyre *et al.*, 1983).

TABLE 4

The effect of enrichment and supplementation on the basic energy and protein intake of a patient with cancer

Meal	Basic intake	Intake with enrichment and supplementation
Breakfast	Porridge with milk and sugar	Porridge with milk and sugar
	$\frac{1}{2}$ Boiled egg	$\frac{1}{2}$ Boiled egg
	$\frac{1}{2}$ Slice toast with butter	$\frac{1}{2}$ Slice toast with butter
	$\frac{1}{2}$ Cup milky coffee	$\frac{1}{2}$ Cup milky coffee
Mid-morning	$\frac{1}{2}$ Cup milky coffee	Glass of Build-Up milk shake
	$\frac{1}{2}$ Biscuit	$\frac{1}{2}$ Biscuit
Lunch	Small bowl of soup	Small bowl of soup with added milk, powder and glucose polymer
	$\frac{1}{2}$ Slice bread	$\frac{1}{2}$ Slice bread
	1 Scoop of ice cream	1 Scoop of ice cream with 'Hycal', sauce
Mid-afternoon	Tea with milk	Tea with milk
	$\frac{1}{2}$ Biscuit	$\frac{1}{2}$ Biscuit
Evening meal	Roast beef (50 g)	Roast beef (50 g)
	Few carrots	Few carrots
	Few peas	Few peas
	$\frac{1}{2}$ Roast potato	$\frac{1}{2}$ Roast potato
	Rice pudding (75 g)	Rice pudding with added milk powder and glucose polymer
Bedtime	Drinking chocolate	Chocolate flavoured Build-Up
	$\frac{1}{2}$ Slice of toast	$\frac{1}{2}$ Slice of toast
	Protein = 43 g	Protein = 82 g
	MJ = 4·79	MJ = 8·4
	kcal = 1140	kcal = 2000

The amounts managed by cancer patients are usually very small.
Enrichment and supplementation will also enhance vitamin and mineral intake.
Compiled from Paul & Southgate (1978).

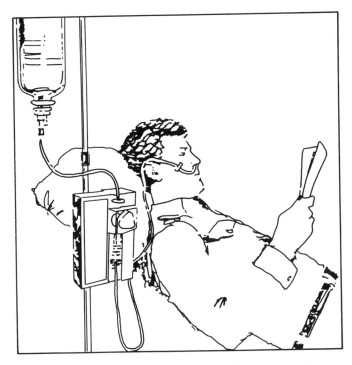

FIG. 5. Some patients may require tube-feeding. Fine bore drip feeding which can be regulated by a pump is the preferred method (Adapted from Whitney & Cataldo, 1983).

COELIAC DISEASE

Coeliac disease is caused by an extreme sensitivity to a protein, gluten, which is found in wheat, oats, rye and barley. The onset of the disease often occurs in early childhood, during weaning, when the sufferer is first exposed to gluten.

As a result of the inflammatory reaction, the mucosa of the small intestine produces a massive secretion of mucus which interferes with nutrient absorption. Typically the child has a distended abdomen and passes large, pale, foamy stools which are very offensive due to the malabsorption of dietary fats. Frequently the condition is complicated by the failure to absorb vitamins, minerals and some carbohydrates. The child therefore fails to thrive, is often anaemic and, if left untreated, can sometimes develop vitamin deficiency conditions such as rickets.

Interestingly, the incidence of coeliac disease in early childhood has been declining in recent years. This is thought to be due to changes in weaning practices, with wheat-based foods now being introduced at a later stage (Stevens *et al.*, 1987). In contrast, the incidence of coeliac disease in adults has been increasing. Between 1983 and 1985 figures from the Coeliac Society (UK) indicated that just 25% of newly diagnosed coeliacs joining the Society were children, the remaining 75% being adults (Thomas, 1988). The symptoms of adult onset coeliac disease are more subtle than in childhood and it is thought that the higher incidence may be due to increased general practitioner awareness resulting in improved levels of diagnosis.

In health, the surface area and consequently the absorptive potential of the gut is greatly increased by the presence of intestinal villi—thousands of finger-like protrusions from the gut lining (Fig. 4(a)). The diagnosis of coeliac disease is confirmed by biopsy of this tissue, showing that the normal convolutions of the intestinal microvilli are completely flattened (Fig. 6(b)). It is the absence of the microvilli which results in severe malabsorption. The symptoms of the disease are a consequence.

The objectives of dietary treatment

The treatment for coeliac disease is dietary, for if gluten can be completely eliminated from the diet, the microvilli will regenerate and the symptoms subside. The exclusion of gluten from the diet is a daunting task, as wheat flour is present in so many foods—bread, cakes, biscuits, breakfast cereals, pasta, processed meats, soups, sauces, etc. To assist in the identification of foods that are free from gluten, every year the Coeliac Society publishes a comprehensive list of the gluten-free products available commercially. Some food manufacturers also print the 'Crossed Grain' symbol (Fig. 7) on their food packets to indicate that the product is free from gluten.

Gluten-free flour, bread and biscuits are available on prescription for coeliacs, (Fig. 8). These products are, in some respects, similar to their low-protein equivalents but as there is no need to restrict protein on a gluten-free diet other proteins are introduced to the gluten-free flour to improve its flavour and texture. In addition to the prescribable products there is a wide range of gluten-free biscuits and cakes that are manufactured for people with coeliac disease. These are considered by the ACBS to be luxury items and are therefore not available on prescription.

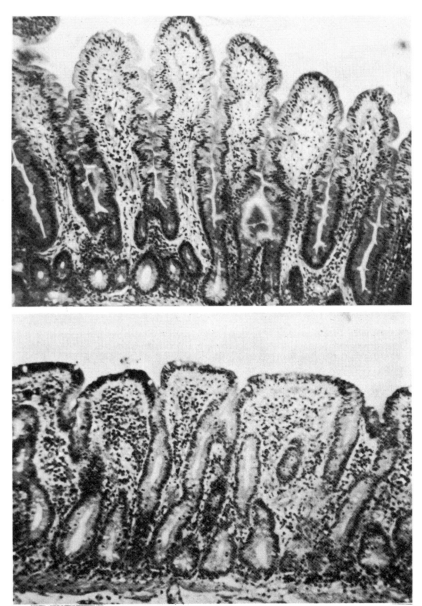

FIG. 6. (a) the normal jejunal mucosa. The epithelial cells are columnar and their nuclei are basally oriented. The villus height-to-crypt-depth ratio is 4:1. There are plasma cells and lymphocytes in the lamina propria (× 180); (b) the gluten sensitive enteropathy mucosa. The epithelial cells are cuboidal and their nuclei are not basally oriented. There are increased numbers of mitoses in the crypts, and the villi are flat. There are increased inflammatory cells present in the lamina (× 180). Reproduced with permission from A.J. Katz & M. Falchuk, Current Concepts in Gluten Sensitive Enteropathy. In *Pediatrics in North America*, Vol. 22, W.B. Saunders, London, 1975.

Kathleen Debenham

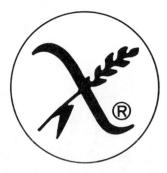

FIG. 7.   The 'Crossed Grain' symbol is printed on the labels of some foods known to be gluten free.

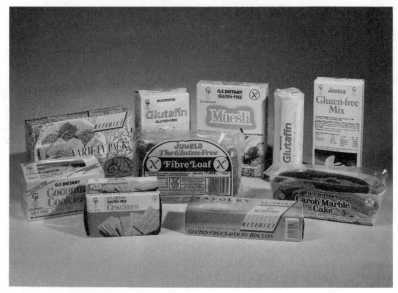

FIG. 8.   In coeliac disease, gluten present in wheat flour needs to be completely eliminated from the diet. Gluten-free flour, bread and biscuits are available on prescription for coeliacs in the United Kingdom. Other products are considered 'luxury' items which the patient may buy over-the-counter.

PHENYLKETONURIA

Phenylketonuria(PKU) is an inherited metabolic disorder. It is caused by a deficiency of phenylalanine hydroxylase, the enzyme that converts the essential amino acid phenylalanine into tyrosine (Fig. 9). As a consequence of this block in the normal metabolic pathway, the blood analysis shows a marked increase in the levels of phenylalanine and its metabolites (Stanbury *et al.*, 1983).

Phenylalanine is neurotoxic, and if the condition is not diagnosed and treated within the first few weeks of life the infant will suffer irreversible brain damage. The prevalance of PKU, between 1 in 12 000 and 1 in 30 000 births, is sufficiently high that all new babies in the UK are screened between the 6th and 14th day of life. In 1968 the Guthrie test, a sensitive

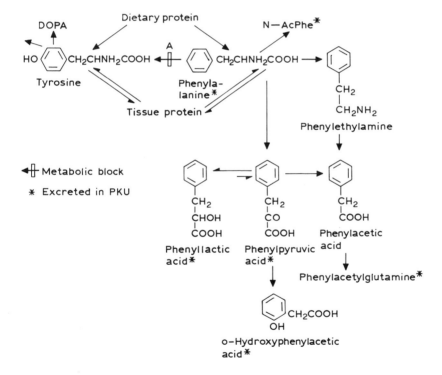

FIG. 9. The metabolism of phenylalanine indicating the metabolic block which leads to the build-up of phenylalanine and the production of phenylketones, (Adapted from Francis, 1987).

blood test, replaced urine testing. This led to improved diagnosis which in turn has been shown to be matched by significantly greater IQ scores in those children whose treatment was initiated at an earlier stage (Smith & Beasley, 1989).

Objectives of dietary treatment

The objective of treatment in PKU is to control blood phenylalanine levels. This is achieved by a very strict dietary control of phenylalanine intake (Francis, 1987). Phenylalanine, a constituent of all dietary proteins, is an essential amino acid. That is, our bodies cannot synthesize it, so to maintain normal growth it must be included in the diet. A balance must therefore be struck such that sufficient dietary phenylalanine is supplied to permit normal development but that the upper level is controlled to prevent mental impairment. In practice the aim is to maintain the blood concentration of phenylalanine between 180 and 480 μ mol/litre. Since phenylalanine is present in all dietary proteins, a very strict diet low in natural protein is given. The actual amount of natural protein allowed is determined by the child's blood phenylalanine level. This will vary according to the age, weight and tolerance of the child but for a 4 year old it is typically about 25 mg/kg body weight. The natural dietary protein is then calculated in terms of 50 mg phenylalanine exchanges. The resulting diet is very low in protein (typically up to 8 g for young children and up to 25 g for teenagers). As this would not permit the child to grow and develop normally because of the low levels of all other amino acids, these are supplied as a mixture of pure amino acids, free from phenylalanine.

The dietary treatment of PKU was first used in 1951 (Bickel et al., 1953). The first protein preparations, based on casein hydrolysates, were crude and extremely unpalatable. Over the years the formula has been refined and the flavour improved. However, it is difficult to disguise the unpleasant taste of free amino acids, so the continual challenge to improve the flavour remains. Happily, babies who have known nothing else since birth will take the formula and thus thrive.

The small amount of protein that is allowed to PKU infants is given as 50 mg phenylalanine exchanges of regular infant formula or breast milk. Older children take their exchanges as 'normal' foods. Typically, exchanges will be given as milk, cereal, potatoes, etc., but when more than 10 exchanges are tolerated some chocolate and other treats may be allowed. This will not jeopardize the intake of amino acids other than phenylalanine, as these will be met from the amino acid supplement anyway. The rest of the diet is made up of very low-protein foods such as fruits and non-legu-

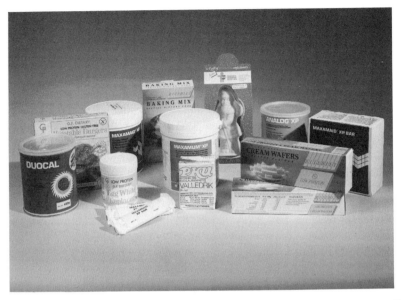

Fig. 10. The amounts of phenylalanine (an essential amino acid found in all dietary proteins) must be strictly controlled in the diets of young children with phenylketonuria. Sufficient dietary proteins are permitted to provide sufficient phenylalanine and the rest of the protein is supplied in the form of a mixture of pure amino acids free from phenylalanine.

minous vegetables. In addition to the amino acid supplements the full range of low-protein and high-energy products is available on prescription in the UK as previously discussed for renal disease. In an attempt to normalize the diet, luxury items such as low protein 'chocolate' Easter eggs and Santa Claus can be purchased (Fig. 10).

Vitamin and mineral supplementation is essential for such an artificial diet and some of the amino acid preparations now contain these supplements within the mix. For those preparations that do not contain vitamins and minerals, separate supplements are available on prescription.

Diet for life

Until about two years ago it was the practice in the UK to relax the diet at the age of about 8 years. The reasoning was that by this age brain development was complete and raised phenylalanine levels would therefore not be detrimental. This allowed children a freer diet which had both nutritional and social benefits (Naughten, 1989). Even so, blood levels of phenylalanine were only allowed to rise from around 480 μmol/ litre up to the 1200 μmol/litre mark so some dietary constraints were still necessary.

However, a growing body of evidence suggesting worsening IQs and behavioural and neurological problems at this age has led to a change in thinking and now most UK centres are adopting a 'diet for life' policy (Naughton, 1985). This poses new nutritional challenges as the adolescent growth spurt, previously managed on the relaxed diet, is now being managed on a stricter diet typically controlling the blood phenylalanine level to about 600 μmol/litre. As PKU children grow into adults another challenge has been faced when PKU women wish to become mothers. In this instance, the blood levels need to be controlled very tightly because of the vulnerability of the developing foetus to high phenylalanine levels. Although there are not many reports in the literature there is sufficient evidence to suggest the necessity for a tightly controlled diet even prior to conception (Brenton, 1989).

CONCLUSION

Within this chapter the wide spectrum of dietary manipulations used in the treatment of disease has been illustrated with four examples. The low-protein renal diet provided an example of a general restriction, whilst the high-energy, high-protein diet used in cancer cachexia was representative of a general addition. The complete exclusion of a dietary factor was illustrated by the gluten-free diet, which contrasted with the very specific restriction but not exclusion of phenylalanine in the PKU diet. Whilst the conditions described can all be greatly helped by strict compliance with the prescribed diet, it should be noted that only in the cases of coeliac disease and PKU can the symptoms be completely controlled by dietary means.

This chapter has also illustrated how technology, applied to the creation and manufacture of specialized dietary products, can make these very difficult diets easier and more palatable for those unfortunate people who require them. The dietitian, whose job it is to interpret the doctor's prescription and translate it into an acceptable diet, is in the best position to communicate patient needs to the food manufacturer. With the advent of microwave cookery and cook chill foods one can look forward to an even wider range of ingenious dietary products to help patients.

ACKNOWLEDGEMENT

Thanks are due to the Photographic Department, University of Reading, for the preparation of Figures 1, 4, 8 and 10.

REFERENCES

Bennett, S.E., Russell, G.I. & Walls, J. (1983). Low-protein diets in uraemia. *British Medical Journal* **287**, 1344–5.

Beutler, B. (1988). Cachexia: A fundamental mechanism. *Nutrition Reviews* **46**, 369–73.

Bickel, H., Gerrard, J. & Hickmans, E.M. (1953). Influence of phenylalanine intake on phenylketonuria. *Lancet* **ii**, 812–3.

Brenton, D.P. (1989). Maternal phenylketonuria. *European Journal of Clinical Nutrition* **43**, suppl. 1, 13–17.

DHSS (1979). *Recommended Daily Amounts of Food Energy and Nutrients for Groups of People in the United Kingdom.* Report on Health and Social Subjects no. 15. London: H.M. Stationery Office.

Francis, D. (1987). *Diets for Sick Children*, 4th ed. Oxford: Blackwell Scientific Publications.

Gregory, J., Foster, K., Tyler, H. & Wiseman, M. (1990). *The Dietary and Nutritional Survey of British Adults.* Office of Population Census and Surveys. Social Survey Division. London: H.M. Stationery Office.

Holmes, S. (1987). Nutrition problems in the cancer patient. *Nursing: The Journal of Clinical Practice, Education and Management* **3**, 733–8.

Kern, H.A. & Norton, J.A. (1988). Reviews—Cancer cachexia. *Journal of Parenteral and Enteral Nutrition* **12**, 286–98.

Lee, H.A., Hadfield, C.M.I., Talbot, S.J. & Jackson, J.M. (1987). Dialamine (essential amino acid powder) as a supplement to low-protein diets in advanced chronic renal failure. *Clinical Nutrition* **6**, 111–16.

MacIntyre, P.B., Wood, S.R., Powell-Tuck, J. & Lennard-Jones, J.E. (1983). Nocturnal nasogastric feeding at home. *Postgraduate Medical Journal* **59**, 767–9.

Naughten, E.R. (1989). Continuation vs discontinuation of diet in phenylketonuria. *European Journal of Clinical Nutrition* **43**, suppl. 1, 7–12.

Parkinson, S.A., Lewis, J., Morris, R., Allbright, A., Plant, H. & Slevin, M.L. (1987). Oral protein and energy supplements in cancer patients. *Human Nutrition: Applied Nutrition* **41**, 233–43.

Paul, A.A. & Southgate, D.A.T. (1978). *McClance and Widdowson's: The Composition of Foods.* London: H.M. Stationery Office.

Smith, I. & Beasley, M. (1989). Intelligence and behaviour in children with early treated phenylketonuria. *European Journal of Clinical Nutrition* **43**, suppl. 1, 1–5.

Stanbury, J.B., Wyngarden, J.B., Fredrickson, D.S., Goldstein, J.L. & Brown, M.S. (1983). *The Metabolic Basis of Inherited Disease*, 5th ed. New York: McGraw-Hill.

Stevens, F.M., Egan-Mitchell, B., Cryan, E., McCarthy, C.F. & McNicholl, B. (1987). *Archives of Diseases in Childhood* **62**, 465–8.

Stubbs, L. (1989). Taste changes in cancer patients. *Nursing Times* **85**, 49–50.

Thomas, B. (1988). *Manual of Dietetic Practice*. Oxford: Blackwell Scientific Publications.

Wardley, B.L. & Taitz, L.S. (1988). Clinical trial of a concentrated amino acid formula for older patients with phenylketonuria (Maxamum XP). *European Journal of Clinical Nutrition* **42**, 81–6.

Whitney, E.N. & Cataldo, C.B. (1983) *Understanding Normal and Clinical Nutrition*. St Paul, MN: West Publishing Company.

10

Viewpoint I: Large Animals as Models for Studies in Human Nutrition

A. Graham Low
AFRC Institute for Grassland and Environmental Research, Reading, UK

INTRODUCTION

Why should we use animal models for studies on human nutrition? It can be argued that only studies on humans are valid and that we should devote all our energies to devising ways of direct studies, and thereby avoid the real possibility of drawing false conclusions from animals. But many investigators know to their cost that human studies are expensive (they may be up to 10 times dearer than pig studies and 100 times dearer than rat studies), that suitably homogeneous subject groups are difficult to find, that long-term compliance to unvarying nutritional regimens is not easy to achieve, that environmental, social and psychological conditions may change during a study and that detailed physiological information is often impossible to obtain because suitable non-invasive techniques do not exist.

Problems of these kinds have made the interpretation of many studies in human nutrition very difficult, and have led researchers to approach research questions initially with the aid of animal models. Such models have been used very successfully, particularly at a physiological level, to provide information that has allowed reasonable hypotheses to be tested and predictions to be made of human responses to nutritional changes, especially in relation to the management or alleviation of the many diseases that have a nutritional component. Animals can be given a wide range of treatments and, because of their greater genetic homogeneity, better statistical designs can be achieved than in human studies. Because of their relatively short generation time, animals can be used to examine life-span or multigeneration topics within an acceptable time span. The use of a variety of animal models for the study of human nutrition has been discussed by Aggett & Davies (1980), Crawford & Frankel (1980), Goss (1980) & Gurr (1980).

One of the advantages of animal models is that they can be given extreme diets, containing highly purified ingredients, permitting studies of between-nutrient interactions and variations in the level of incorporation of individual nutrients. Such diets are, however, unlike normal diets in various respects. They may lead to adverse effects if extreme concentrations of nutrients are used, which would not normally occur and hence under- or over-estimation of adverse effects could occur. Such adverse effects could include both disturbances of the gut microflora and of metabolism. If extreme diets are being used, it is essential to provide a range of levels of inclusion of the nutrient of interest: linearity of response must not be assumed, and extrapolation from one species to another must be done with great caution. The basis of such extrapolation may be on the basis of relative intakes of energy or per unit of metabolic body weight (frequently the animal weight$^{0.75}$).

SUITABLE MODELS

Although animals are unlikely ever to provide an exact quantitative picture of the responses by humans to a nutritional regimen, they may provide an initial screening prior to critical direct testing. At all times caution has to be a keynote in the extrapolation and interpretation of animal studies, tempering the enthusiasm that basic studies in animals may generate in the experimenter. At a time of increasing public concern about the use of animals for research purposes it is appropriate to note that it is customary only to run experiments that have potential to contribute useful knowledge, using the minimum number of animals consistent with achieving the objectives of the study and with particular emphasis on the avoidance of any stress, however caused. While great hopes are placed upon the possibility of using alternatives to live animals or humans, e.g. tissue culture, nutritional responses are the result of very complex interactions of the whole organism with its diet and as such can only be studied at this level.

When the nutritionist has exhausted all possible means of investigating his or her problem in direct human studies, he or she is faced with the question of which animal model to choose: although a very large number have been considered, rats, rabbits and dogs have been the most widely used for many years. Nevertheless there have often been difficulties in selecting the most appropriate species for use as a model. In certain cases suitable models have not been used because the experimenter has been unfamiliar with the appropriate techniques required for their successful breeding, housing and handling in relation to the human nutrition problem being studied. Furthermore, limitations on research funds have often led to the use of small animal models in spite of their known deficiencies: a number of people have pointed out that those who control research funds have not always provided sufficient support for the breeding, maintenance and use of models that have the greatest chance of providing sound experimental results, partly at least because scientists have sometimes made an inadequate case for the use of the best model.

In considering the most suitable animal model, investigators need to consider very carefully both similarities and differences between the animal and humans in terms of anatomy, (especially of the digestive system and the liver), physiology (especially hormonal regulation of growth and metabolism), susceptibility to and aetiology of nutritional diseases, similarity of immunological responses, qualitative requirements for essential nutrients and patterns of growth in relation to the topic being studied. The best model will vary according to the topic. At the same time availability, cost, number and type of breeding lines available as well as provision of suitably skilled staff and satisfactory housing conditions are important factors. Clearly no model will satisfy all these criteria, but the experience of many research groups in recent years shows that large domesticated animals such as pigs are particularly useful in nutritional research. An obvious question which may be raised is: why not use primates? Clearly for some purposes there may be no satisfactory alternative but they are very expensive, difficult to house and major problems can arise in handling when physiological measurements are required. By contrast, laboratory animals do have considerable value for some types of studies, as discussed by Eggum & Beames (1986).

The value of pigs as models for nutritional research is that they are very similar to humans both anatomically and physiologically (Table 1). Furthermore, their size and docility make them suitable for a wide range of studies that involve taking samples of sufficient size for detailed physical, chemical and biochemical analysis, and surgical intervention is practicable using a very wide range of techniques analogous to those used in human surgery. Other benefits of pigs are the diversity of the genetic lines available, their relatively short reproductive cycle (115 days), large litter size

TABLE 1
Similarities between pigs and man

Dental characteristics
Renal morphology and physiology
Eye structure and visual acuity
Skin morphology and physiology
Cardiovascular anatomy and physiology
Digestive anatomy and physiology
Proportions of fat-free body at common stages of life

(allowing within-litter studies with correspondingly low variation), their wide availability from commercial sources, their ability to eat a very wide range of foods over long periods of time, and the remarkable similarity of many aspects of their metabolism with that of man at a biochemical level. Some of these issues were discussed in detail by Pond & Houpt (1978), Dodds (1982), Low et al. (1982) and Miller & Ullrey (1987).

In the remaining part of this chapter, the potential of pigs as models will be described in relation to some human diseases of major importance, which have a nutritional component in their aetiology. It is worth noting at this point that such studies may often also lead to improved understanding of the nutrition and physiology of pigs, which can be applied in practical pig production for meat.

A VALUABLE MODEL FOR THE STUDY OF TWO DIET-RELATED DISEASES

Many studies published during the last 20 years or so have shown that pigs appear to be valuable models for studying spontaneous and induced atherosclerosis, both of which follow patterns closely similar to those found in man. The morphology and the biochemistry of atherosclerotic lesions in pigs are very similar to those seen in man and severe experimental lesions can be induced by diet faster than occurs during the atherogenic process in the human population. At the same time it has been shown that serum low density lipoproteins, which appear to be important in the development of atherosclerosis in man, are similar in physicochemical structure and properties in pigs and humans, and are the main vehicle for cholesterol transport in both species. The other major serum lipoproteins (very low density and high density lipoproteins) are also similar in the two species. It is also of interest to note that von Willebrand's disease (an inherited impairment in the adherence of platelets to damaged vascular

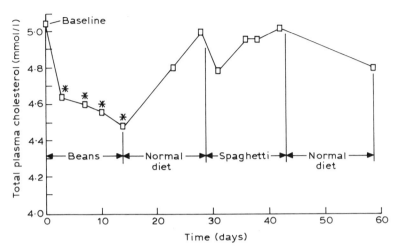

FIG. 1.   Change in plasma cholesterol level of healthy young men during daily consumption of 450 g of canned baked beans or spaghetti. *, significantly different from baseline. (Modified from Shutler *et al.*, 1989.)

tissue, thought to be a factor in the development of atherosclerosis) can be induced in pigs: such animals show reduced diet-induced atherogenesis and may thus be valuable models for clarifying the role of platelets in atherogenesis. Numerous recent studies have confirmed the utility of the pig model in detailed studies of diet-related atherogenesis, with differences between the species being largely confined to matters of detail. The possible role of *trans* fatty acids in human atherogenesis is of considerable current interest and studies using pigs as a model may be of value. Similarly, dietary protein and amino acid levels and/or ratios, excessive vitamin D levels and deficiencies in vitamin E, selenium and copper have also been implicated in human atherosclerosis but their significance is not yet clearly proven. Again, studies with pigs may provide a useful lead.

An example of the value of pigs for studies on nutritional influences on cholesterol metabolism in man comes from an initial demonstration that baked beans, peas, lentils and butter beans could all reduce plasma total cholesterol levels in hypercholesterolaemic pigs; butter beans and baked beans were particularly effective. Subsequently baked beans were given to human volunteers and they also led to significantly reduced plasma cholesterol levels (Shutler *et al.* 1989; Fig 1).

Finally, it is clear that although most, if not all, strains and breeds of pigs tested are susceptible to atherosclerosis there are clear genetic differences between lines and these may be the result of mechanisms which if understood could throw light on some of the immensely complex factors that appear to be involved in the development of human atherosclerosis. A very large literature exists on the suitability of pigs, of both normal and miniature lines, for studies on cardiovascular disease, especially in relation to diet-induced aspects (Bustard & McClellan, 1966; Roberts & Dodds, 1982; Tumbleson, 1986).

Diabetes is a highly complex disease whose incidence is increasing in many countries. It has no known cure, but careful nutritional management is an essential feature of its treatment. In recent years it has become clear that certain types of dietary fibre are of particular value in diabetic control, but their mode of action has not been clearly elucidated because of the difficulty of appropriate direct studies on the function of the digestive system in man. It is clear from human studies that responses to dietary fibre differ greatly among different types but so far it has not been possible to specify suitable therapeutic doses and types of dietary fibre with any accuracy. Furthermore, the most effective types of dietary fibre so far used for diabetic therapy, e.g. guar gum and pectin, are soluble and have the property of increasing meal viscosity, with the result that palatability is reduced. Several ingenious attempts to overcome this problem have been made by incorporating guar gum directly into foods rather than by separate administration and these have met with success. Studies with pigs (which respond to guar gum and pectin in the same way as man) have shown that such forms of dietary fibre modify gastro-duodenal motility, delay the emptying of the liquid phase of digesta (but not glucose) from the stomach and reduce the rate of glucose absorption from the small intestine. Each of these observations provides insight into the mode of action of guar gum; this information can now be used as a basis for novel and rational approaches to designing new approches to diabetic therapy.

It might be argued that the studies described above could have been done in man or in small animal models, and indeed some research groups have attempted to do this. However, in the case of gastric emptying, the methods used in man do not allow accurate measurement of the movement of different fractions of digesta from the stomach and do not permit reliable sampling of normal foods during their digestion in the gut. Quantitative measurements of motility and absorption in man are also very difficult to achieve; this is of considerable importance because detailed understanding of the physicochemical events during digestion is likely to be of paramount importance in future developments of diabetic therapy. Small animals can be used for such studies but their use is limited by the small sample volumes which can be obtained and by the difficulty of long-term complex physiological studies on the whole animal under relatively normal conditions because of their small size. Such animals can, however, provide useful information about cell, tissue and organ function which can form the basis for studies with larger animals (Eggum & Beames, 1986).

This brief review is only an introduction to the value of large animal models, and in particular pigs, for studies on human nutrition and related disease states. The literature on the use of pigs for such studies includes well over 1,000 papers covering almost every aspect of human nutrition and the attention of interested readers is drawn to the reviews cited above.

CONCLUSION

The problems of nutritional studies in man include high cost, unreliable long-term compliance with sometimes spartan and unvarying dietary regimens, recruitment of suitable volunteers and the difficulty of making detailed physiological studies. The need to ensure that an animal model responds at least as qualitatively as man to nutritional regimens must be established. Small animals may have limited value for long-term physiological studies but larger, domesticated animals such as pigs are useful and appropriate because of their many close similarities to man as well as their sufficient size for physiological studies and availability. The uses of pigs for research into nutritional aspects of atherosclerosis and diabetes are described as examples of their current widespread role in nutritional and medical research.

REFERENCES

Aggett, P.J. & Davies, N.T. (1980). Animal models for the study of trace metal requirements. *Proceedings of the Nutrition Society* **39**, 241–8.

Bustard, L.K. & McClellan, R.O. (Editors) (1966). *Swine in Biomedical Research.* Richland, WA: Pacific Northwest Laboratory.

Crawford, M.A. & Frankel, T. (1980). Models for the human brain. *Proceedings of the Nutrition Society* **39**, 233–40.

Dodds, W.H.J. (1982). The pig model for biomedical research. *Federation Proceedings* **41**, 247–56.

Eggum, B.O. & Beames, R.M. (1986). Use of laboratory animals for studies on nutrition of domestic animals. In *Laboratory Animals*, pp. 265–90 [E.J. Ruitenbeg and P.W.J. Peters, editors]. Amsterdam: Elsevier Science Publishers B.V.

Goss, R.J. (1980). Animal models for growth. *Proceedings of the Nutrition Society* **39**, 213–7.

Gurr, M.I. (1980). Animal models for the study of energy balance. *Proceedings of the Nutrition Society* **39**, 219–25.

Low, A.G., Rainbird, A.L. & Gurr, M.I. (1982). Animal models for studying the effect of fibre on gastrointestinal function. *Journal of Plant Foods* **4**, 29–32.

Miller, E.R. & Ullrey, D.E. (1987). The pig as a model for human nutrition. *Annual Review of Nutrition* **7**, 361–82.

Pond, W.G. & Houpt, K.A. (1978). *The Biology of the Pig*. Ithaca, NY: Comstock.

Roberts, H.R. & Dodds, W.J. (Editors) (1982). *Pig Model for Biomedical Research*. Taiwan: Pig Research Institute.

Shutler, S.M., Bircher, G.M., Tredger, J.A., Morgan, L.M., Walker, A.F. & Low, A.G. (1989). The effect of daily baked bean (*Phaseolus vulgaris*) consumption on the plasma lipid levels of young, normo-cholesterolaemic men. *British Journal of Nutrition* **61**, 257–65.

Tumbleson, M.E. (Editor) (1986). *Swine in Biomedical Research*. Vols 1, 2 and 3. New York: Plenum Press.

Whitehead, R.G. (1980). Animal models for the study of protein–energy malnutrition. *Proceedings of the Nutrition Society* **39**, 227–31.

11

Viewpoint II: Small Animals as Models for Studies on Human Nutrition

GEOFFREY WEBB

The Polytechnic of East London, London, UK

INTRODUCTION

The consumer may be confronted with two opposing and non-overlapping views concerning the usefulness of animal experiments in human biology.

The anti-vivisectionist's view is that animal experiments are of little value because of the differences between experimental species and man: an hypothesis which, if proved, would make the ethical case against them overwhelming. Such statements are often coupled with logically contradictory suggestions that, given resources and commitment, most experimentation could be switched to models that are even further divorced from humans, e.g. computer models, microorganisms and cultured cells.

The scientist's view is that animal experiments are essential if much practically useful research in the medical sciences is to continue. Most research workers share the concern of anti-vivisectionists for animal welfare but have concluded that the benefits that accrue from properly regulated, humanely conducted animal experiments outweigh any infringement of animal rights. Scientists tend to emphasize only the positive benefits of animal experiments, usually by focusing upon anecdotal examples of individual (but often spectacular) advances in medical or surgical treatment that have resulted from animal experiments, e.g. insulin therapy for diabetes and open heart surgery. It is not often that the consumer is offered a reasoned case for animal experiments coupled with constructive criticism of them and their interpretation. The rather defensive and uncritical posture of many scientists is not surprising given the hostile and distorted nature of much material aimed at undermining public and political support for animal-dependent research. However, an increased level of constructively critical debate about the role and validity of a animal experiments might not only lead to improvements in the design and interpretation of such experiments, but perhaps also help reassure public opinion that they are not lightly or wastefully undertaken.

The thesis presented here is that animal experiments have played a vital role in human biological research (including human nutrition) and that they will remain essential in the foreseeable future if much research is to continue. However, it is also argued that these experiments have a large potential to mislead, particularly if the results are extrapolated to humans with little experimental confirmation in people and with inadequate consideration of biological factors that make such projections unsafe.

Are there examples in human nutrition where animal experiments have encouraged important errors?

A positive response to this question would result from a convincing demonstration that animal experiments played a significant role in generating a once popular but now discredited theory.

Webb (1989) has argued that the 'protein gap' is just such an example —the now largely discredited concept of a huge and increasing shortfall in world protein supplies, with primary protein deficiency as the most serious and widespread cause of worldwide malnutrition. Three dubious assumptions underpinned this theory:

(i) children required a high dietary protein: energy ratio;
(ii) kwashiorkor resulted from a low protein: energy ratio; and
(iii) kwashiorkor was the most widespread form of worldwide malnutrition but represented only an extreme manifestation of an even larger problem.

According to Hegsted (1959) cross-species generalizations played an important part in setting the then very high estimates of children's protein requirements. However, human infants are atypical in their protein requirements compared with common laboratory, domestic and agricultural species. Milk of cows, sheep, rabbits, rats, cats and mice has 20–25% of the energy as protein whereas human milk has only around 6%. Hegsted's paper was part of a symposium entitled 'Protein requirement and its assessment in man' and yet Webb (1989) points out that two-thirds of the tables and figures in this symposium presented animal data.

Oedema is a characteristic symptom of kwashiorkor and is generally believed to result from hypoalbuminaemia; the induction of hypoalbuminaemia in animals by protein restriction may have reinforced the view that kwashiorkor was due to protein deficiency.

The detrimental repercussions of this probably erroneous theory were widespread and long-lasting (McClaren, 1974; Webb, 1989).

Valid use of animal experiments
The only strictly valid use of animal models in human biology is to generate testable hypotheses about humans; before projecting from animal experiments to humans, two things need to be considered.

(i) Biological differences between the model species and the species being modelled. There may be clear reasons why results obtained with one species would not be expected to predict the effect in another, e.g. poikilotherms would be poor models of homeotherms when investigating the effects of cold on metabolic rate and food consumption.

(ii) Differences between the circumstances of the experiment and the proposed projection. It may be that laboratory results would not even accurately predict the response of free-living wild animals of the same species, let alone the response of people.

Consideration of these factors should occur during the experimental design and prior to model selection as well as during interpretation of the results, although in practice model selection may be limited by more practical considerations, such as cost. The hypothesis generated is now ideally tested with the modelled species. This may not always be practical; indeed, animals may have been used initially because the topic is refractory to investigation using human subjects for ethical or technical reasons. Under such circumstances, one may be limited to checking observations that are obtainable in people for consistency with the animal-generated hypothesis, and also looking for consistency of the response obtained in several non-human species.

Logical basis and extent of animal use
Evolution from a common ancestor is the theoretical thread that links all the biological sciences. It implies commonality between different life-forms—e.g. all independently viable organisms have their genetic blueprint encoded in a common, triplet code of DNA nucleotide sequences. Thus much of our understanding of the molecular processes of genetics are derived from studies with microorganisms. Even in human nutrition, microbial models have their uses: mutagenesis in bacteria is used as a

TABLE 1

The percentage of Nobel prizewinners in physiology and medicine ($n = 139$) between 1901 and 1984 who used different categories of experimental subjects in their research.

Years	Experimental subjects					
	Humans	Primates	Other mammals	Other vertebrates	Other metazoa	Micro-organisms
1901–1984	22[a]	6	47	26	11	24
1901–1942	29	2	48	40	12	7
1942–1984	20	8	46	20	10	31

[a] This figure for humans is halved if those using only humans are counted.
Totals are more than 100% because many winners used more than one category.
Calculated from data in Morowitz (1985).

screen for carcinogenic potential of food additives because DNA damage is involved in both processes.

The closer two species are phylogenetically then the more areas of commonality one would expect and thus the logical case for use would be enhanced.

Paradoxically, evolution also implies diversity and distinctiveness of individual species—it produces an array of life-forms capable of exploiting various habitats, environmental conditions and potential food sources. It is thus necessary to consciously avoid the temptation to regard small mammals as scale models of people.

Home Office returns (HMSO, 1990) indicate that 3·3 million live vertebrates were used for experiments in the UK in 1989, a figure that has been steadily falling from a peak of around 5·5 million in the mid 1970s. Just over half this total was mice and a quarter rats. If rabbits and rodents are combined they account for 90% of all animals used, with a substantial majority of the remainder being non-mammalian vertebrates.

Most justifications of the usefulness of animal experiments in the human biological sciences rely upon anecdotal examples which—no matter how persuasive—fail to convey the impression of those teaching in the field that experiments with non-human species have played a part in creating most knowledge in human biology, and thus the practical benefits that result from it. Nobel prizes in physiology and medicine represent landmark achievements that have withstood critical scrutiny for some time prior to the award. Table 1 shows a breakdown of prizewinners over an 80 year period according to the nature of the experimental subjects used in their work. This analysis shows that around 90% of all such prizewinners have made use of species other than man and that the trend since 1942 has been to use species more phylogenetically distant from man, reflecting in particular the growth of molecular biology. This simple analysis gives a realistic impression of the contribution of animal experiments to physiology and medicine and also complements the logical case for the use of non-human models for the study of man.

Why are animal experiments so useful?

Animal experiments are likely to be more repeatable than those done with human subjects, and 'one of the basic assumptions of science is that experiments should be repeatable' (Festing, 1979). It is often possible to make precise measurements in animals of variables that can only be inaccurately estimated in people and controllability of experiments is also more achievable.

The range of experiments that are possible is extended by the use of animals. Rodents are small, have a short generation time and large litter size, which reduces cost of experiments. Their widespread use over many decades should mean a good background knowledge of their biology and thus facilitates the interpretation of new findings. There are fewer ethical restrictions on what can be done with animals than with people and one is less likely to be hampered by technical limitations when one is using small animals than when using people or even large animals.

All of these factors make animal experiments likely to be technically better and more reliable than human experiments as well as extending the range of experiments that it is possible to attempt. However, a whole new dimension is added to the problem of validity when results from controlled experiments on small laboratory animals are extrapolated to free-living people.

Nutrition measurements in small animals and people

Measurement of certain variables is fundamental to the study of nutrition: intake of energy and nutrients, body composition and pool of nutrients, energy expenditure and rate of metabolism and excretion of nutrients.

Webb (1990) illustrated the problems of measuring such variables in people by the observation that a quarter of all communications presented to the Nutrition Society in 1988 involving the use of human subjects were directed towards improving these measurements. Given care and commitment, these variables can usually be measured with some precision and often relative simplicity in experimental animals.

Webb and Jakobson (1980) exemplified such problems by a discussion of the relative problems of assessing body fat content in mice and man. In mice, the absolute measure of chemical analysis offers a high precision option. It also provides a standard against which other, less rigorous, methods can be calibrated and validated. In humans, the only measures are indirect estimates. Not only is the high precision option excluded, but more significantly there is no absolute standard against which to validate or calibrate those methods that are feasible.

Laboratory animals in controlled experiments as models for free-living people
Controlled experiments are an essential feature of biological research. The aim in such experiments is to make the imposed variable(s) the only difference between control and experimental groups. In laboratory animal experiments, these two groups can be kept under identical environmental conditions, be fed on identical diets or be maintained pathogen-free; even genetic variability can be practically eliminated by the use of inbred stains.

Such controlled experiments have played an important part in the identification of essential nutrients. Animals can be fed on purified diets, devoid of a suspected nutrient, and then fractions or extracts of particular foods, and ultimately the purified nutrient, can be tested for their curative effect on any resultant symptoms of deficiency. The requirement for essential fatty acids was demonstrated in the rat several decades before unequivocal confirmation in man (Webb, 1990). Four of the Nobel prize-winners discussed earlier were awarded their prizes for work on the identification of vitamins that included the use of non-human species.

Controlled animal experiments are the principal method of trying to ensure the long-term safety of food additives (critically discussed by Millstone, 1985). The range of additives and the difficulty of assessing individual intakes make it improbable that epidemiological methods could detect relatively small, long-term, harmful effects of individual additives.

It is possible in animal experiments to administer high doses of single additives over the whole life-span and to compare the morbidity and mortality of the test animals with other animals that have been otherwise identically maintained. Such single-variable experiments preclude the possibility of detecting interactions, not only the more obvious additive–additive interactions but also the possibility that harmful effects of an additive will occur, e.g. in nutrient deficiency, in smokers, when particular drugs or alcohol are taken or with particular genotypes. There is a well known interaction between monamine oxidase inhibitors (anti-depressants) and tyramine containing foods (e.g. cheese).

The circumstances of testing—on small numbers of genetically, relatively homogeneous, animals—contrast with those of use, when large numbers of genetically diverse people will be exposed. This raises the possibility that a small harmful effect will be obscured by background noise in the tests but will adversely affect significant numbers of people when in use. Such possibilities are hopefully minimized by testing on several animal species, identifying a level that produces no detectable effect in a sensitive species and then dividing this by a large safety factor to decide upon what is an acceptable daily intake for people.

Sibling matings over many generations produce strains of rodents that are said to be syngeneic and homozygous for all traits: tissue can be transplanted between members of such strains without risk of rejection as is only possible between human monozygotic twins. Such reductions in genetic variability are considered a major advantage because they greatly enhance repeatability of experiments (Festing, 1979). There is a need, however, for extreme caution when extrapolating from a narrow gene pool to a more diverse genetic population, especially when quantitative observations like nutrient requirements or drug sensitivity are involved. One would be cautious of assuming that results obtained in a single inbred strain of mice would be predictive of the response of mice generally, especially as inbreeding (whilst it reduces within-strain variation) increases between-strain variation (Festing, 1979). Webb (1990) poses the question of whether an experiment performed on an individual from an isolated and highly inbred human tribe would be necessarily representative of what would happen with people in general, let alone to phylogenetically distant species, like rats or mice.

If one were assessing the relative importance of thirst in controlling water balance then observations on laboratory rats fed on dry, salty food and given bland tap water to drink *ad libitum* do not model the human situation. Much human food has high water content, people drink highly palatable and drug-containing fluids, and there are strong cultural and social pressures that not only tend to increase consumption but also encourage consumption at particular times.

Similar arguments could be made about the seemingly more complex mechanisms regulating energy balances. Laboratory rats have long been regarded as model regulators of food intake and energy balance, but it is quite apparent that given access to a wide variety of palatable, energy-dense foods ('cafeteria' feeding), they are, like people, prone to over-eat and become obese (Rothwell & Stock, 1979).

Experimental animals may have different nutrient requirements from people
Animal experiments played an important part in establishing protein and certain amino acids as essential nutrients. It has, however, been argued earlier that these same sorts of experiments may have misled nutritionists quantitatively, encouraging inflated estimates of protein requirements in children.

Amongst the common laboratory animals, only guinea-pigs share the primates' dietary requirement for vitamin C. Thus, studies on scurvy and vitamin C are usually confined to this species. However, Pauling (1972) has used estimates of the rat's daily synthesis of vitamin C, scaled up on a weight-to-weight basis, to support his view that gram quantities are needed in people to ensure optimal health. This is an example of a species being selected as a model because of, rather than in spite of, its differences from man.

Differences in the nature of the diet and pattern of feeding between species
If an animal is exposed to a mode of feeding or type of diet to which it is not phylogenetically adapted, this may have limited relevance to a species that is so adapted. Results generated by feeding an herbivorous species with dietary components that are confined to foods of animal origin might have limited applicability to omnivores or carnivores. Gorging or meal-feeding of species known to be 'nibblers' (i.e. eating spread over long periods) might give a false or exaggerated impression of the effect in a species more adapted to meal feeding.

An analysis of the literature (e.g. Constantinides, 1965; Frantz & Moore, 1969) suggests that rabbit experiments helped promote the idea that dietary cholesterol was very important in raising serum cholesterol and consequently in accelerating atherogenesis. However, recent UK dietary guidelines (NACNE, 1983) give low priority to reducing dietary cholesterol intake. Selye (1970) went as far as to suggest that had om-nivorous rats rather than rabbits been the favoured experimental animals at the start of the century, the phenomenon of cholesterol-induced atherosclerosis might never have been discovered because of the rats' resistance to this method of induction. Even though this discussion may seriously undermine the validity of using rabbit experiments to assess the significance of dietary cholesterol in human atherogenesis, they may nevertheless be useful in supporting epidemiological evidence of an aetiological link between high serum cholesterol and atherosclerosis, and perhaps also in providing a convenient model to study the process of atherogenesis.

SCALING

Widdowson (1976), quoting earlier writings of Haldane, suggests that size is an obvious but often inadequately considered difference between species. Expressing dosages, or nutrient requirements, per unit of body-weight is a widely used practice when making within, or between, species comparisons. The principal merit of this procedure seems to be convenience, rather than any convincing evidence that it is a reliable guide. This problem of scaling is complex and multi-faceted and pervades all aspects of species comparison; it is particularly important and difficult for nutritionists in the field of energetics.

Scaling of dosages and nutrient requirements
Schmidt-Nielsen (1972) demonstrated the immense capacity for producing variation when scaling dosages between species of different sizes. He produced a range of 0·5–300 mg of LSD as the likely suitable dose for an elephant depending on whether he scaled from the dose effective in people or cats and depending on whether he used relative weight, relative metabolic rate or relative brain size as the criterion of scaling. This exercise undermines confidence in Pauling's earlier weight-to-weight extrapolation of vitamin C production in the rat to produce an indication of the optimal intake for people.

Scaling the energy costs of exercise
Miller & Mumford (1966) calculated the percentage increase in the maintenance energy requirement that would result from undertaking a 10 km walk in three species and they produced figures of 22%, 10% and 3% respectively for an elephant, a man and a rat. They made the seemingly reasonable assumption that the energy costs of walking would be directly related to body-weight (i.e. $0·5\,kcal\,kg^{-1}\,km^{-1}$). These figures are striking because of the small calculated impact on the metabolism of the rat despite the fact that it represents a much more considerable walk for a rat than the other two species. Webb (1990) recalculated these percentages using a regression equation relating minimum energy costs of running to body-

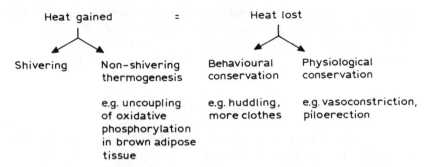

FIG. 1.   The range of responses that can be employed by homeothermic animals
to maintain heat balance in a cold environment.

weight, derived experimentally by Taylor *et al.* (1970); he produced figures
of 5·5%, 22% and 22% respectively for the elephant, man and rat. The
whole perspective is changed when different assumptions are made about
scaling. Note that the figure produced from the equation for the man has
been doubled, in line with the empirical observations of Taylor *et al.*
(1970), and which they suggest might reflect the extra energy costs of
bipedal locomotion.

Scaling and metabolic rate
Absolute metabolic rate obviously will tend to increase with increasing size
but when metabolic rate is expressed per unit weight then this relative
metabolic rate declines with increasing body size. The empirically derived
regression equation

$$\text{Metabolic rate} = k \text{ weight}^{3/4}$$

is widely used to scale or compare metabolic rates both within, or between
species. It is widely assumed that this inverse relationship between relative
metabolic rate and body size is a reflection of the greater surface area to
volume ratio in small mammals making the energy costs of homeothermy
increase with decreasing size. However, Bligh (1973) suggested that a plot
of log body-weight against log metabolic-rate also produces a linear
regression in poikilotherms, where presumably such arguments would not
apply.

Scaling and the energy costs of homeothermy
Figure 1 shows four potential strategies that animals can employ to
maintain heat balance in a cold environment. Heat conservation by vaso-

constriction supplemented by shivering is the predominant physiological response in humans. People have a capacity to increase thermal insulation by several fold in response to cold stress (Kleiber, 1975). Small mammals have a very limited capacity to physiologically increase their thermal insulation (Jakobson, 1981) and in most laboratory experiments, after acclimatization, will rely principally on non-shivering thermogenesis. Heldmaier (1971) suggested that mice have a capacity to increase oxygen consumption by up to four fold by non-shivering mechanisms. Foster & Frydman (1979) showed that the major site of this non-shivering thermogenesis in rodents is brown adipose tissue. Heldmaier (1971) found a negative association between size and non-shivering thermogenic capacity and Joy (1963) estimated a maximum 10–20% capacity to increase oxygen consumption by non-shivering mechanisms in adult man. Brown adipose tissue has traditionally been regarded as vestigial or even absent in adult man but human babies do employ non-shivering thermogenesis in thermoregulating and do have active brown adipose tissue (Aherne & Hull, 1966).

Some mammals abandon energy-expensive homeothermy when adverse climatic or food supply conditions prevail. Some mammals, like hamsters, hibernate but this phenomenon is so well known and so apparent that the dangers of it resulting in misinterpreted experimental results is probably only theoretical. Some other small mammals are said to be heterothermic; they become torpid in response to food deprivation (Hudson, 1978). Several relatively recent studies have clearly shown that mice can become torpid when fasted (Hudson & Scott, 1979; Webb *et al.* 1980 and 1982). During bouts of torpor, core temperature drops to a minimum of around 20°C for several hours, presumably representing a significant energy saving and thus a survival advantage for wild mice. Webb *et al.* (1982) showed that even at ambient temperatures close to freezing, core temperature did not fall below about 20°C. They discussed a number of other observations that led them to classify this as an adaptive response rather than a failure of thermoregulation. Figure 2 shows sample core temperature profiles of mice during a 72 h period that included a 48 h fast. These mice became torpid during the first day of the fast, aroused spontaneously and re-entered torpor on the second day. Torpor is a fundamental aspect of the biology of the most widely used of all the laboratory animals which might affect the interpretation of results using mice, especially in energy balance studies. Many experimenters using mice would, in the past, have been unaware of the heterothermic nature of mice and perhaps many still are.

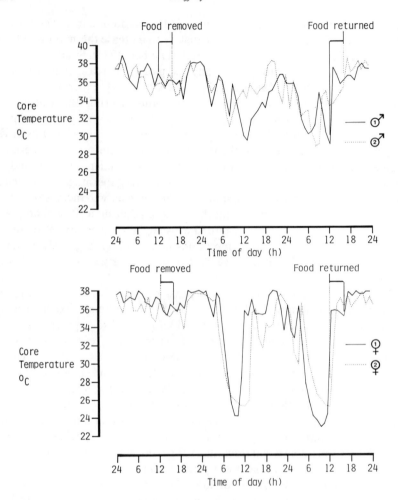

Fig. 2. Sample core temperature profiles of four C57Bl/6 mice over a 3 day period that included a 48 h fast. Temperature was monitored by radiotelemetry pills implanted within the abdominal cavity. Ambient temperature about 20°C. Taken from previously unpublished results of Jakobson & Webb, using the method outlined in Jakobson & Webb (1984).

Scaling the nutritional burden of pregnancy and lactation

Table 2 gives an indication of the relative metabolic demands of pregnancy and lactation in several small mammals and in women. Widdowson (1976) in reviewing such comparisons concluded that total offspring weight forms

TABLE 2

Relationship between maternal mass, offspring mass, gestation length and time to double birth mass in several species, to illustrate variation in the relative burdens of pregnancy and lactation

Species	Mass of mother (kg)	Mass of average litter as % of maternal mass	Gestation length (day)	Time to double birth mass (day)
Mouse	0·025	40	21	5
Rat	0·200	25	21	6
Guinea-pig	0·560	68	67	14
Rabbit	1·175	19	28	6
Cat	2·75	16	64	7
Woman	56	6	280	120–180

Data taken largely from Widdowson (1976) and Blaxter (1961).

a much higher percentage of mother's weight in small species than in large ones, and that because of the short gestation periods of small mammals, the differences in the rate of prenatal growth of offspring compared with maternal weight is even greater. Payne & Wheeler (1968) suggested that primates have small offspring and long gestation lengths compared even with comparably sized non-primates. These observations indicate that the metabolic stresses of pregnancy are relatively low in women compared with small mammals; there is also evidence of reduced activity and resting metabolism in pregnant women (DHSS, 1969; Prentice, 1989) as well as increased efficiency of absorption of calcium and iron (Passmore & Eastwood, 1986). Thus, the extra nutritional requirements of pregnant women are likely to be very small, a suggestion that is consistent with measurements of food intake in pregnant women (Morgan, 1988).

The young of small species grow much more rapidly than babies, as indicated by the times taken to double birth weights shown in Table 2. Webb (1990) makes the comparison of a female mouse and a woman. The former produces a litter of 40% of maternal weight in 21 days of pregnancy and then supplies milk to enable this litter to double its birth weight in 5 days. The latter produces a baby that represents 6% of her pre-pregnant weight in 9 months and then provides milk to enable this infant to double its birth weight in 4–6 months.

Differences like those discussed indicate the need for extreme caution in extrapolating observations made in small mammals to women in this field. Trayhurn (1985) found suppression of brown adipose tissue thermogenesis in rats and mice during lactation, a predictable finding given the

expected reduction in thermogenic drive consequent upon the raised
metabolic expenditure for lactogenesis. It would, however, be premature
to use these findings to explain the less than expected energy costs of
lactation in women, as brown adipose tissue thermoregulatory thermogenesis will be a small or non-existent component of total human
energy expenditure.

Animal models of human obesity
Webb (1987) reports a quinquennial survey between 1935 and 1985 of
entries in *Biological Abstracts* under the heading obese/obesity. This
survey demonstrates a huge absolute and relative growth in published
papers in this field. Rat and mouse models predominate amongst the
papers in which animal subjects were used—all other species account for
less than 10% of these papers. Crude numbers indicate that papers using
human subjects consistently outnumber those using animal subjects, but
only a minority (about a quarter) of these human papers are experimental
studies investigating aetiology of obesity or metabolic characteristics of
the obese—most are concerned with the consequences of obesity or
obesity therapy and its complications. Thus, experiments with rats and
mice make up a substantial proportion of studies investigating the causes
of obesity and thus presumably they have played a part in influencing
fluctuating opinions as to the causes of human obesity. Less than 0·3% of
papers sampled reported results from both animal and human studies, and
only around 7% of the animal papers used more than one model. This
raises the possibility that the characteristics of individual animal models
of obesity may have unduly influenced views as to the cause(s) of human
obesity. Webb (1990) quotes a survey of nutritionists and obesity workers
on the relevance of animal models to improving the understanding and
treatment of human obesity. There was a clear divergence of views
between those researching with animals (markedly skewed towards the
very relevant end of the scale) and clinicians or researchers using only
human subjects (moderately skewed towards the not relevant end of the
scale). Those who work with animal models have much more faith in their
usefulness than those whose experience is with obese people.
    Early work with animal models (from 1940) focused attention on the
hypothalamic mechanisms that regulated food intake—stereootaxic or
chemically induced lesions in areas of the hypothalamus could induce
obesity (usually attributed to hyperphagia) or a cessation of eating (and
drinking) behaviour (reviewed by Brobeck, 1948; Mayer, 1956). The
concept of discrete nuclei within the hypothalamus regulating hunger and

satiety to produce a metered supply of energy to maintain energy balance became very prominent in nutrition textbooks (e.g. Davidson & Passmore, 1963): some defect in this regulating mechanism or hedonistic overriding of it would be the cause of obesity. The idea of obesity caused by a physiological defect in the hyothalamic mechanisms regulating food intake has now become unfashionable. Webb & Geissler (1990) underlined the current eclipse of this theory when they reported that in a survey of people with a professional interest in obesity, variation in the efficiency of physiological intake-regulating mechanisms rated easily the least popular of six suggested causes of obesity.

The mutant obese-hyperglycaemic mouse (*ob/ob*) played an important part in encouraging the metabolic view of obesity. This theory suggests that variations in capacity to regulate energy expenditure in response to excess energy intake (diet-induced thermogenesis, DIT) may be significant in predisposing some individuals to obesity. The ready availability of palatable, energy-dense food and the low requirement for physical work in industrialized countries would allow expression of this variable, inherited metabolic tendency towards corpulence. Mayer (1960) classified *ob/ob* mice as having metabolic obesity because pair-feeding with genetically lean litter-mates did not prevent obesity. According to Festing (1979) *ob/ob* became the second most widely used of all the mammalian mutants, and thus we have a widely used and unequivocally metabolic experimental obesity, which must surely have had a persuasive influence on attitudes to human obesity causation.

Ob/ob mice have a low body temperature and poor cold tolerance; they are extremely inactive and do exhibit hyperphagia when fed *ad libitum*. Their 'defective thermoregulation' has been widely assumed to contribute to, if not cause, their obesity. Rothwell & Stock (1979) demonstrated that diet-induced thermogenesis in very hyperphagic cafeteria-fed rats could prevent or limit obesity and they suggested that the mechanism of this DIT was by uncoupling of oxidative phosphorylation in brown adipose tissue initiated via the sympathetic innervation, i.e. a mechanism analogous to non-shivering thermogenesis. This relationship between thermoregulatory thermogenesis and the thermogenic mechanisms involved in maintaining energy balance provided a clarification of how the 'defective thermoregulation' of *ob/ob* mice could produce their severe obesity. Notwithstanding the minor role of brown adipose tissue thermogenesis in human thermoregulation, these observations provided a major stimulus to the metabolic view of human obesity. It also encouraged the idea that pharmacological intervention might one day compensate for the metabolic defect in obese people, i.e. by mimicking the action of central or local nerve transmitters that normally induce brown fat thermogenesis. Rothwell & Stock (1979) did provide preliminary evidence of active brown fat in adult people, a question reviewed by Lean & James (1986).

It is possible that the usual interpretation of the imperfect homeothermy of *ob/ob* mice as an impaired thermogenic potential or a defect in the switching mechanism may be anthropocentric and would be modified by a more biological consideration of the heterothermic nature of mice. Webb *et al.* (1982) suggested that if *ob/ob* mice had a defective satiety mechanism, then physiologically they should respond as if in a permanently food-restricted state. One might expect to find inactivity, reduced thermoregulatory and dietary thermogenesis and increased food consumption —the very characteristics described earlier. Webb *et al.* (1982) and Jagot *et al.* (1983) reported occasional frank torpor in ad-libitum fed *ob/ob* mice, but if torpor is loosely defined as a state of profound inactivity, reduced thermogenesis and reduced core temperature, torpidity is the usual state of *ob/ob* mice. Their poor cold tolerance and the abnormal ultrastructure of their brown fat (see Himms-Hagen, 1985) could represent a sort of disuse atrophy—their cold tolerance does seem to be improvable by cold acclimatization (Hogan & Himms-Hagen, 1980) and by intermittent feeding (Webb *et al.*, 1982). Himms-Hagen (1985) has gone so far as to argue that the basic defect in *ob/ob* mice probably lies in a centrally determined high propensity for entry into torpor.

Knittle & Hirsch (1969) reported that early overfeeding of rats (by reducing litter size) resulted in increased adipocyte number in their epididymal fat pads. Hirsch & Han (1969) suggested that these fat pads initially grew by hypertrophy and hyperplasia, but after 6 weeks of age adipocyte numbers were fixed. These results have had immense practical impact in human nutrition, encouraging the belief that early overfeeding of children increased adipocyte number and thus predisposed to obesity —the fat cell theory (Pond, 1987). Pond argues that in primates relatively little capacity exists for increasing fat cell size, but that hyperplasia is not limited and thus that extrapolation from rats to humans is invalid. Pond argues that the fat cell theory depended upon acceptance of the growth of the rat epididymal fat pad as a good model of human adipose tissue development and she shows good grounds for believing it to be, in fact, a poor model.

CONCLUDING REMARKS

The choice of examples here has been made to illustrate potential difficulties in relating results from experiments using small animals to man. Despite these difficulties, the opportunity to do good controlled experiments in many areas is only available if animals are used. The limitations when using humans are such that the experimenter is often limited to naturalistic observation and correlation. This approach is dependent upon quality measurement, but in human nutrition it is not possible to make precise and representative measurements of many key variables.

REFERENCES

Aherne, W. & Hull, D. (1966). Brown adipose tissue and heat production in the newborn infant. *Journal of Pathology and Bacteriology* **91**, 223–30.

Blaxter, K.L. (1961). Lactation and the growth of the young. In *Milk: The Mammary Gland and its Secretion*, vol. II [S.K. Kon and A.T. Cowie, editors]. Academic Press, New York.

Bligh, J. (1973) *Temperature Regulation in Mammals and other Vertebrates*. North-Holland Publishing Company, Amsterdam.

Brobeck, J.R. (1948). Mechanism of the development of obesity in animals with hypothalamic lesions. *Physiological Reviews* **26**, 541–59.

Constantinides, P. (1965). *Experimental Atherosclerosis*. Amsterdam: Elsevier.

Davidson, S. & Passmore, R. (1963). *Human Nutrition and Dietetics, 2nd ed.* Edinburgh: Churchill Livingstone.

DHSS (1969). *Recommended intakes of nutrients for the United Kingdom*. Report on Public Health and Medical Subjects, no. 120 London: H.M. Stationery Office.

Festing, M.W.F. (1979). The inheritance of obesity in animal models of obesity. In *Animal Models of Obesity*, pp. 15–37 [M.W.F. Festing, editor]. London, Macmillan.

Foster, D.O. & Frydman, M.L. (1979). Tissue distribution of cold-induced thermogenesis in conscious warm or cold-acclimated rats re-evaluated from changes in tissue blood flow: the dominant role of brown adipose tissue in the replacement of shivering by non-shivering thermogenesis. *Canadian Journal of Physiology and Pharmacology* **57**, 257–70.

Frantz, I.D. & Moore, R.B. (1969). The sterol hypothesis in atherogenesis. *American Journal of Medicine* **46**, 684–90.

Hegsted, D.M. (1959). Protein requirement in man. *Federation Proceedings* **18**, 1130–6.

Heldmaier, G. (1971). The relationship between non-shivering thermogenesis and body size. In *Proceedings of International Symposium on Energy Balance*, pp. 73–80 [L. Jansky editor]. Prague: Academia.

Himms-Hagen, J. (1985). Brown adipose tissue metabolism and thermogenesis. *Annual Reviews of Nutrition* **5**, 69–94.

Hirsch, J. & Han, P.W. (1969). Cellularity of rat adipose tissue: effects of growth, starvation and obesity. *Journal of Lipid Research* **10**, 77–82.

HMSO (1990). *Statistics of experiments on living animals.* Great Britain 1989. London: H.M. Stationery Office.

Hogan, S. & Himms-Hagen, J. (1980). Abnormal brown adipose tissue in obese (ob/ob) mice; response to acclimation to cold. *American Journal of Physiology* **239**, E301–9.

Hudson, J.W. (1978). Shallow, daily torpor: A thermoregulatory adaptation. In *Strategies in Cold: Natural Torpidity and Thermogenesis*, pp. 67–108 [L.C.H. Wang & J.W. Hudson, editors]. New York: Academic Press.

Hudson, J.W. & Scott, I.M. (1979). Daily torpor in the laboratory mouse, *Mus musculus* var. albino. *Physiological Zoology* **52**, 205–18.

Jagot, S.A., Jakobson, M.E. & Webb, G.P. (1983). Torpor in genetically obese mice. *Proceedings of the Nutrition Society* **42**, 19A.

Jakobson, M.E. (1981). Physiological adaptability: the response of the house mouse to variations in the environment. *Symposium of the Zoological Society of London* **47**, 301–35.

Jakobson, M.E. & Webb, G.P. (1984). Torpor in laboratory mice. *International Journal of Obesity* **8**, 469.

Joy, R.J.T. (1963). Responses of cold-acclimatized men to infused norepinephrine. *Journal of Applied Physiology* **18**, 1209–12.

Kleiber, M. (1975). *The fire of life. An Introduction to Animal Energetics*, 2nd ed. John Wiley: New York.

Knittle, J.L. & Hirsch, J. (1969). Effect of early nutrition on the development of rat epididymal fat pads: cellularity and metabolism. *Journal of Clinical Investigation* **47**, 2091–8.

Lean, M.E.J. & James, W.P.T. (1986). Brown adipose tissue in man. In *Brown Adipose Tissue*, pp. 339–65 [P. Trayhurn & D.G. Nicholls, editors]. London: Edward Arnold.

Mayer, J. (1956). Appetite and obesity. *Scientific American* **195**(5), 108–16.

Mayer, J. (1960). The obese hyperglycaemic syndrome of mice as an example of 'metabolic' obesity. *American Journal of Clinical Nutrition* **8**, 712–18.

McClaren, D.S. (1974). The great protein fiasco. *Lancet* **ii**, 93–6.

Miller, D.S. & Mumford, P. (1966). Obesity: physical activity and nutrition. *Proceedings of the Nutrition Society* **25**, 100–6.

Millstone, E. (1985). Food additive regulation in the UK. *Food Policy* **10**, 237–52.

Morgan, J.B. (1988). Nutrition for and during pregnancy. In *Nutrition in the Clinical Management of Disease*, 2nd ed, pp. 1–29 [J.W.T. Dickerson & H.A. Lee, editors]. London: Edward Arnold.

Morowitz, H. (1985). *Models for biomedical research. A new perspective.* Report of the Committee on Models for Biological Research. Washington: National Academy Press.

NACNE (National Advisory Committee on Nutrition Education), (1983). *A Discussion Paper on Proposals for Nutrition Guidelines for Health Education in Britain.* London: Health Education Council.

Passmore, R. & Eastwood, M.A. (1986). Human Nutrition and Dietetics, 8th ed. Edinburgh: Churchill Livingstone.

Pauling, L. (1972). *Vitamin C and the Common Cold.* London: Ballantine Books.

Payne, P.R. & Wheeler, E.F. (1968). Comparative nutrition in pregnancy and lactation. *Proceedings of the Nutrition Society* **27**, 129–38.

Pond, C. (1987). Fat and figures. *New Scientist* 4 June, 62–6.

Prentice, A.M. (1989). Energy expenditure in human pregnancy. British Nutrition Foundation *Nutrition Bulletin* **14**, 9–22.

Rothwell, N.J. & Stock, M.J. (1979). A role for brown adipose tissue in diet-induced thermogenesis. *Nature* **281**, 31–5.

Schmidt-Nielsen, K. (1972). *How Animals Work*. Cambridge: Cambridge University Press.

Selye, H. (1970). *Experimental Cardiovascular Disease*. Berlin: Springer-Verlag.

Taylor, C.R., Schmidt-Nielsen, K. & Raab, J.L. (1970). Scaling of the energetic cost of running to body size in mammals. *American Journal of Physiology* **219**, 1104–7.

Trayhurn, P. (1985). Brown adipose tissue thermogenesis and the energetics of lactation in rodents. *International Journal of Obesity* **9**, 81–8.

Webb, G.P. (1987). A critique of animal use in human nutrition research, MSc Thesis, University of London.

Webb, G.P. (1989). The significance of protein in human nutrition. *Journal of Biological Education* **23**(2), 119–24.

Webb, G.P. (1990). A selective critique of animal experiments in human-orientated biological research. *Journal of Biological Education* **24**(3), 191–7.

Webb, G.P. & Jakobson, M.E. (1980). Body fat of mice and men: a class exercise in theory or practice. *Journal of Biological Education* **14**, 318–24.

Webb, G.P. & Geissler, C.A. (1990). What YOU think causes obesity. *Proceedings of the Nutrition Society* **49**, 43A.

Webb, G.P., Jagot, S.A., Rogers, P.D. & Jakobson, M.E. (1980). The effects of fasting on thermoregulation in normal and obese mice. *IRCS Medical Sciences* **8**, 163–4.

Webb, G.P., Jagot, S.A. & Jakobson, M.E., (1982). Fasting-induced torpor in *Mus musculus* and its implications in the use of murine models for human obesity studies. *Comparative Biochemistry and Physiology* **72A**, 211–19.

Widdowson, E.M. (1976). Pregnancy and lactation: the comparative point of view. *In Early Nutrition and Later Development*, pp. 1–10 [A.W. Wilkinson, editor]. Tunbridge Wells: Pitman Medical.

Index